Cardiac Disorders

MMD Managing Major Diseases

Cardiac Disorders

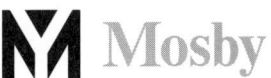

Mosby

St. Louis Baltimore Boston Carlsbad Chicago Minneapolis New York Philadelphia Portland
London Milan Sydney Tokyo Toronto

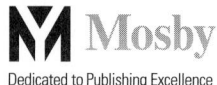
Dedicated to Publishing Excellence

Publisher Stanley Loeb
Editorial Director William J. Kelly
Clinical Director Cindy Tryniszewski, RN, MSN
Editor Catherine E. Harold
Clinical Editors Heather A. Butler, RN, MSN, CNS, CCRN; Marcy Caplin, RN, MSN, CS;
Eva McCaully, RN, MSN, BCLS; Karen E. Michael, RN, MSN;
Aleesa M. Mobley, RN, MS, CS, CCRN; Colleen Seeber-Combs, RN, MSN, CCRN
Copy Editor Stacey Ann Follin
Production Coordinator Marie C. Fusco
Manufacturing Manager William A. Winneberger, Jr.
Art and Design Manager Guy Jacobs
Designers Lynn Foulk, Jennifer Marmarinos
Illustrators Todd Buck, Rolin Graphics, Inc.
Composition Mosby Electronic Publishing

Printed in the United States of America
Printing and binding by R.R. Donnelley & Sons, Inc./CTP

Mosby, Inc.
11830 Westline Industrial Drive
St. Louis, Missouri 63146

Library of Congress Cataloging-in-Publication Data
Cardiac disorders.
        p.   cm. — (Managing major diseases)
    Includes bibliographical references and index.
    ISBN 0-323-00741-4
    1. Heart—Diseases. I. C.V. Mosby Company. II. Series.
    [DNLM: 1. Cardiovascular Diseases. WG 120 C2665 1999]
RC681.C1777 1999
616.1'2—dc21
DNLM/DLC
for Library of Congress   98-40594
                                                                          CIP

99 00 01 02 03 04 / 9 8 7 6 5 4 3 2 1

Contents

Contributors

Linda S. Baas, RN, PhD, CCRN
Associate Professor
College of Nursing and Health
University of Cincinnati Medical Center
Cincinnati, Ohio

Theresa A. Beery, RN, PhD, CCRN
Assistant Professor
College of Nursing and Health
University of Cincinnati Medical Center
Cincinnati, Ohio

Sandra J. Bixler, RN, MSN
Clinical Nurse Specialist
Berks Cardiologists
Reading, Pa.

Mary Evangelista Dietmann, RN,CS, MSN, APRN
Associate Professor of Nursing
St. Vincent's College
Bridgeport, Conn.

Darren Flaherty-Thompson, RN, MSN, NP, CCRN
Director of Nursing
North Medical Urgent Care
Liverpool, N.Y.

Joyce A. Fontana, RN, MS, PhD, CS
Assistant Professor of Nursing
College of Nursing and Health
University of Cincinnati Medical Center
Cincinnati, Ohio

Mary Jo Gerlach, RN, MSNEd
Assistant Professor in Adult Nursing
Medical College of Georgia School of Nursing
Athens, Ga.

Carla Coggins Gilroy, RPh, BS, PharmD
Clinical Pharmacy Specialist
Birmingham Baptist Medical Centers-Montclair Hospital
Birmingham, Ala.

Kimberly Lacey, RN, MSN
Cardiovascular Clinical Nurse Specialist
Section of Cardiology
Yale University, School of Nursing, School of Medicine
Clinical Supervisor
VNA of South Central Connecticut
New Haven, Conn.

Sharon A. Lobert, RN, MSN, PhD
Professor of Nursing and Biochemistry
University of Mississippi Medical Center
Jackson, Miss.

Sally M. Sikora, RN, MSN, CNS,C, CCRN, CNA
Administrative Director of Nursing
Atlantic Gastroenterology Associates
Advanced Practice Nurse
Shore Memorial Hospital
Somers Point, N.J.

Ruth Stanley, PharmD
Associate Director of Pharmacy Services
Birmingham Baptist Medical Centers-Montclair Hospital
Birmingham, Ala.

Consultants

Lynne T. Braun, RN, PhD
Associate Professor
Rush University College of Nursing
Rush University
Chicago, Ill.

Flerida Imperial-Perez, RN, MN
Clinical Nurse Specialist, Cardiothoracic ICU
UCLA Medical Center
Assistant Clinical Professor
UCLA School of Nursing
Los Angeles, Calif.

CARDIAC ESSENTIALS

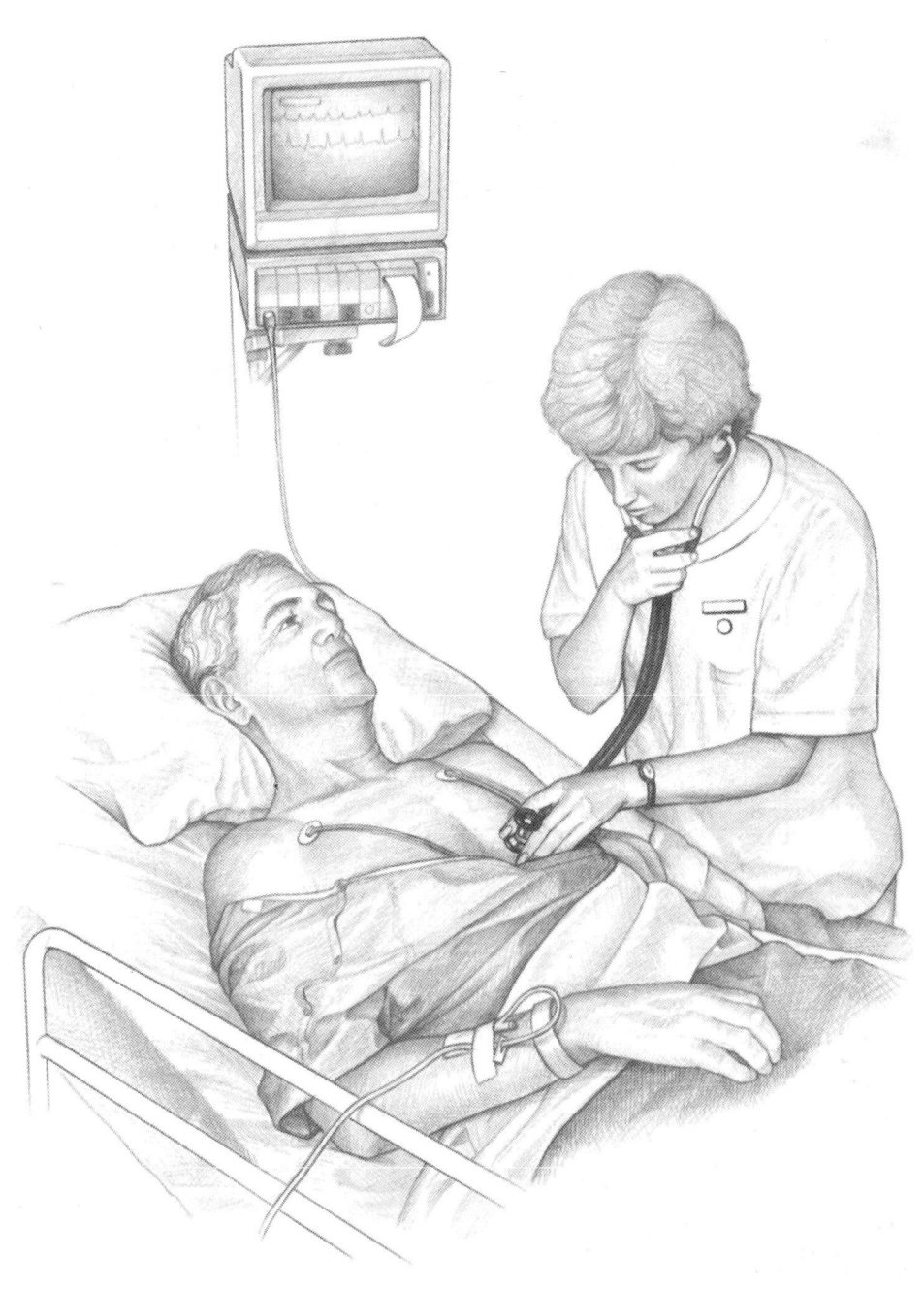

CARDIAC ESSENTIALS

Anatomy and Physiology Review

Across the broad spectrum of patients in your care, a remarkable number have some form of cardiovascular disease. Indeed, American Heart Association statistics suggest that one American in four is affected to some degree by a cardiovascular disease. At the very least, these diseases threaten the quality of life; commonly, they threaten life itself.

Clearly, you must be ready to manage cardiac disorders in a wide range of patients—even those in your care for other reasons. This chapter gives you a quick refresher on the anatomy and physiology you must know to deliver that care with accuracy and expertise.

Structures of the heart

The heart is a hollow muscular organ that lies in the thoracic cage, between the lungs and just above the diaphragm. In front of the heart lie the sternum and the costal cartilages of the third, fourth, and fifth ribs. Behind it lie the esophagus, thoracic aorta, and spinal column. From the front, the heart looks as though it's tipped to the side, with about two-thirds of its bulk extending from the sternum toward the patient's left arm.

An adult's heart measures about 12 cm from top (the base) to bottom (the apex). It spans about 6 cm from front to back, 8 to 9 cm at its widest point. Although the weight and size vary

with age, sex, height, epicardial fat volume, and nutritional status, the heart typically weighs between 250 and 350 grams—a figure that corresponds to about 0.45% of a man's body weight and 0.40% of a woman's. You can visualize the average adult heart as being about the size of a man's fist.

Chambers

As you know, the heart contains four chambers: two atria and two ventricles (see *Reviewing the anatomy of the heart,* page 2). The atria are smaller and thinner-walled than the ventricles. That's because they collect blood under low pressure and act mainly as holding tanks, channeling an appropriate volume of blood into the ventricles with each heartbeat.

The right atrium lies to the right and in front of the left atrium, and above, behind, and to the right of the right ventricle. Its wall is about 2 mm thick.

The left atrium lies above and behind the other cardiac chambers, in the center of the chest. At 3 mm, its wall is slightly thicker than that of the right atrium. The esophagus touches the posterior surface of the left atrium.

The ventricles have thicker walls than the atria because they must pump blood against higher pressures and contract with a greater force to circulate blood to the lungs and the body's tissues.

Reviewing the anatomy of the heart

Use these illustrations to review the position of the heart in the chest and the heart's external and internal structures.

Position of the heart

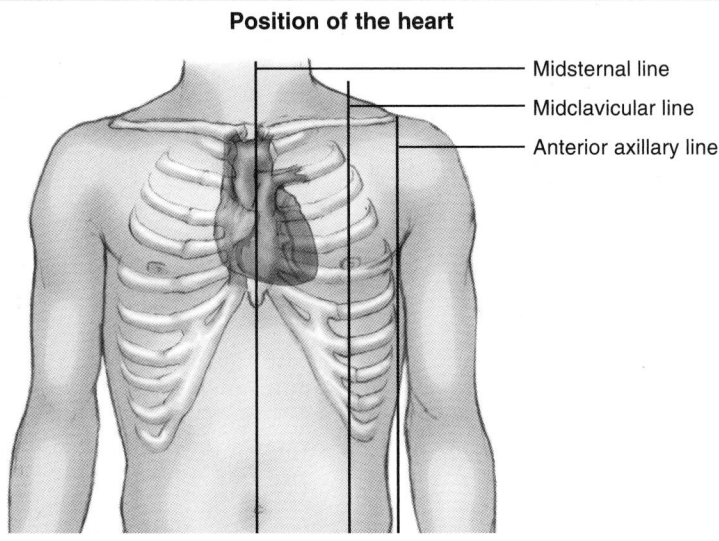

- Midsternal line
- Midclavicular line
- Anterior axillary line

Cross-sectional view

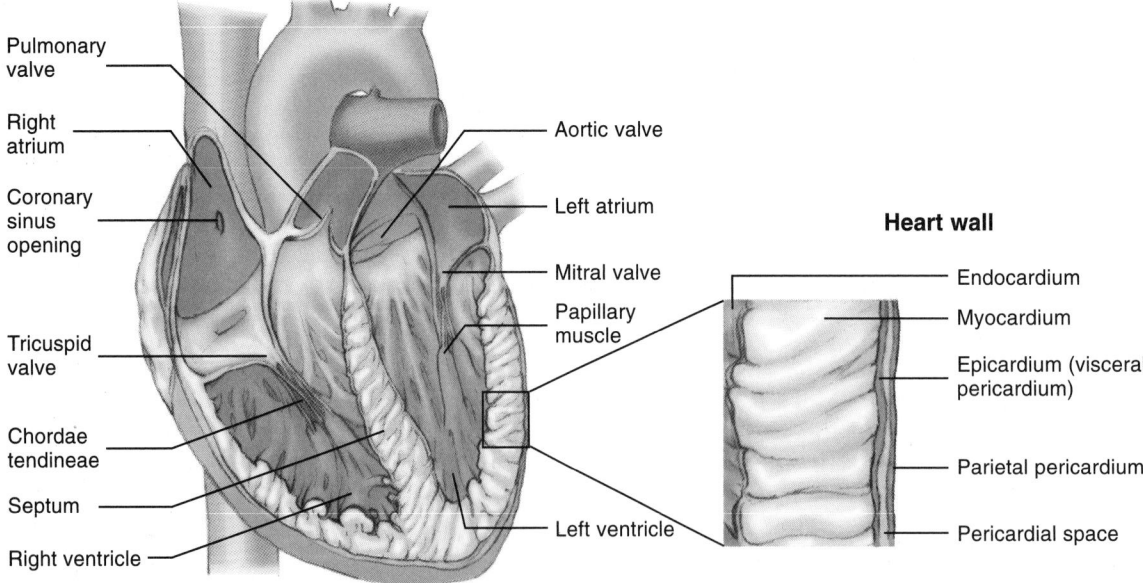

Pulmonary valve

Right atrium

Coronary sinus opening

Tricuspid valve

Chordae tendineae

Septum

Right ventricle

Aortic valve

Left atrium

Mitral valve

Papillary muscle

Left ventricle

Heart wall

Endocardium

Myocardium

Epicardium (visceral pericardium)

Parietal pericardium

Pericardial space

The right ventricle, the heart's most anterior chamber, lies just beneath the sternum, partly below and in front of the right atrium and in front of and to the right of the left ventricle. Shaped like a crescent, the right ventricle curves around the left ventricle. The chamber ejects blood when its anterior free wall shortens, moving inward toward the left ventricle in a bellows movement. Of the two ventricles, the right has much thinner walls. They span 4 to 5 mm.

The oval-shaped left ventricle points downward, forward, and to the left. It lies mainly toward the back of the heart, to the left of and below the right ventricle, in front and to the left of the left atrium. The left ventricle is the largest and thickest of the heart's four chambers because it works the hardest. Blood pumped from the left ventricle must circulate to all parts of the body. Consequently, its muscular wall spans 8 to 15 mm.

A septum separates the left ventricle from the right ventricle. Part of the left ventricular wall makes up part of this septum. The portion of the ventricular wall that doesn't contribute to the septum is commonly called the free ventricular wall.

Layers and walls

The heart wall contains three tissue layers:
- the endocardium or innermost layer
- the myocardium or middle muscular layer
- the epicardium or outer layer.

The endocardium, a thin layer of epithelium and connective tissue, lines the heart's inner chambers, valves, chordae tendineae, and papillary muscles. This layer is continuous with the endothelial lining of the arteries.

Made up of cardiac muscle cells with connective tissue and small blood vessels scattered throughout, the myocardium is responsible for pumping blood through the atria and ventricles and for conducting electrical impulses. Some of the myocardium's fibers are anchored to the heart's fibrous skeleton—four rings of dense fibrous connective tissue called anuli fibrosi. These rings provide secure attachments for the heart's valves and chambers.

The epicardium, a thin transparent tissue, adheres to the heart and forms the outer layer of the heart muscle. It contains coronary arteries, nerves, and fat and covers a portion of the great vessels. The visceral portion of the epicardium lies directly against the heart and is known as the visceral pericardium (inner wall). The epicardium folds back upon itself to form one continuous membrane called the pericardial sac. The outer portion of the membrane is known as the parietal pericardium (outer wall).

The parietal pericardium is made up of tough, fibrous tissue that surrounds the heart without attaching to it. On the anterior side, it attaches to the great vessels, the manubrium, and the xiphoid process. On the heart's ventral and posterior sides, it connects to the diaphragm and the spine.

Between the visceral and parietal membranes is a potential space called the pericardial space. It typically contains 10 to 30 ml of thin, clear, serous fluid—pericardial fluid—that lubricates the membrane surfaces and prevents friction as the heart beats. The pericardium also helps to prevent ventricular dilation, hold the heart in place, and block the spread of infections and neoplasms.

Valves

At the base of the heart are four one-way valves that function in pairs to keep blood flowing smoothly forward through the heart, lungs, and systemic vasculature. One pair is called atrioventricular (AV); the other is called semilunar (see *Viewing the valves,* page 4).

Atrioventricular valves
Also known as AV valves, these structures act as conduits for blood flowing out of the atria and into the ventricles. The tricuspid valve lies between the right atrium and ventricle; the mitral valve lies between the left atrium and ventricle. Several important structures work together to make the AV valves open and shut properly:
- fibrous rings (anuli fibrosi)
- valvular tissue (leaflets, or cusps)
- chordae tendineae
- papillary muscles.

The heart's fibrous skeleton divides the atria from the ventricles and provides a point of attachment and support for valvular tissue. Between the valves and the ventricle wall are fibrous bands called chordae tendineae and muscle bundles called papillary muscles anchored to the ventricle wall. Chordae tendineae connect

Viewing the valves

The main illustration shows a cross-sectional view from above the heart. The pulmonary and aortic valves are closed during diastole and open during systole. The mitral and tricuspid valves are closed during systole and open during diastole.

The close-ups of the open and closed mitral valve show the supporting chordae tendineae and papillary muscles.

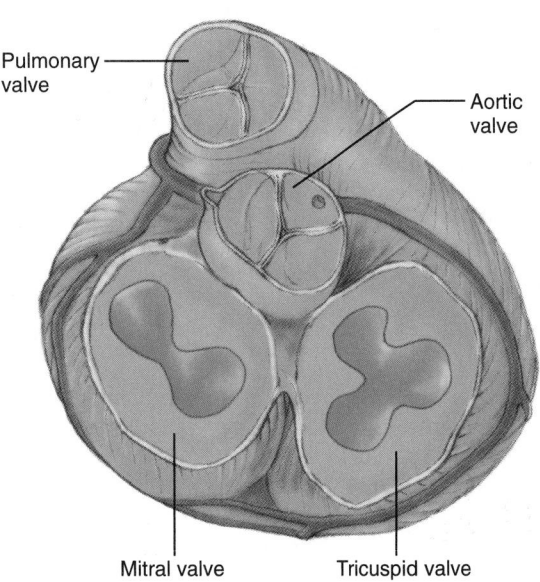

Pulmonary valve

Aortic valve

Mitral valve   Tricuspid valve

Open mitral valve   **Closed mitral valve**

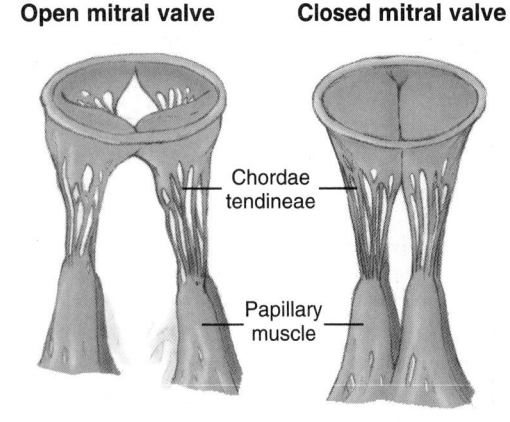

Chordae tendineae

Papillary muscle

the free edges of the leaflets with the papillary muscles. Contraction of the papillary muscles pulls the chordae tendineae taut to prevent the valve leaflets from prolapsing into the atria.

The tricuspid valve, which is larger than the mitral valve, has three leaflets: the anterior, septal, and posterior leaflets. These tricuspid leaflets are thinner, more translucent, and harder to separate than the mitral leaflets. The anterior leaflet is the largest, and the posterior is the smallest.

The mitral valve (sometimes called the bicuspid valve) has two major leaflets: the anterior and posterior. The anterior leaflet extends into the left ventricle during diastole; the posterior leaflet is less mobile.

Semilunar valves

The semilunar valves act as conduits for blood flowing out of the ventricles and into the pulmonary artery and aorta. The pulmonary valve lies between the right ventricle and the pulmonary artery, the aortic valve between the left ventricle and the aorta.

Semilunar valves have smaller, thicker leaflets than the AV valves. The three cup-shaped leaflets of each valve curve down into the ventricle. The base of each leaflet attaches to the outflow tract of the pulmonary artery or aorta; thus, these valves don't have all the supporting structures that AV valves do. Also, in contrast to AV valves, the semilunar leaflets don't overlap.

The pulmonary valve has right anterior, left anterior, and posterior leaflets. The aortic valve has right coronary aortic, left coronary aortic, and noncoronary aortic leaflets. The leaflets of the aortic valve are thicker than those of the pulmonary valve. In fact, they form a bulge at the base of the aorta called the sinus of Valsalva.

Surfaces of the heart

On the anterior surface of the heart, the right and left ventricles are separated by the anterior interventricular groove (also known as a sulcus). On the posterior surface, they're separated by the posterior interventricular groove. On both surfaces, the AV groove marks the separation between atria and ventricles. The crux is the point on the posterior surface where the posterior interventricular and AV grooves cross. The crux also marks the spot where the interatrial septum meets the interventricular septum.

How blood moves through the heart

| Isovolumetric ventricular relaxation | Ventricular filling and atrial contraction | Isovolumetric ventricular contraction | Rapid ventricular ejection |

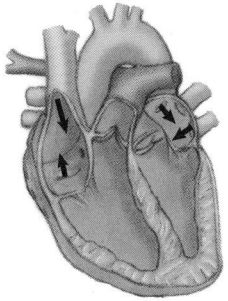 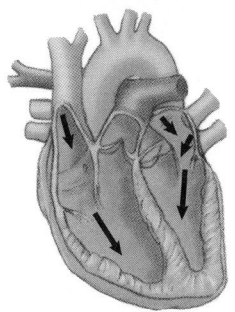 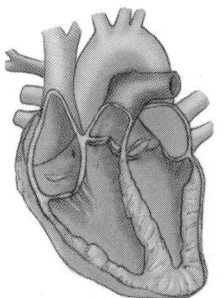 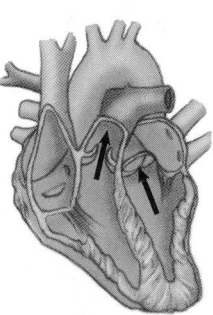

Heart function

As you know, proper heart function involves a coordinated set of electrical and muscular activities, all regulated by the autonomic nervous system. The repeating pattern of contraction and relaxation created by these forces is known as the cardiac cycle.

Cardiac cycle

In a synchronized, two-stage process that includes diastole and systole, blood moves through the atria, ventricles, and valves to the lungs and systemic circulation (see *How blood moves through the heart*).

Keep in mind that your understanding of this cycle offers more than simply theoretical knowledge; rather, it arms you with the practical information you need to accurately interpret your patient's heart sounds, a crucial assessment skill.

Diastole

During ventricular diastole, or relaxation, pressure in the atria rises as they receive blood from the venae cavae and pulmonary veins. When atrial pressure becomes greater than ventricular pressure, the AV valves open. Blood empties rapidly into the ventricles. During this period of rapid ventricular filling, pressure in the atria remains higher than that in the ventricles because the ventricles are still in a period of relaxation. In late diastole, after rapid ventricular filling, the AV valves are still open and pressures in the atria and ventricles are essentially equal. At this point, the atria contract—an event commonly known as atrial kick—forcing a small percentage of additional blood into the ventricles. This step marks the beginning of ventricular systole.

Systole

Immediately before the ventricles contract, pressure in the left ventricle rises rapidly. This rise in pressure causes the AV valves to close, and for a moment just before the ventricles contract, all four valves are closed. During this period, called isovolumetric ventricular contraction, the volume in the ventricles remains constant; no blood flows into or out of them.

As the ventricles contract, however, pressure inside rises beyond the pressure in the aorta and pulmonary artery. Consequently, the semilunar valves open, and blood is ejected into the aorta and pulmonary artery. This action is called rapid ventricular ejection.

As ventricular pressure declines below that in the aorta and pulmonary artery, the flow of blood from the ventricles slows down. The ventricles begin to relax, reducing the pressure inside and allowing blood to begin flowing backward toward the heart. The semilunar valves close against this backward flow of blood, and for a moment, all four valves are closed. Called

On the path of cardiac conduction

The heart's conduction pathway begins at the sino-atrial (SA) node in the right atrium. It then splits into the internodal tracts and Bachmann's bundle before merging again at the atrioventricular (AV) node. From there, the pathway splits into two bundle branches running down the interventricular septum. The left bundle branch splits again into anterior and posterior branches. Purkinje fibers form the tips of all the branches.

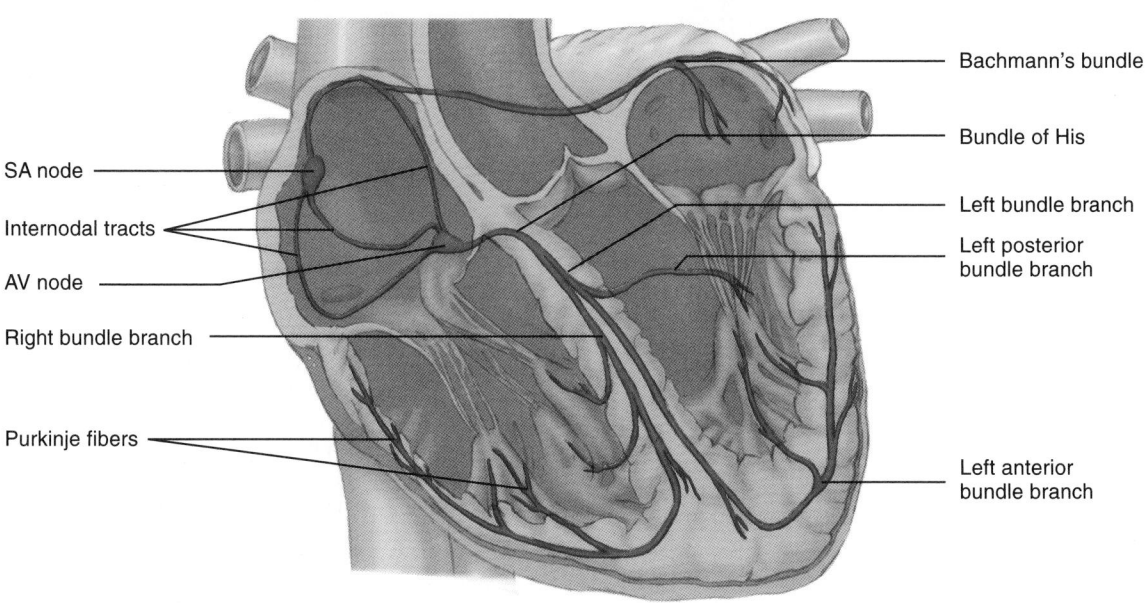

isovolumetric ventricular relaxation, this moment marks the beginning of ventricular diastole.

Cardiac conduction

The cardiac cycle occurs—and continues—only because electrical impulses move through the heart muscle and prompt it to contract. These impulses flow in a predictable pattern across the myocardium because of the action potential of groups of specialized muscle cells arranged in nodes and conduction pathways throughout the heart (see *On the path of cardiac conduction*).

Cardiac muscle cells
The heart has two types of muscle cells: pacemaker cells and working myocardial cells. Pacemaker cells can generate their own rhythmic electrical impulses or action potentials. These electrical impulses are then conducted to the working myocardial cells, which rapidly conduct the impulse throughout the myocardium. Under normal conditions, working myocardial cells don't spontaneously produce electrical impulses.

Sinoatrial node
In the right atrium near the superior vena cava is a small, oval-shaped area of specialized muscle and pacemaker cells called the sinoatrial (SA) node. Also called the heart's pacemaker, the SA node generates electrical impulses at a rate of 60 to 100 beats per minute.

This is where the heart's spontaneous rhythmic electrical impulse—or action potential—begins. This impulse then spreads to the working cardiac muscle cells, travels through the specialized conduction pathways, and stimulates contraction of the atria and ventricles. On their own, the cells of the SA node have little ability to contract.

Internodal pathways
When electrical impulses leave the SA node, they spread over the atria by way of three internodal pathways—the anterior, middle, and posterior—that can conduct impulses across the atria faster than atrial muscle can. Bachmann's bundle, a branch of the anterior internodal pathway, conducts impulses to the left atrium. As each impulse spreads across the atria, it prompts them to contract.

Atrioventricular node
The internodal pathways merge in the lower septal wall of the right atrium, just behind the tricuspid valve and near the opening of the coronary sinus. Here they join another oval-shaped cluster of pacemaker cells called the AV node. When an electrical impulse arrives at the AV node, it pauses, which allows time for blood to flow from the atria to the ventricles before the ventricles contract. After this pause, the impulse spreads to the bundle of His, a continuation of the AV node located on the right side of the interatrial septum.

Bundle branches
The impulse travels quickly across the bundle of His and then simultaneously down the left and right bundle branches in the interventricular septum. The left branch splits into anterior and posterior bundle branches (or fasciculi). The left anterior branch travels to the anterior papillary muscle of the left ventricle and then to the apex of the left ventricle. The left posterior branch travels to the posterior papillary muscle of the left ventricle. Meanwhile, the right bundle branch travels on the right side of the interventricular septum to the anterior papillary muscle of the right ventricle.

Purkinje fibers
The ends of the bundle branches have fingerlike projections called Purkinje fibers that conduct the electrical impulse toward the apex of the heart and then upward toward the base. In some circumstances, the Purkinje fibers can act as a pacemaker for the heart, but they can only generate impulses at a rate of 20 to 40 beats per minute.

Action potential
Electrical impulses flow along the pathways in the myocardium because changes in the permeability of the cell membrane alter the rate of ion passage across the membrane. This phenomenon, called the cell's action potential, involves primarily sodium, potassium, and calcium ions. Movement of potassium and sodium ions into and out of cardiac muscle cells produces an electrical difference across the membrane, called a membrane potential.

In a resting (or polarized) state, the cell has equal negative and positive charges inside and outside. When the cell is stimulated by an electrical impulse, however, an action potential occurs. In other words, the cell membrane potential enters a two-phase change: depolarization and repolarization.

Depolarization permits sodium ions to move rapidly into the cell, making the inside more positive than the outside. This change creates an impulse that travels from cell to cell throughout the heart, causing muscle contraction. After depolarization and contraction, potassium ions move slowly back into the cell, restoring it to its polarized state in a process called repolarization. In this state, the cardiac muscle is relaxed.

Cardiac muscle cells have a refractory period during which they can't respond to a stimulus or initiate an action potential. This refractory period prevents abnormally rapid contractions that could be life threatening.

Autonomic regulation of the heart

The autonomic nervous system, consisting of the sympathetic and parasympathetic nervous systems, regulates cardiac function by affecting the rate at which the SA node generates impulses, the speed at which those impulses are conducted, and the strength of the myocardial contraction.

Sympathetic nerve fibers innervate all parts of the atria and ventricles. When stimulated, they release the neurotransmitter norepinephrine, which increases heart rate and contractility. Parasympathetic nerve fibers, which enter the heart through the vagus nerve, innervate the SA node, AV node, and atrial muscle. When stimulated, they release acetylcholine, which decreases heart rate and contractility. Thus, the sympathetic and parasympathetic systems provide opposing, balancing influences.

The sympathetic and parasympathetic nervous systems respond to information sent to the medulla from baroreceptors and chemoreceptors. Baroreceptors, also called pressoreceptors, are pressure-sensitive structures embedded in the aortic arch and the walls of the carotid sinuses in the internal carotid arteries. When stimulated, they cause a reflex response in either the sympathetic or the parasympathetic nervous system. A decrease in systolic blood pressure, for example, will trigger a reflex sympathetic response that increases heart rate, contractility, and vasoconstriction—all of which contribute to an increase in blood pressure.

Chemoreceptors are sensitive to chemical changes in the body. They're found in carotid bodies located at the bifurcation of the carotid arteries and in aortic bodies along the aortic arch. Chemoreceptors respond to changes in blood pH (hydrogen ion concentration), carbon dioxide levels, and oxygen levels. As with baroreceptors, the response can be sympathetic or parasympathetic. For example, a decrease in blood pH or partial pressure of arterial oxygen triggers a reflex sympathetic response that increases heart rate, vasoconstriction, and contractility. This response increases perfusion to the heart and lungs in an effort to increase the exchange of carbon dioxide for oxygen.

Circulation

When neurologic, electrical, and muscular forces function normally, blood flows at an adequate pace from the heart to all areas of the body through the systemic and pulmonary circulations.

Systemic circulation

The systemic circulation carries blood to all parts of the body except the lungs. The left atrium receives newly oxygenated blood from the lungs via the two pulmonary veins located on each side the left atrium. As blood enters the left atrium, pressure rises enough to open the mitral valve, allow-

ing blood to enter the left ventricle. The atrium contracts when the ventricle is about 75% full. As pressure in the ventricle rises, the mitral valve closes against backflow into the atrium, and the aortic valve opens. Freshly oxygenated blood then flows through the aortic valve, into the aorta, and throughout the body.

Cardiac circulation

Two main coronary arteries—the left and right—branch from the aorta just beyond the aortic valve. The first blood vessels to branch off the aorta, they fill mainly during diastole, when the heart is relaxed. During systole, myocardial contractions compress these arteries, preventing them from filling.

Left coronary artery

The left coronary artery, sometimes called the left main coronary artery, emerges from the aorta just behind the left cusp of the aortic valve and travels between the left atrial appendage and the pulmonary artery. Then it splits into two branches, the left anterior descending artery and the left circumflex artery (see *Two views of the coronary arteries*).

The left anterior descending artery travels down the anterior interventricular groove between the two ventricles toward the apex of the heart. In most people, it then circles the apex before ending in the lower portion of the posterior interventricular groove. This artery supplies blood to parts of the left and right ventricles and much of the interventricular septum.

The left anterior descending artery has several branches, including the diagonal and septal perforator branches. Several diagonal branches supply blood to the free wall of the left ventricle as well as the anterior left ventricular papillary muscle. The septal branches perfuse blood to a portion of the anterior interventricular septum, the anterior papillary muscle of the left ventricle, and the right and left bundle branches.

The left circumflex artery branches from the left coronary artery and travels around the left side of the heart in the left AV groove. In about 15% of people, it continues to the crux of the heart and becomes the posterior descending artery. You may hear these people called left dominant. In others, the right coronary artery reaches the crux. They are called right dominant.

The left circumflex artery supplies blood to parts of the left atrium and left ventricle and to the

Two views of the coronary arteries

The right and left coronary arteries, which carry oxygenated blood to the myocardium itself, branch from the aorta just past the aortic valve. The right coronary artery supplies the right atrium, right ventricle, and a portion of the posterior wall of the left ventricle. The left coronary artery supplies the left atrium and the thick walls of the left ventricle.

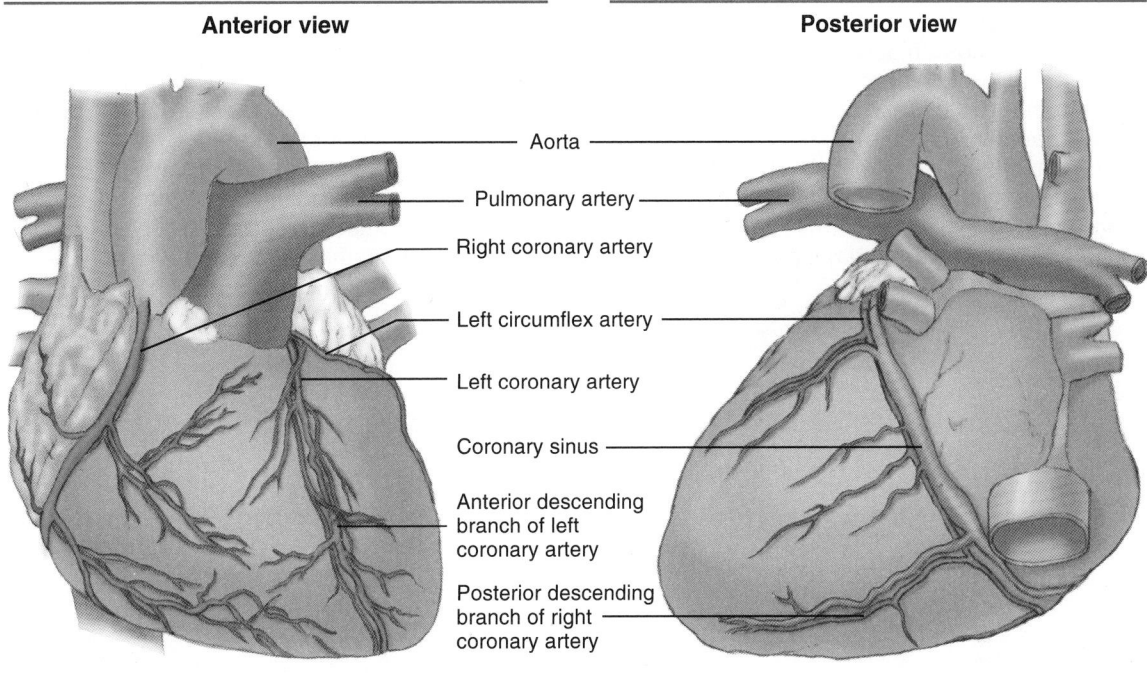

Anterior view   **Posterior view**

Aorta

Pulmonary artery

Right coronary artery

Left circumflex artery

Left coronary artery

Coronary sinus

Anterior descending branch of left coronary artery

Posterior descending branch of right coronary artery

papillary muscles. In 40% to 45% of people, the left circumflex artery also supplies the SA node. In 10%, it perfuses the AV node. The left circumflex artery has several branches, including marginal branches that supply parts of the left ventricle.

Right coronary artery
The right coronary artery begins behind the right aortic cusp and travels behind the pulmonary artery, down into the right AV groove, and around the right side to the back of the heart. This artery and its many branches supply the right atrium, right ventricle, posterior papillary muscle of the left ventricle, and the lower left ventricle.

The posterior descending branch of the right coronary artery follows the posterior interventricular groove and perfuses the rear portion of the interventricular septum. In about half of the population, the right coronary artery supplies blood to the SA node and, in most people, it supplies the AV node and bundle of His. In others, the left circumflex artery provides blood to the SA and AV nodes.

Pulmonary circulation

Pulmonary circulation refers to the flow of blood through the right ventricle, pulmonary artery, lungs, pulmonary veins, and back to the left atrium. As you know, deoxygenated blood returns to the right atrium by way of the superior and inferior venae cavae. The superior vena cava returns deoxygenated blood from the head, neck, and arms. The inferior vena cava returns blood from organs in the trunk, such as the liver and kidneys, and from the legs. Blood from the coronary arteries that has been used to nourish the heart muscle returns to the right atrium through the coronary sinus. Commonly, the blood that is returned to the right side of the heart is called venous return.

As deoxygenated blood enters the right atrium, pressure increases enough to open the tricuspid valve, which allows blood to flow passively into the right ventricle. When the right atrium contracts, it empties the remainder of its blood into the right ventricle. As blood fills the right ventricle, pressure increases above that in the right atrium, the tricuspid valve closes, and the pulmonary valve is forced open. When the right ventricle contracts, blood flows through the pulmonary valve, into the pulmonary artery, and toward the lungs.

In the lungs, the pulmonary artery branches into smaller and smaller vessels. Eventually, this repeated branching leads to the pulmonary capillary bed, where gas exchange takes place. Carbon dioxide in venous blood diffuses from the capillaries into the alveoli, and oxygen from the alveoli enters the capillaries. Beyond the pulmonary capillaries, the newly oxygenated blood flows into pulmonary venules. Eventually, these venules merge to form the four pulmonary veins that transport oxygenated blood from the lungs to the left atrium.

Clearly, many forces come to bear on the heart's ability to function smoothly and circulate appropriate amounts of blood through the systemic, cardiac, and pulmonary vessels. But commonly, the cardiac vessels themselves underlie patients' cardiac disorders.

CARDIAC ESSENTIALS

Assessment

Sound ongoing assessment can point the way toward accurate diagnosis and successful treatment of cardiac disorders. In this chapter, you'll find a thorough discussion of the essential assessment techniques you need when evaluating a patient who has or may have a cardiac disorder.

As you'd expect, you'll also find discussions of many diagnostic tests, some of which involve high-tech procedures and monitoring systems. But keep in mind that even high-tech tests depend on human interpretation of a patient's signs, symptoms, and other test results. What's more, the selection of high-tech, typically costly, testing methods relies largely on the accurate findings of a traditional health history and physical examination.

Consequently, even in a high-tech environment, your keen assessment skills are as important as ever in gathering information and making appropriate decisions about your patient's care. The health history and physical examination continue to be essential components of a complete cardiac assessment.

Health history

For many of the patients in your care, your ability to detect cardiac problems may have as much to do with your communication skills as your advanced cardiac expertise. Even for a patient already diagnosed with a cardiac problem, your ability to provide ongoing accurate assessments and patient care depends largely on your communication skills.

Before you can conduct a comprehensive and holistic interview, you must be relaxed and focused. To minimize distractions, try to conduct the interview in a private area. Be aware that subtle cues, environmental factors, and your intuition can influence the data you collect and the conclusions you reach.

During the interview, convey an attitude of sincere interest. Start by explaining the purpose of your assessment. Ask all your questions with caring and concern; make sure all your responses are nonjudgmental. Throughout the interview, make note of your patient's nonverbal behaviors, such as facial grimacing and hand-wringing. If you observe such behaviors, mention them and encourage your patient to discuss any concerns he may have. Also, note the level of your patient's language skills and tailor your questions and teaching accordingly.

Also, consider your patient's ability to participate in the interview. If he is critically ill or easily fatigued, you'll need to prioritize your assessment needs, gathering as much essential information as you can before giving the patient a chance to rest. If you need more information, plan another time to assess the patient within the needed time frame.

By adopting this general approach, you'll be well on your way to obtaining an accurate, detailed history that contains the data you need for completing your cardiac assessment.

Current health status

Begin the health history by assessing your patient's perception of his current health. To start this process, try asking him a general question, such as, "What brought you here today?" By

Deciphering your patient's chest pain

Because the experience of chest pain varies widely among patients, sometimes you may have trouble pinpointing the origin and implications of such pain. The clues presented below may help you better decipher your patient's descriptions.
- **Angina.** Many patients describe angina as aching, squeezing, burning, tightness in the chest, or a choking sensation. Nitroglycerin, rest, and oxygen usually relieve the symptoms.
- **Myocardial infarction.** The pain of a myocardial infarction (MI) may be mild or severe. Usually, it waxes and wanes. Many patients describe it as burning, heaviness, tightness, or constriction. Mild pain may seem like indigestion. Severe pain may be crushing. Nitroglycerin typically doesn't relieve the pain of an MI. Indeed, the patient may need morphine to relieve it.
- **Pericarditis.** Patients typically describe the pain of pericarditis as sharp, dull, or aching. You can distinguish it from ischemic pain because it worsens with specific movements—such as lying down, turning in bed, coughing, or breathing deeply. Taking anti-inflammatory drugs and sitting up and leaning forward may relieve the pain.

Keep in mind that many types of chest pain—including angina, the pain of an MI, and the pain of pericarditis—radiate to other locations, including the shoulders, arms, neck, and jaw.

having the patient describe events in his own words, you allow him to set the tone for the interview, and you gather information that he feels is important. This information arms you with what you need to ask your next question.

For instance, if the patient offers little verbal information, ask broader, multiple-choice questions to help trigger his memory and guide the conversation. If he offers too much extraneous information, focus him by asking more specific questions.

In either case, try to elicit information about the patient's signs and symptoms in the order

that they occurred. Most cardiac patients have evidence of cardiac ischemia or insufficiency, such as chest discomfort, syncope, dyspnea, heart rate or rhythm disturbances, or changes in blood pressure.

If your patient reports that he had chest discomfort or pain, thoroughly assess its characteristics. Begin by asking him to describe it. Find out when, where, and under what circumstances it occurred. Ask about the pain's location in the patient's chest—and any other signs or symptoms that appeared with the pain. Have him describe the quality, quantity, and duration of the pain as well any aggravating and alleviating factors (see *Deciphering your patient's chest pain*).

Keep in mind that chest discomfort can stem from many problems, some cardiac, some not. In many cases, its characteristics can help you predict its cause. For example, substernal pain or pressure that arises with exertion and subsides with rest or nitroglycerin probably stems from angina. If it occurs with food intake and responds to antacids rather than nitroglycerin, it probably stems from indigestion or esophageal spasms, especially if the patient has a history of gastritis.

Related signs and symptoms

After you've determined the character of your patient's current signs and symptoms, check for the following additional problems that could stem from cardiac disease.
- *Dyspnea.* Ask if the patient ever has trouble breathing or catching his breath. If so, does it happen at rest or with exertion? How far can he walk before he feels short of breath? How many flights of stairs can he climb?
- *Orthopnea.* Find out if the patient needs to sit upright for adequate ventilation. Can he lay flat without becoming short of breath? Does he sleep in a chair? How many pillows does he sleep on?
- *Paroxysmal nocturnal dyspnea.* Ask if the patient ever has sudden episodes of shortness of breath while he's resting or sleeping.
- *Weight gain.* Question the patient about recent, rapid increases in his weight. If he confirms them, ask him to describe what happened. Remember that a gain of 2 pounds in 1 day or 5 pounds in 1 week usually results from fluid retention—commonly from heart failure. It also

can stem from other factors, such as a high-sodium diet, poor nutrition, renal failure, or noncompliance with diuretic therapy.

- *Cough.* Does the patient have a cough? If so, ask about its frequency, duration, and quality. Is it a dry hack or loose and productive? If productive, is it ever frothy or bloody? Does it interfere with his breathing? Keep in mind that patients with severe pulmonary edema may develop a frequent, productive, loose, frothy cough with occasional hemoptysis.
- *Peripheral edema.* Ask if the patient ever notices that his hands, ankles, or feet are swollen. If so, are both hands, ankles, or feet affected? Is the swelling most noticeable after sitting up for several hours or after walking? Does it disappear after he elevates his feet? Remember that peripheral edema may stem from cellulitis, poor circulation, or right ventricular heart failure.
- *Syncope.* Find out if the patient ever feels light-headed or dizzy, as though he has vertigo. If so, when does he feel this way? What happens when he moves from a lying to a sitting or standing position? Does the light-headedness ever occur with palpitations? Keep in mind that syncope may signal cardiac rhythm disturbances or orthostatic hypotension, especially in older adults. Other causes include the use of diuretics or vasodilators. What's more, aging reduces the body's ability to respond to changes in cardiac output (CO), which poses an increased risk of a myocardial infarction (MI) from decreased blood flow to the heart.
- *Fatigue.* Ask the patient if he is easily fatigued. Has he noticed a change in the amount of energy or effort it takes to perform routine tasks?
- *Intermittent claudication.* Does the patient get leg cramps after walking or during the night?
- *Nocturia.* Does the patient have to urinate frequently during the night? Is it a large amount? Does he have pain when urinating or blood in his urine? Is his urine concentrated or dark amber in color?
- *Falls.* Ask whether the patient has fallen recently. If so, does he remember what caused the fall? Did it occur at night? Remember that syncope, fatigue, and nocturia all predispose patients to falling. If your patient is admitted after a fall, keep in mind that the fall could be an early sign of an underlying cardiac problem.

Previous health problems

To assemble a complete health history, you'll need to obtain information about all the patient's previous health problems, including illnesses, hospitalizations, treatments, blood transfusions, and surgeries. Identify any history of heart problems, including cardiac enlargement, heart failure, murmurs, an MI, arrhythmias, cardiomyopathy, and heart infections. If your patient had cardiac or vascular surgery in the past, have him describe the purpose and type of surgery, its postoperative course, its effectiveness, and any complications.

Next, ask about past illnesses that could lead to cardiac problems, including rheumatic fever, scarlet fever, glomerulonephritis, and viral or bacterial infections. Determine whether your patient has a history of peripheral vascular disease, hypertension, or other circulatory problems.

Naturally, if your patient has had an illness that commonly leads to cardiac problems, you'll need to investigate. For example, if a patient with chest discomfort has a history of coronary artery disease (CAD), an MI, or heart failure, gather specific information about similar episodes in the past. Investigate how the current problem is similar to and different from the previous one. Ask about previous treatments and their effects.

Likewise, as you review each of the patient's body systems, ask specifically about a history of any of the following conditions that could contribute to cardiac disease.

- For the respiratory system, ask about tuberculosis, asthma, pneumonia, bronchitis, lung cancer, and pneumothorax.
- For the renal and endocrine systems, ask about any renal diseases (such as kidney stones, trauma, tumors, or infections); hyperthyroidism, hypothyroidism, or thyroidectomy; any current signs or symptoms of thyroid abnormalities, such as intolerance to heat or cold and weight gain or loss; diabetes mellitus; and any signs or symptoms that may suggest diabetes, such as polyuria, polydipsia, or polyphagia.
- For the neurologic and cardiovascular systems, ask about any history of vertigo, fainting, strokes, or high blood pressure.

Finally, because an effective treatment plan depends on adequate functioning in all body systems, ask about past liver, gallbladder, gastrointestinal (GI), or genitourinary problems.

Checklist of family risk factors

A family history of any of the following conditions may increase your patient's risk of cardiac disorders:
- arthritis
- cardiac conduction disturbances
- cardiomyopathy
- cerebrovascular disease, including cerebrovascular accident
- diabetes mellitus
- hematologic abnormalities
- hypercholesterolemia
- hyperlipidemia
- hypertension
- peripheral vascular disease
- rheumatic fever
- sickle cell anemia
- sudden death
- thyroid disease.

Family history

Your patient's family history contributes important information about cardiovascular risk factors. Ask about the age, sex, and health status of living and deceased family members, including parents, siblings, children, and spouses. Pay close attention to whether any close family members have or had conditions that could increase your patient's risk of cardiac disease (see *Checklist of family risk factors*). Also, investigate for genetic conditions known to increase the risk of cardiac complications, such as Marfan syndrome or Down syndrome.

Cardiac risk factors

Numerous risk factors have been correlated with cardiovascular disease. Typically they're classified as nonmodifiable or modifiable. During your assessment, make careful note of both types.

Nonmodifiable factors

Examples of nonmodifiable cardiac risk factors include the patient's age, sex, and race; a family history of cardiovascular disease; and the presence of certain incurable diseases. Clearly, even if your patient wanted to alter these factors, he

couldn't. For example, he can't change the fact that increasing age increases the risk of an MI, nor can he change the fact that diabetes mellitus contributes to CAD.

Modifiable factors

However, several cardiac risk factors can be reduced through changes in behavior. Question your patient to see if he has any of these risk factors. Also, assess his understanding of these factors as a threat to his cardiac health.

Smoking

Cigarette smoking is the most significant modifiable risk factor for heart disease. During your assessment, ask your patient if he smokes or ever did. If so, find out how much and for how long.

Lifestyle

Sedentary lifestyles and high levels of stress also put people at risk for CAD. Question your patient about activity, rest, stress, and coping mechanisms, not only to assess his risk level but also to help develop a treatment plan that includes appropriate discharge goals.

Alcohol intake

Excessive alcohol intake may lead to dilated or alcoholic cardiomyopathy, which can lead to heart failure. Alcohol also contributes to a poor nutritional state and an unhealthy lifestyle, which may affect the functioning of all body systems over time. Ask your patient about current and past alcohol intake, amount, and frequency. Consider the possibility of alcohol abuse.

Nutrition

Your patient's nutritional status can have a profound impact on the course of his illness and recovery. Plus, certain kinds of foods can raise his risk of CAD and predispose him to having an MI. To assess your patient's nutritional status as it relates to his cardiac risk, ask if he's now on a low-sodium, low-fat, or low-cholesterol diet—or any other special diet. Ask if his dietary habits have changed recently. And ask about his bowel and bladder habits and his use of laxatives or diuretics.

Also, ask about any lifestyle habits, such as exercise, that may affect his dietary intake. Determine whether your patient is now taking any vitamin, mineral, herbal, or other supplements. Ask him to describe what he ate during the previous 24 hours and ask about the types of foods he likes and dislikes. Finally, identify any mechanical problems with chewing or swallowing that could affect his nutritional status. From your comprehensive nutritional assessment, you'll be able to formulate an appropriate educational plan.

Obesity

Obesity causes an increased risk of CAD, angina, and sudden death because of its adverse effect on blood pressure and lipids and its role in increasing the risk of diabetes. What's more, obesity raises the patient's risk of heart failure or an MI by increasing myocardial workload.

Estrogen level

After natural or artificial menopause, women who aren't using estrogen replacement therapy have a higher risk of CAD and MI than premenopausal women. Because estrogen may play an important role in protecting women from heart disease, you should ask your female patients about their use of oral contraceptives or hormone replacement therapy, the cessation of menses, and the start of menopause.

Drug history

Ask your patient for a list of all the drugs he takes. Verify the name of each drug, its purpose and dosage, the length of time the patient has taken it, and any adverse effects he has experienced. Ask about both prescription and over-the-counter (OTC) drugs, including aspirin, acetaminophen, ibuprofen, laxatives, sleeping pills, cold medications, vitamins, and appetite suppressants.

Keep in mind that OTC drugs may interact with prescription drugs—including cardiac drugs. For example, nasal decongestants can increase blood pressure, which may decrease the effect of antihypertensive drugs. Some OTC antihistamines, in combination with certain antibiotics or antifungal drugs, may produce cardiac arrhythmias.

A drug history is especially useful with older patients who may be seeing several physicians for several different medical problems. The resulting combination of prescription drugs, along with advanced age, lack of information, and possible noncompliance, can put your patient at increased risk for drug interactions. If your patient can't recall which drugs he's taking or why, you may need to contact his family, his health care provider, or his place of residence (a skilled nursing facility, for instance) to obtain recent medical records.

Allergies

Ask your patient whether he has any drug, food, environmental, chemical, or other allergies. As appropriate, ask specifically about allergic reactions to latex, dye, or tape. If he reports having an allergic reaction, investigate the circumstances surrounding its onset, the signs and symptoms he experienced, the duration of the event, and any treatments he needed.

Also, investigate whether your patient is sensitive to any drugs or other substances. Although sensitivity isn't as life threatening as anaphylaxis, it is an adverse reaction. This information is essential in planning treatment and avoiding serious complications of therapy.

Self-care and activity tolerance

Information about your patient's activity tolerance, self-care abilities, limitations, exercise habits, and leisure activities can be used to support a diagnosis, establish therapeutic goals, and develop a realistic discharge plan.

Begin by evaluating your patient's ability to perform self-care. Include eating, swallowing, bathing, grooming, dressing, maintaining a satisfactory appearance, and using the toilet or commode. Ask your patient about any limitations in his physical mobility. Can he get into and out of a chair or bed? Has he noticed a decrease in muscle size, tone, strength, or control?

To assess his activity tolerance, begin by having your patient describe the kinds of activities he performs in a typical day. Ask if any of them cause him discomfort; mention such activities as climbing stairs, performing household chores, working outdoors, or pursuing recreational activities. How far can he walk before becoming fatigued? Does he feel constantly tired, weak, or exhausted? Which activities cause him to become short of breath or develop chest discomfort? (Patients with heart failure may report shortness of breath; those with angina may report chest pain.) Are there activities that he can no longer perform? Has he noticed a change in endurance or a decrease in strength? Finally, has he noticed an increase in irritability or listless-

Understanding advance directives

The Patient Self-Determination Act of 1991 requires that nearly every American health care facility (including hospitals, skilled nursing facilities, home-health agencies, and hospices) advise new patients of their right to accept or refuse treatment if they become gravely ill.

Your patient is entitled by law to state his treatment wishes in documents known as advance directives. The most common type of advanced directive is a living will, which outlines the life-prolonging treatments the patient wants or doesn't want if he becomes unable to make his own medical decisions. With another type of advance directive, the health care power of attorney, the patient appoints a proxy to make medical decisions for him if he becomes unable to do so.

Depending on your facility's policy, you may be responsible for informing patients of their right to prepare advance directives. If so, make sure you understand your state's statute and the forms and procedures needed to uphold it. Then, be sure to discuss all the options with the patient, his family, and the patient's physician as early in the hospitalization as possible.

ness or an inability to concentrate or maintain his usual routines?

Determine if your patient is involved in a regular exercise program. Ask about the type of program, the number of times he exercises each week, and the duration of each session. Ask if he has difficulty maintaining his usual activity level; keep in mind that patients who spend several hours a week in an aerobic exercise program may find exertional angina devastating.

After evaluating the patient's activity tolerance, ask about his ability to rest. Inquire about the patient's usual activities before bedtime, the number of hours he sleeps each night, and the kinds of rest periods he observes during the day. Does he use sleep aids, such a warm shower, alcohol, hypnotics, tranquilizers, music, or food? Does he have trouble falling asleep? Does he awaken frequently during the night? Does he feel that he gets adequate rest? This information will give you a baseline for establishing a plan for activities and exercises designed for your patient's individual level of tolerance.

Psychosocial history

As part of a thorough history, you'll want to assess your patient's psychological health, including perceived stress, emotional integrity, and spiritual concerns. These factors can exert a profound influence on your patient's ability to cope with illness and therefore may affect the outcome of his treatment. Also, factors that act as stressors for patients with compromised cardiac function can prompt or aggravate the signs and symptoms of illness.

Ask the patient if he has experienced any stressful events lately, including family, financial, or work-related problems. Ask if these events have caused him anxiety, fear, or grief. Anxiety may arise if your patient faces an altered self-concept, a threat of death, or changes in his health or socioeconomic status, role function, or environment. He may express fear as feelings of dread, but he may not be able to identify the source of these feelings. Finally, the patient may be feeling a real or anticipated sense of loss that he experiences as grieving.

Ask your patient to describe what his illness means to him, bearing in mind that feelings of hopelessness, powerlessness, or frustration can profoundly affect its outcome. As much as possible, have the patient participate in making decisions about his care.

To assess the role of spirituality in your patient's life, start by asking him if he has a religious preference. Ask him how important religion or spirituality is to him and whether it affects his daily life. Ask if he'd like to talk to a clergy member or if he'd like any religious items with him in the hospital. Also, ask about any religious beliefs and practices that could affect his treatment. Finally, find out if the patient has an advance directive that specifies his wishes for future treatment (see *Understanding advance directives*).

Culture, roles, and relationships

Cultural heritage is an important aspect of your patient's identity and may influence his roles and relationships during periods of illness. Cultural beliefs also may render some treatments unacceptable or require the patient's participation in alternative forms of therapy. To assess your patient fully and plan appropriate care, you'll want to investigate the influence of your patient's cultural background.

Keep in mind that culture and roles may affect the patient's manner of communication, both in spoken language and in silence and nonverbal signals, such as eye contact and touch. Throughout your interview, continually assess verbal and nonverbal behaviors that help provide information. If a language barrier hampers your assessment ability, consider using an interpreter. Be aware, however, that using a family member rather than another staff member or professional interpreter may introduce errors or unwanted emotions into your discussion of medical conditions and their treatments. Using gestures and pictures may aid communication.

Because role changes can decrease a patient's coping ability, take time to investigate your patient's roles. For example, ask about his marital status and family situation, including the ages and health status of his family members. If the patient has a job, find out how his illness, hospitalization, and treatment will likely affect it. Find out if the patient is the main source of financial support for his family and, if so, to what degree his illness will affect the family's income. Naturally, anxiety caused by a financial crisis brought on by illness can produce or aggravate the signs and symptoms of a cardiac disorder.

Also, try to determine the effect of your patient's occupation on his health. Ask him to describe his occupation. Find out how many hours he works each week and whether his job produces physical or mental stress. Psychological stress raises the risk of angina, CAD, and an MI.

Is your patient responsible for running the home and caring for children or older adults? If so, assess his level of concern about fulfilling that role, both during hospitalization and after discharge.

Identify and address any sexual concerns the patient may have. Cardiovascular illness, angina, or heart failure can affect your patient's interest in sexual activity and his ability to engage in it. Thus, his illness may profoundly influence his intimate relationships, which may contribute to his anxiety and feelings of loss.

Previous diagnostic reports

Previous diagnostic studies can provide you with valuable information about your patient. Thus, if he has a chronic cardiac problem, such as CAD or heart failure, be sure to ask if he has ever had electrocardiography (ECG), echocardiography, thallium studies, cardiac catheterization, or other cardiac diagnostic tests. Even if he has just been diagnosed with angina, ask if he has had a baseline ECG or stress test.

Ask about the location and date of any previous diagnostic tests. Also, find out if the patient had any recent blood work to check his complete blood count, coagulation time, thyroid function, or electrolyte, cholesterol, triglyceride, serum isoenzyme, or troponin levels. Even if the patient doesn't know the reason for recent blood work, you may want to look at his medical records to examine the results and compare them with those of any new tests he undergoes.

Physical examination

After completing the patient's cardiac health history, you'll perform a systematic physical examination focused on areas that reflect cardiac health and disease. These areas include the patient's height, weight, and vital signs; the precordium; selected arteries and veins; the respiratory system; the abdomen; and the skin, hair, and nails.

Before beginning your physical examination, take steps to provide privacy for your patient. Plan your examination so that you'll obtain essential data first. To minimize the patient's anxiety and promote trust, explain each part of the physical examination before performing it. Reassure the patient that you'll expose only the areas of his body that you're examining. Once you and your patient are comfortable, you can begin.

Height, weight, and vital signs

A cardiac patient's height and weight are essential measurements for establishing the proper dosages of heparin, antibiotics, vasoactive drugs, and other drugs. Ask your patient his height and his most recent weight; compare it to his present weight. A recent weight gain may suggest fluid retention from heart failure, electrolyte imbalances, or renal insufficiency. If your patient is being admitted to an intensive care unit, height and weight measurements are also needed to determine his body surface area when monitoring his CO.

Obtain the patient's pulse rate using both the radial and apical sites. Determine whether his heart rate is rapid or slow and whether his rhythm is regular or irregular. Make note of any radial-apical discrepancies (such as if the apical rate exceeds the radial rate). A difference between the two pulses may reveal cardiac arrhythmias, such as premature systoles or atrial arrhythmias.

Observe the patient's respiratory rate. An accelerated or irregular rate may indicate cardiac decompensation.

Obtain his body temperature. An elevation above 101°F (38.3°C) usually indicates a bacterial infection and should be reported right away. Cardiorespiratory causes of fever could include pneumonia, pericarditis, and endocarditis, especially if your cardiac patient has a valve disorder or mechanical valve. Don't ignore a low body temperature either because it could warn of poor perfusion or a metabolic disorder.

Before taking the patient's blood pressure, remember to ask about conditions that could affect the result, including a history of a mastectomy, cerebrovascular accident (CVA), vascular surgery (such as an arteriovenous shunt in one or both arms), or a circulatory disorder, such as subclavian steal syndrome. If any of these conditions exists, checking blood pressure in the affected arm may not give you an accurate reading.

Normal blood pressure values vary with age, sex, and race. Normally, however, blood pressure in large arteries, such as the brachial artery, ranges from 100 to 140 mm Hg systolic and from 60 to 90 mm Hg diastolic. The difference between systolic and diastolic pressures, called the pulse pressure, represents the range of pressure in the arteries.

To obtain an accurate blood pressure, make sure you have the right size cuff for your patient. The distal margin of the cuff should be at least 2.5 cm above his antecubital fossa, the cuff width should be 40% of the circumference of his arm, and the bladder should encircle his arm one and a half times. Obtain blood pressure readings in both arms, if possible. A difference of 5 to 10 mm Hg between arms is common; a larger difference may reflect mechanical or pathologic problems in arterial blood flow.

In older adults, postural hypotension commonly causes syncope and falls, and it may contribute to an MI by decreasing myocardial blood flow. To assess for this problem, measure your patient's blood pressure while he's supine, and then remeasure it after he has been standing for more than 1 minute, preferably 2 to 3 minutes. If his systolic pressure declines by 20 mm Hg or his diastolic declines by 10 mm Hg in the standing position, consider the test results abnormal.

Consider using a Doppler system to assess blood pressure during low-flow, hypotensive periods in patients who have heart failure or in whom you can't clearly auscultate Korotkoff sounds. To do so, palpate your patient's antecubital fossa for his brachial artery. Place the cuff around his arm and conduction gel on the Doppler probe. Then place the probe over the patient's brachial artery, inflate the cuff, and deflate it until you hear the systolic pressure.

Precordial assessment

After gathering your patient's vital signs, turn to the precordial assessment. As you know, the anterior surface of the patient's chest, closest to his heart and aorta, is called the precordium. By understanding the landmarks of this area and by applying appropriate assessment techniques, you can gain crucial information about your patient's cardiac status (see *Reviewing thoracic landmarks*).

Inspection and palpation
Inspect the precordium for pulsations, lifts, heaves, or retractions and record their locations using anatomic landmarks as reference points. The patient's point of maximal impulse may be visible between the fourth and sixth intercostal spaces, medial to the left midclavicular line, where the anterior wall of the heart lies closest to the chest.

Next, palpate the chest, especially over areas where you observed pulsations. Use the palmar surface of your hand at the bases of your fingers because it's most sensitive to vibrations. Also, palpate the heart valve auscultation sites:
- For the aortic area, palpate the second intercostal space at the right sternal border.
- For the pulmonic area, palpate the second intercostal space at the left sternal border.

Reviewing thoracic landmarks

Your ability to assess your patient's cardiac status accurately depends in part on your ability to use thoracic landmarks precisely. The illustration below shows the key thoracic landmarks and the locations of the heart valves and auscultation sites. Use it to refresh your memory and refine your technique.

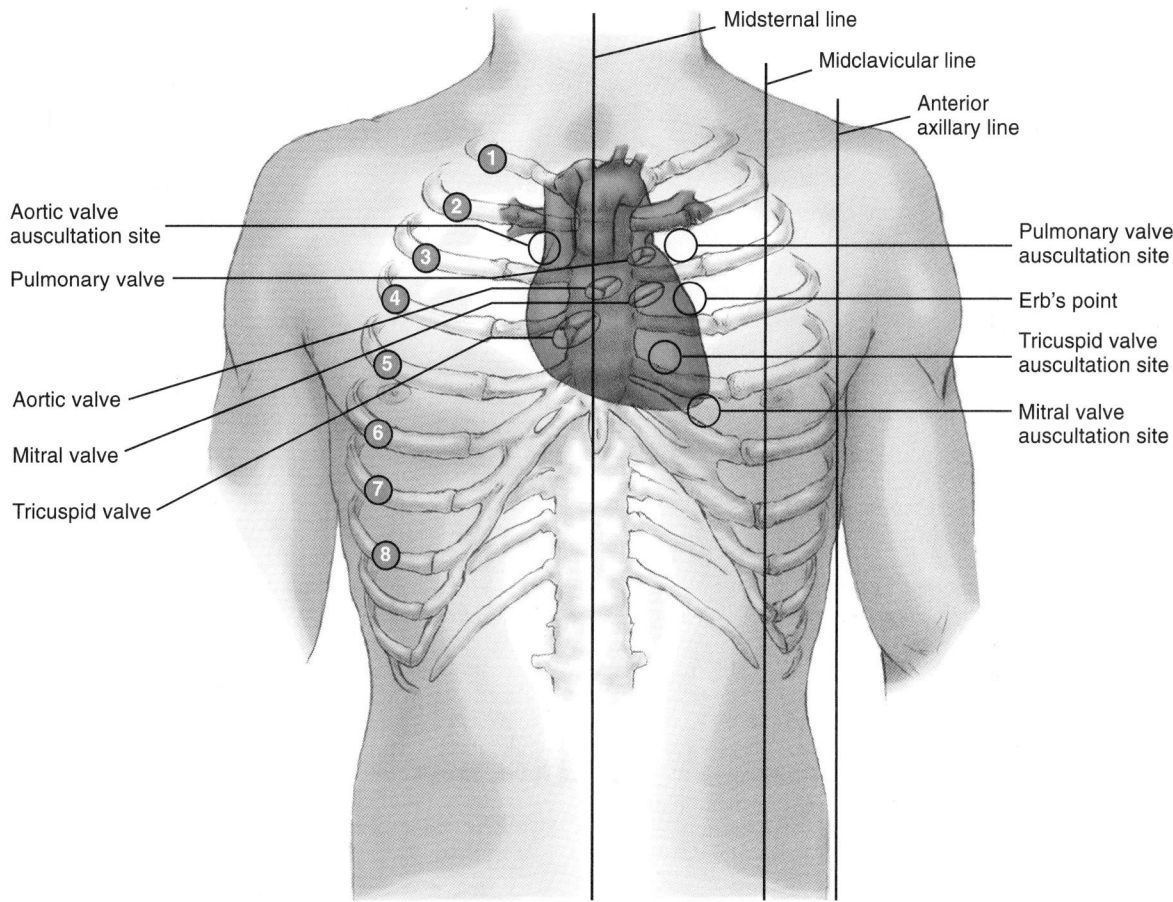

- For the mitral area, palpate the fifth left intercostal space just medial to the midclavicular line.
- For the tricuspid area, palpate the fourth intercostal space at the left sternal border. A lift or heave palpated at the left sternal border may suggest right ventricular hypertrophy.
    Finally, palpate the epigastric area at the base of the sternum, avoiding the xiphoid process.

Pulsations from the abdominal aorta may be felt here. Also, palpate all areas for vibrations, thrills (very rapid, fine vibrations), or pulsations. Note the locations of your findings.

Auscultation
The movement of valves and the flow of blood through the chambers of the heart produce sounds that you can hear with a stethoscope—

Interpreting heart sounds

When you auscultate your patient's chest, you may hear a number of heart sounds, both normal and abnormal. Here's a brief review.

First heart sound
The *lubb* of the normal *lubb-dupp*, the first heart sound (S_1) results from closure of the mitral and tricuspid valves at the onset of systole. It's synchronous with the apical pulse and heard best at the tricuspid valve area or apex.

Second heart sound
The *dupp* of the normal *lubb-dupp*, the second heart sound (S_2) results from closure of the aortic and pulmonary valves at the onset of diastole. It's heard best at the aortic valve area or base of the heart.

When a patient inhales, S_2 may split into two sounds because inspiration prompts an increased blood return to the right side of the heart and a decreased return to the left side (because inflated lungs hold more blood). The sound splits because the aortic valve closes before the pulmonary valve. During expiration, you'll hear only one sound because both valves close at the same time.

Third heart sound
In young children, you may hear a third heart sound (S_3), also called a ventricular gallop, early in diastole during rapid ventricular filling. You'll hear it best at the apex with your patient in the left lateral decubitus position. Only rarely will you hear an S_3 in a healthy patient over age 40. Usually, in an older patient, it results from heart failure or another cardiac disorder.

Fourth heart sound
A fourth heart sound (S_4), also called an atrial gallop, may arise late in diastole. You'll hear it best at the apex. In elderly patients, it may be a normal sound caused by decreased ventricular compliance. Usually, however, it reflects hypertensive cardiovascular disease, coronary artery disease, cardiomyopathy, or aortic stenosis.

Summation gallop
In adults with severe heart disease and tachycardia, S_3 and S_4 may merge into one sound called a summation gallop.

Click
When pressure in the ventricles exceeds that in the aorta, you may hear a click as the aortic valve opens. This click is also called an aortic ejection sound. You can hear it best at the base and the apex. It may result from aortic stenosis, dilation of the aorta, or hypertension. If you hear it just after S_1, it's called an early systolic ejection sound. If you hear it in the middle of systole, it's called a midsystolic click and probably results from damage to the mitral valve's chordae tendineae.

Opening snap
Changes in the mitral or tricuspid valve can result in an opening snap early in diastole. An opening snap in the mitral valve sounds higher pitched than S_3 and occurs earlier in diastole.

Rub
Pericardial inflammation or inadequate lubricating fluid between the visceral and parietal pericardial layers may produce a creaking or grating sound called a pericardial friction rub. It may arise after cardiac surgery or from a myocardial infarction or renal failure.

---

sounds that you can use to assess heart function (see *Interpreting heart sounds*).

As you systematically auscultate over your patient's precordium, first use the diaphragm of your stethoscope (for high-pitched sounds), and then the bell (for lower-pitched sounds). Listen over the four valve auscultation sites and Erb's point.

Normal heart sounds
In a patient with normal heart function, you'll hear two sounds: S_1 and S_2. The first, S_1, results from closure of the mitral and tricuspid valves; S_2 results from closure of the aortic and pulmonary valves.

Because pressure on the left side of the heart exceeds that on the right side, the aortic and mitral valves close a few milliseconds before the pulmonary and tricuspid valves do. Consequently, you may sometimes hear what's called a split S_1 or S_2, especially over the tricuspid area. (To better hear a split S_2, have your patient hold his breath while you listen.) This split sound results from the following:
- normal inspiration (because pulmonary vascular capacity increases and less blood reaches

Characteristics of heart murmurs

When you detect a heart murmur, use its characteristics to help determine its cause.

Timing	Quality and shape	Pitch	Location of maximum intensity	Possible cause
• systolic (ejection)	• harsh • rough • crescendo-decrescendo	• variable	• apex • second right intercostal space	• aortic stenosis
• diastolic	• blowing • decrescendo • loudest just after S_2, diminishing during diastole	• high	• second right intercostal space • third left intercostal space or left sternal border when patient leans forward and holds breath	• aortic regurgitation
• diastolic	• rumbling • presystolic emphasis in sinus rhythm • decrescendo-crescendo	• low	• apex • heard best with patient in left lateral decubitus position	• mitral stenosis
• holosystolic	• blowing • plateau	• high	• apex • heard best with patient in left lateral decubitus position	• mitral regurgitation
• variable	• whooping • honking • crescendo-decrescendo	• high	• apex • heard best with patient in left lateral decubitus position	• mitral valve prolapse with decreased venous return (early systole) or increased venous return (late systole)

the left ventricle)
- increased venous return to the heart during inspiration
- delayed pulmonary valve closure caused by right ventricular systole being slightly more prolonged than left ventricular systole.

Abnormal heart sounds
Extra, usually abnormal, sounds include a third heart sound (S_3), a fourth heart sound (S_4), clicks, snaps, rubs, and murmurs. Use the bell of your stethoscope to auscultate low-pitched sounds, such as S_3, S_4, and diastolic murmurs.

Murmurs are produced by turbulent blood flow through a narrowed, stenotic, or insufficient heart valve. They also can be caused by blood flow through atrial or ventricular septal defects or by other structural problems, such as ruptured pap-

illary muscles or ruptured chordae tendineae (see *Characteristics of heart murmurs*). Valve insufficiency can decrease your patient's activity tolerance and increase his risk of CVA, endocarditis, and heart failure.

Evaluate all murmurs carefully and describe them fully, noting timing, intensity, quality, shape, pitch, location, and radiation.

Timing: Determine whether the murmur occurs during systole or diastole. A systolic murmur occurs with S_1, just after you feel the pulse and just before S_2. It may sound like *lubb-shh-dupp*. A diastolic murmur begins with or just after S_2 and may sound like *lubb-dupp-shh*. If the murmur occurs throughout systole, it's termed *holosystolic* (or *pansystolic*). If it occurs throughout diastole, it's termed *holodiastolic* (or *pandiastolic*).

Intensity: Describe the intensity of the murmur by using a grading system like this one.
- Grade I—a faint murmur heard after listening carefully.
- Grade II—a faint murmur heard right away.
- Grade III—a loud murmur.
- Grade IV—a loud murmur with a thrill.
- Grade V—a very loud murmur that can't be heard without using a stethoscope and an easily palpated thrill.
- Grade VI—a very loud murmur that can be heard without using a stethoscope and an easily palpated and visible thrill.

Keep in mind that a murmur's intensity doesn't always correlate with your patient's condition. For example, a small ventricular septal defect may produce a loud murmur because blood must travel through a small hole under high pressure. If the defect enlarges, the murmur will become softer even as your patient's hemodynamic status declines.

Quality and shape: Describe the sound you hear using such terms as *harsh, blowing,* or *rumbling.* Also, describe the murmur's shape using one of the following four options:
- crescendo, when the murmur starts soft and grows louder
- decrescendo, when it starts loud and grows softer
- crescendo-decrescendo, when it grows louder then softer
- plateau, when the volume remains the same.

Pitch: Identify the pitch of the murmur as either high, medium, or low. If you can hear the murmur best with the diaphragm of your stethoscope, call it high-pitched. If you can hear it best with the bell, call it low-pitched. If you can hear it equally well with diaphragm and bell, call it medium-pitched.

Location: Describe where you can best hear the murmur in relation to the precordial valve areas and other landmarks, such as the sternum, midclavicular lines, and intercostal spaces. Listen over each intercostal space between the second and fifth ribs because heart sounds may not be directed in exactly the same location with every patient. Also, left or right ventricular hypertrophy may shift the angle of the heart in the chest, which may displace the best location to listen to the tricuspid and mitral valves.

Radiation: Document whether the murmur radiates to the chest, axilla, neck, or down the left sternal border. As you listen, follow the direction of the sound. Remember that where you hear it the loudest is not necessarily over the affected valve.

Finally, keep in mind that the patient's position and respirations may alter the characteristics of his murmur. Having him exhale, hold his breath, or sit up and lean forward may help to accentuate aortic murmurs. Mitral murmurs are best heard by placing him in a left lateral recumbent position.

Carotid arteries

To assess your patient's carotid arteries, begin by inspecting both sides of his neck, just below the angle of his jaw. Note whether you can see any pulsations and, if so, whether they're symmetrical.

Then auscultate over each carotid artery with the diaphragm of your stethoscope. Listen for bruits—sounds caused by turbulent blood flow through a vessel narrowed or made irregular by constriction, stenosis, or partial obstruction. Ask your patient to exhale and then to hold his breath while you listen; this will prevent respiratory sounds from obscuring a bruit. Remember that murmurs of aortic stenosis, severe aortic regurgitation, or ruptured chordae tendineae may radiate to the carotid arteries and be mistaken for bruits.

Next, palpate one carotid artery with the distal pads of your index and middle fingers. If you heard a bruit in that artery, press lightly. Never palpate the carotid arteries simultaneously because you could compromise blood flow to the patient's brain or slow his heart by stimulating the vagus nerve. Determine the rate and rhythm of carotid pulses on both sides of his neck, along with their amplitude (or strength) and symmetry.

Jugular veins

Pulsations of the internal and external jugular veins can give you information about right atrial function. To assess these veins, place your patient on his back with the head of the bed raised 45 degrees. Then watch the pulsations. You'll see them as a series of undulating waves, called the a, c, and v waves, and the x and y descent (see *Observing the jugular venous pulse*).

Observing the jugular venous pulse

If you watch your patient's jugular venous pulse closely, you'll see that it's actually a series of undulating waves—not one sharp impulse. These waves result largely from the effects of the heart's mechanical movements, as described below and shown on the waveform.

The jugular venous pulse consists of three upward waves and two major descents. The first upward wave, the *a* wave, reaches its peak just before the first heart sound (S_1). It results from retrograde transmission to the jugular veins after atrial contraction. In fact, if you palpate the carotid artery on the other side of the patient's neck, you'll see the *a* wave just before you feel the carotid pulsation. If your patient's atrial pressure is elevated, as in right ventricular heart failure, the *a* wave will be more pronounced than usual.

Just after S_1, you'll see the *c* wave. It's caused by forceful closure of the tricuspid valve. After the *a* and *c* waves, you'll see a downward movement of the jugular venous pulse called the *x* descent. It results from atrial diastole.

Just after the second heart sound (S_2) comes the *v* wave, which results from the increase in right atrial pressure during ventricular contraction, while the tricuspid valve is closed. After the tricuspid valve opens and right atrial pressure drops, you'll see what's called the *y* descent. Just before S_1, the *a* wave will rise to start the process all over again.

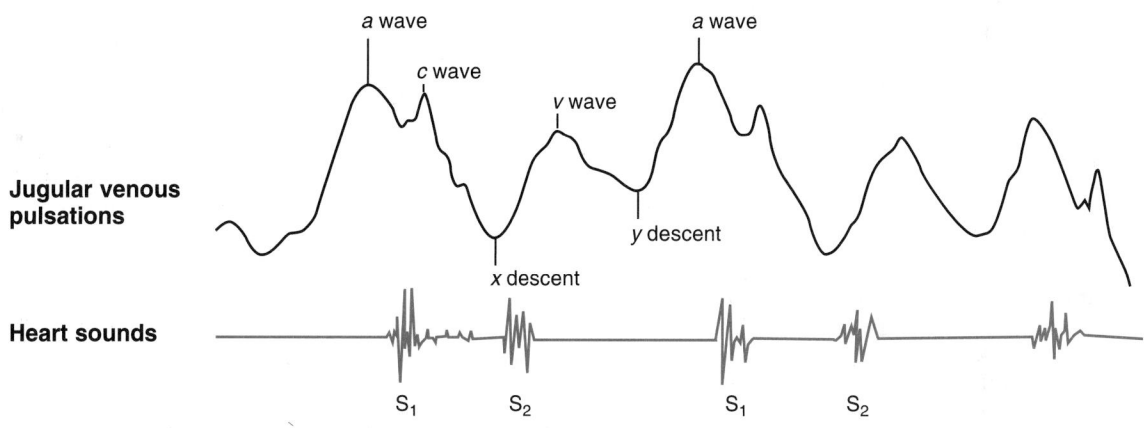

Venous pulse waves may be easier to observe in the external jugular veins. Plus, because the internal jugular veins run close to the carotid arteries, you might confuse the two. (Venous pulsations are easier to obliterate than arterial ones. Just press at the base of the patient's neck; the pulsations that disappear are venous.)

Several factors can affect jugular vein waves. One is patient position. With your patient supine, the waves will be accentuated. If he sits up, they'll be less prominent. Another factor is venous pressure. Normally, venous pressure decreases with inspiration; however, the amplitude of the waves you see may increase because thoracic vein capacity increases during inspiration, with a resulting increase in blood returning to the right side of the heart. A third factor is the application of pressure on the patient's abdomen. Applying firm pressure to the right upper quadrant of the patient's abdomen for about 30 seconds can make his jugular veins more visible even if he has normal heart function. If he has right ventricular heart failure, the waves will become yet more prominent.

You can assess your patient's central venous pressure (CVP) by holding a centimeter ruler in a vertical position with the bottom at the patient's manubriosternal junction (angle of Louis). Then hold another ruler in a horizontal position so that one end rests at the highest level of jugular filling and the other intersects the centimeter ruler. The vertical distance on the centimeter ruler equals your patient's CVP.

Normally, CVP is 1 to 2 cm above the angle of Louis with your patient lying at a 45-degree angle. A larger measurement, which indicates that pulsations rise higher in the neck, may result from heart failure, constrictive pericarditis, or obstruction of the superior vena cava.

Keep in mind that, in older adults, using the left jugular veins to measure CVP may not give you a reliable result. That's because with increasing age, the aorta stiffens, dilates, and elongates—changes that may compress veins on the left side of the neck and obliterate the pulsations, thus giving you a falsely low reading and masking one of the signs of heart failure.

Arterial pulses

Palpating your patient's peripheral pulses will give you an indication of the sufficiency of his arterial circulation. Palpate bilateral radial and pedal pulses and compare the intensity and symmetry between limbs and between the upper and lower limbs. Determine the rate, rhythm, contour, and amplitude of each pulse. Assess rate and rhythm by palpating for at least 30 seconds if the pulse is regular and 1 to 2 minutes if it's irregular.

The contour of the pulses should be rounded and smooth (dome shaped) in healthy arteries, with a sharp upstroke and more gradual downstroke. Increased arterial pressure may produce a large, bounding pulse with a rapid upstroke and fast downstroke; it may result from exercise, anxiety, fear, anemia, aortic regurgitation, hypertension, or CAD. Decreased pressure may produce a small, weak pulse; it may result from decreased left ventricular output in heart failure or from aortic stenosis, where blood is ejected slowly over a stenosed valve. If your patient has weak pulses, you may need to use a Doppler ultrasound device to assess them.

Describe your patient's pulse amplitude on a scale of 0 to 4:
- 0 = not palpable
- +1 = faintly palpable but diminished
- +2 = normal
- +3 = increased
- +4 = bounding.

If you notice that the strength or amplitude of your patient's pulses changes in a pattern, you'll want to assess for alternating pulse and paradoxical pulse. In alternating pulse, the patient has a regular pulse that alternates in size and intensity; it stems from heart failure.

In paradoxical pulse, the pulse diminishes in amplitude with normal inspiration. This abnormality results from wide swings in intrathoracic pressure during breathing. To check for paradoxical pulse, use the following procedure:
- Explain the procedure to your patient and ask him to breathe normally.
- Inflate the blood pressure cuff to 20 to 30 mm Hg above his usual systolic level.
- Deflate the cuff until you hear the first clear Korotkoff sound, then stop deflating. Make note of this reading.
- If the Korotkoff sound disappears when the patient takes a breath, then reappears when he exhales, continue with the steps listed below.
- Begin deflating again, but only 2 mm Hg at a time. After each 2 mm Hg, stop and assess your readings again as the patient breathes.
- Continue this procedure until you can hear Korotkoff sounds during both inspiration and expiration. The difference between the first sound you heard and the sound unaffected by breathing is the paradoxical pulse. If it's more than 10 mm Hg, the patient may have pericardial tamponade, adhesive pericarditis, severe lung disease, or advanced heart failure.

Peripheral veins

Inspect your patient's peripheral veins for signs of thrombosis, varicosities, or edema. Bilateral dependent edema results from increased fluid pressure in the extracellular spaces from poor circulation or heart failure.

To assess your patient for peripheral edema, press over a bony prominence in his ankles or feet. If he's bedridden, press over the sacral area. Watch for pitting, or an indentation, when you release the pressure, and use this scale to record your findings:
- 0 = no edema
- +1 = trace edema; indentation disappears rapidly
- +2 = moderate edema; indentation disappears in 10 to 15 seconds
- +3 = deep edema; indentation disappears in 1 to 2 minutes
- +4 = very deep edema; indentation still present after 5 minutes.

If your patient has peripheral edema but no pitting, he may have arterial disease rather than venous disease. In general, arterial insufficiency or occlusion causes a dull ache called claudication that results from ischemia. Claudication is brought on by exercise, increases with the intensity and duration of exercise, and resolves with rest. Eventually, if the occlusion progresses, the patient will have pain even at rest.

Pain caused by venous occlusion begins during or possibly several hours after exercise and tends to be constant. Although relieved by rest, it may take several hours or days to disappear. Pain from venous insufficiency doesn't correlate directly with the intensity or duration of exercise.

Respiratory assessment

To assess your patient's cardiac function adequately, you also must assess his respiratory function. That's because cardiac problems may produce respiratory problems. Heart failure commonly causes pulmonary edema, for instance.

Begin your assessment by determining the rate, rhythm, and depth of your patient's respirations. Adults normally breathe 16 to 20 times per minute. Observe whether his breathing is shallow, moderate, or deep. Also, note whether he's using accessory muscles to breathe and whether his chest expands symmetrically. When you ask him to take a deep breath, does he show a poor respiratory effort? Is his breathing noisy? Does he flare his nostrils? Does he purse his lips when breathing? Are his lips pink, dusky, or cyanotic? Is he using diaphragmatic or abdominal breathing? As you continue to observe his breathing, watch for these abnormal variations that could have a cardiac origin:
• bradypnea
• Cheyne-Stokes respirations
• dyspnea
• hyperventilation
• obstructive breathing
• orthopnea
• tachypnea.

Then, observe the shape and symmetry of his chest. After palpating and percussing the lung fields and measuring diaphragmatic excursion, auscultate the patient's lung fields using the diaphragm of your stethoscope. Begin with the upper fields and work your way down to the diaphragm. Remember to assess two lobes on the left and three on the right, noting any abnormal or adventitious breath sounds, such as crackles, wheezes, rhonchi, rubs, or diminished, absent, or referred breath sounds.

Crackles, also known as rales, are abnormal sounds produced when air passes over fluid. You can simulate the sound of fine crackles by rubbing a few strands of hair between your fingers next to your ear. Lower-pitched, medium crackles sound like crackling plastic wrap.

Crackles may result from left ventricular heart failure, in which fluid accumulates in the alveoli. In the early stages of heart failure, you'll hear fine crackles in dependent areas of the lung bases. As the condition progresses, they'll become more moist and more coarse. Usually, they don't clear with coughing.

If you hear a low-pitched, coarse, creaking sound when your patient inhales, it could be either a pleural rub or a pericardial friction rub. To differentiate between the two, ask your patient to stop breathing for a moment while you keep listening. If the sound stops, it's a pleural rub. If you continue to hear it with each heartbeat, it's a pericardial friction rub.

Abdominal assessment

A thorough cardiac assessment also should include the patient's abdomen because some cardiac problems produce abdominal problems and vice versa. For example, increased abdominal pressure will elevate the patient's CVP. Fluid overload from hepatic or renal dysfunction can cause cardiac decompensation and heart failure. And severe right ventricular heart failure can lead to liver congestion and fluid in the peritoneal space, causing ascites.

With your patient in the supine position, begin by inspecting his abdomen from the costal margins down to the pubic symphysis. Inspect the skin for color changes, which may suggest jaundice or cyanosis; taut, shiny skin, which suggests ascites; and marked pulsations, which may indicate an abdominal aneurysm or increased pressure in the vessel.

After a thorough inspection, auscultate the abdomen using the diaphragm of your stethoscope. Listen in all four quadrants for bowel sounds.

Recognizing clubbed fingers

A patient with normal nail bed angles will have a diamond-shaped opening when he places his fingertips nail to nail because the normal nail bed angle is about 160 degrees.

In contrast, a patient with chronically poor oxygenation develops clubbed fingers, in which the nail bed angle increases to more than 180 degrees. When he places his fingertips nail to nail, he has no open space.

Common causes of clubbed fingers include respiratory disease, cardiovascular disease, cirrhosis, thyroid disease, and heavy smoking.

Normal fingers	Clubbed fingers

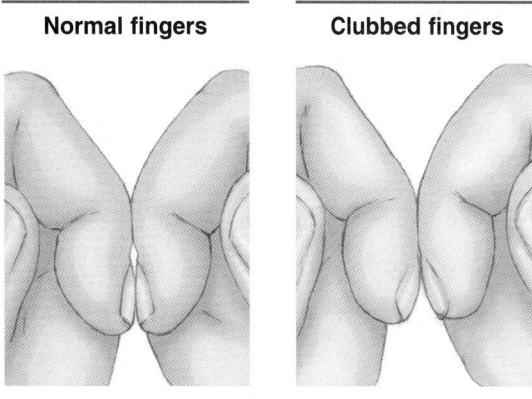

Then use the bell of your stethoscope to listen in the epigastric area and all four quadrants for bruits arising from the abdominal aorta and the renal, iliac, and femoral arteries.

Integumentary assessment

Now examine your patient's skin, hair, and nails, each of which offers information about the patient's circulation. Observe the patient's skin for mottling, cyanosis, or pallor, which suggests diminished or altered blood flow. Note the color of his lips and nail beds; peripheral cyanosis will be most evident in these areas. Also, watch for clubbing of the fingers, a classic sign of chronically poor tissue oxygenation (see *Recognizing clubbed fingers*).

Check your patient's skin turgor to assess hydration, but don't use the back of his hand be-cause the skin is too loose and too thin. To check turgor, squeeze a portion of skin between your thumb and forefingers so that it stands up, and then let it go. It should spring immediately back into place. If it returns slowly or remains pinched together, your patient has poor turgor, which could result from illness, dehydration, or decreased circulation. Keep in mind that skin thickness varies with location and that skin atrophies and becomes thinner with chronically diminished blood flow, as in arterial insufficiency.

Skin temperature, capillary refill time, and hair distribution can tell you about blood supply as well. Chronically cool skin suggests decreased blood flow. In heart failure with low CO, the skin may be cool, moist, and pale. To assess capillary refill time, press the nail bed of your patient's thumb or great toe for about 5 seconds, until it blanches. Then let it go and watch how long it takes for blood to return. With adequate blood flow, color returns within 2 seconds.

To find additional signs of circulatory problems, check your patient's legs. In chronic arterial insufficiency, the skin will be pale and cool, and hair will be diminished or absent (because the follicles need blood to survive). The skin also will look thin and shiny. In a dependent position, the limb may become dusky red. The nails thicken and become ridged. In chronic venous insufficiency, the skin becomes rough, thick, and edematous. Hair loss may not occur, skin temperature may be normal, and skin color may be normal, cyanotic, or brown and pigmented.

As the final step in your assessment of the patient's skin, hair, and nails, make note of any edema. It may result from cellulitis, inadequate circulation, heart failure, malnutrition, lymphatic problems, or electrolyte imbalances.

Diagnostic tests

Along with the health history and focused physical examination, diagnostic tests play a vital role in helping to diagnose and treat your cardiac patient. The following section provides an overview of tests commonly used in cardiac assessment.

Blood tests

These tests include analyses of a patient's serum electrolytes, cardiac enzymes and isoenzymes, lipids and lipoproteins, protein and its metabolites, arterial blood gases (ABGs), and coagulation.

Electrolytes

Typically, you'll check your patient's sodium, potassium, chloride, calcium, and magnesium levels (see *Reviewing normal electrolyte levels*).

Serum sodium levels reflect the patient's fluid balance. They may decrease from the hemodilution caused by heart failure or from diuretic therapy used for hypertension and heart failure. They may increase from dehydration, poor nutrition, and overuse of diuretics.

Potassium imbalances can have serious adverse effects on heart rhythm. Hypokalemia can cause cardiac irritability, ECG changes, and ventricular arrhythmias. It commonly results from using potassium-wasting diuretics to treat heart failure, and it may raise your patient's risk of digitalis toxicity. Hypokalemic alkalosis may persist if you fail to supply chloride with the patient's potassium supplement. Hyperkalemia, on the other hand, can cause myocardial depression, ECG changes, and ventricular irritability, which may lead to ventricular arrhythmias or asystole. It usually stems from renal or endocrine disorders.

Decreased serum chloride levels may result from diuretic therapy; increased levels may result from cardiac decompensation. Although they're seldom a primary problem for the cardiac patient, you'll need to monitor his serum chloride levels if he's receiving potassium supplements to treat hypokalemia.

Decreased calcium levels may cause ventricular arrhythmias, ECG changes, and cardiac arrest; elevated calcium levels may cause atrioventricular (AV) block, ECG changes, digitalis glycoside hypersensitivity, and cardiac arrest.

Because magnesium assists in calcium absorption and metabolism, a deficiency of either one has a significant effect on the metabolism of the other. Consequently, decreased magnesium levels can lead to hypocalcemia or hypokalemia, ECG changes, premature ventricular contractions, ventricular tachycardia, and ventricular fibrillation. Such a decrease may result from diuretic therapy. Increased magnesium levels may cause ECG changes and bradycardia.

Nursing considerations

- Assess your cardiac patient regularly for signs and symptoms of electrolyte disturbances, such as lethargy, leg or abdominal cramps,

Reviewing normal electrolyte levels

Electrolyte	Normal range
Sodium	135–145 mEq/L
Potassium	3.5–5.0 mEq/L
Chloride	95–105 mEq/L
Calcium	4.5–5.5 mEq/L or 9–11 mg/dl
Magnesium	1.2–2.6 mEq/L

confusion, palpitations, and numbness or tingling of the lips or fingers.
- If you suspect an electrolyte disorder, weigh the patient daily and keep accurate fluid intake and output records. Also, watch his ECG carefully for changes.
- If your patient has heart failure, monitoring his electrolyte levels will give you valuable information about his response to treatment.
- If he's receiving diuretic therapy, you'll need to assess his electrolyte levels at regular intervals to avoid complications from excessive or long-term therapy.
- If the patient takes a digitalis glycoside or a diuretic, monitor him closely for arrhythmias. Decreased potassium levels can increase the risk of digitalis toxicity.
- Treatment of electrolyte deficiencies includes electrolyte replacement by oral or I.V. administration.
- Electrolyte excesses can be treated with hypertonic ion exchange resins or hemodialysis.

Cardiac enzymes and isoenzymes

Intracellular enzymes released by damaged cardiac tissue offer key information in the diagnosis of an MI. Those commonly used to detect an MI include creatine kinase (CK), lactate dehydrogenase (LD), and aspartate aminotransferase (AST). After an MI, plasma levels of these enzymes rise in a predictable pattern and then slowly return nearly to baseline levels. Keep in mind that the magnitude by which cardiac enzyme levels rise tells you nothing about the location of cardiac

Measuring myoglobin and troponin T levels

If your patient may be having a myocardial infarction (MI), his physician may order myoglobin or troponin T tests in addition to the usual cardiac isoenzyme testing. That's because myoglobin and troponin T levels rise soon after an MI, and the test results can help ensure that appropriate patients receive thrombolytic therapy as quickly as possible.

Myoglobin is an oxygen-binding protein found in cardiac and skeletal muscle. After an MI, myoglobin levels rise even faster than those of the cardiac isoenzyme creatine kinase (CK-MB). In fact, elevated levels can be detected as soon as 1 hour after an acute MI; they peak 4 to 12 hours after an MI. Because injury to skeletal muscle can increase myoglobin levels as well, this test isn't as specific as a CK-MB measurement, however.

Many emergency departments now measure an isotype of troponin to aid in diagnosing an MI. Troponin, a protein complex found in the ultrastructure of myocardial cells, has three isotypes: T, I, and C. Troponin T is cardiac specific and is elevated for 3.5 hours to 10 days after an MI.

damage. It does, however, provide information about the magnitude of cardiac damage.

Because CK and LD are found in other organs besides the heart, a diagnosis of an MI usually must rely on the measurement of isoenzymes specific to cardiac tissue. CK has three isoenzymes: CK-BB appears in the lungs, intestines, bladder, and brain; CK-MB appears almost exclusively in cardiac muscle; and CK-MM appears in skeletal muscle.

The CK-MB level rises 3 to 8 hours after an MI, peaks between 10 and 24 hours, and returns to baseline after 3 to 4 days. CK-MM can also be found in the serum of all patients for 48 hours after a transmural MI, but it may be elevated with crescendo or unstable angina even in the absence of an MI.

LD has five isoenzymes. Trends in LD_1 and LD_2 provide the most useful information when diagnosing an MI. Normally, serum levels of LD_2 are higher than those of LD_1. After acute myocardial damage or infarction, however, levels of LD_1 (a cardiac-specific isoenzyme) rise above those of LD_2. You'll hear this change called a flipped LD, and it's diagnostic for an MI.

Nursing considerations

- If your patient is admitted through the emergency department within 6 hours after a suspected MI, tell him that his blood will be tested for trends in certain enzyme levels and possibly also for proteins called myoglobin and troponin T (see *Measuring myoglobin and troponin T levels*).
- Tell your patient and his family that you'll need to draw blood in a set sequence to evaluate the trends in his enzyme levels. Usually, you'll take blood samples as soon as an MI is suspected, and again after 12, 24, and 48 hours.
- Heparin may falsely elevate LD and AST levels.
- Avoid giving intramuscular (I.M.) injections if your patient may have had an MI; they can raise CK levels threefold.
- After thrombolytic therapy or percutaneous transluminal coronary angioplasty (PTCA), a rapid, early peak in CK-MB suggests successful coronary artery reperfusion.

Lipids and lipoproteins

Levels of cholesterol, triglycerides, and lipoproteins can help you evaluate your patient's risk of developing CAD. As you know, cholesterol is consumed in the diet and made by the liver. Its metabolism varies with dietary intake and heredity. A total serum cholesterol level above 200 mg/dl may increase your patient's risk of CAD. Triglycerides, another lipid group that provides energy for the body, are also derived from diet and produced by the liver. Lipoproteins, or protein-bound phospholipids, help transport cholesterol into and out of body cells. Two classes of lipoproteins have implications for cardiac disease.

Low-density lipoproteins (LDLs) are 50% cholesterol and have a clear correlation with CAD. They transport endogenous cholesterol to the body's cells. Because they have the highest concentration of cholesterol, LDLs are commonly referred to as bad cholesterol. In general, patients should strive to keep LDL levels below 130 mg/dl; those with CAD should aim for levels below 100 mg/dl.

High-density lipoproteins (HDLs) are mostly

protein with some cholesterol and phospho-lipids. HDLs may help move cholesterol from pe-ripheral cells back to the liver. They also may help to decrease the uptake of cholesterol and lipids into cells. This would account for the pro-tective role attributed to HDLs. They reduce the risk of CAD by preventing an accumulation of lipids in the arterial walls. Normal values range from 35 to 70 mg/dl for men and 35 to 85 mg/dl for women.

A ratio of total cholesterol levels and HDL cho-lesterol levels can help identify an increased risk of heart disease. To determine this ratio, divide your patient's total cholesterol level by his HDL level. The higher the total cholesterol to HDL ra-tio, the greater his risk.

Nursing considerations
- Instruct your patient to fast for 12 hours be-fore having a lipid profile. Tell him he may have water.
- Also, tell him to avoid alcohol or smoking for 12 hours before the test because both may in-terfere with the measurement of HDL levels.
- Before the test, have your patient avoid drugs that alter lipid levels, including oral contracep-tives, corticosteroids, estrogen, and salicylates.
- Initial treatment for patients with high choles-terol levels includes a low-fat, low-cholesterol diet and increased activity. Exercise increases HDL levels, while reducing dietary fat intake decreases LDL levels.
- If levels don't improve with diet and exercise, then the patient may need a lipid-lowering drug and regular monitoring of serum lipid levels.
- Repeated tests of cholesterol, triglyceride, and lipoprotein levels can help evaluate the pa-tient's response to treatment.
- If a lipid-lowering drug is prescribed, teach the patient about it.
- Also, teach the patient about the low-fat, low-cholesterol diet. If he has further questions or special dietary needs, arrange a consultation with a dietitian.

Protein and its metabolites
Cardiac disorders that reduce renal circulation or perfusion, such as heart failure and cardio-genic shock, can increase blood urea nitrogen (BUN) and creatinine levels. That's why you may need to measure BUN and creatinine levels in a patient with a cardiac disorder.

Levels of BUN reflect the kidneys' ability to ex-crete urea, the end product of protein metabo-lism. Normal levels range from 8 to 25 mg/dl. Cre-atinine, produced by the breakdown of muscle tis-sue, is also excreted by the kidneys. Normal levels range from 0.6 to 1.2 mg/dl.

Nursing considerations
- Tell your patient that BUN and creatinine lev-els are measured with simple blood tests to help determine kidney function.
- If decreased renal perfusion results from poor CO, one of the goals of treatment will be to im-prove cardiac function. As CO increases, renal perfusion should improve, and BUN and creati-nine levels should return to baseline.
- Because many drugs are excreted through the kidneys, impaired renal function may affect the dosage for some cardiac drugs.
- A high-protein diet, drugs, blood in the GI tract, injury, infection, fever, poor nutrition, and fluid status can influence BUN levels.
- Creatinine and BUN levels should be moni-tored carefully during long-term use of poten-tially nephrotoxic drugs, such as diuretics, to treat heart failure or hypertension.

Arterial blood gases
Arterial blood gas levels show the adequacy of oxygenation, ventilation, and acid-base balance in the patient's body. Although normal values may vary by facility, here are typical normal ranges:
- pH, 7.35 to 7.45
- partial pressure of arterial oxygen, 80 to 100 mm Hg
- partial pressure of arterial carbon dioxide ($Paco_2$), 35 to 45 mm Hg
- bicarbonate, 24 to 28 mEq/L
- base excess, +1 to −1 mEq/L.

Because many factors influence ABG interpre-tation, consider the patient's signs, symptoms, and diagnosis carefully. Usually, you'll look first at the pH, which indicates the acid-base balance in the patient's blood. If it's high (> 7.45), your pa-tient has alkalosis. If it's low (< 7.35), your patient has acidosis. Now, based on what the pH told you, you can go further (see *Interpreting arterial blood gas values,* pages 30 and 31).

If your patient has acidosis, determine whether it's respiratory or metabolic. If it's respiratory, ex-pect to see an elevated $Paco_2$, which means that your patient isn't eliminating carbon dioxide effi-

Interpreting arterial blood gas values

Use this table to review the characteristic findings for respiratory acidosis, respiratory alkalosis, metabolic acidosis, and metabolic alkalosis.

Acid-base imbalance	pH	Arterial carbon dioxide	Bicarbonate	Nursing considerations
Respiratory acidosis				
Uncompensated	< 7.35	Increased	Normal	• Causes include pneumonia, chronic obstructive pulmonary disease, respiratory depression, and narcotic overdose. • Patient may be restless, disoriented, lethargic, and hypoxic. • Give respiratory therapy, oxygen, and bicarbonate (HCO_3^-) as ordered.
Partially compensated	< 7.35, but moving toward normal	Increased	Increasing	• Body conserves HCO_3^- to increase pH. • Give respiratory therapy, oxygen, and HCO_3^-, as ordered.
Compensated	Normal	Increased, but may start decreasing	Increased	• Occurs in pulmonary diseases that have decreased alveolar ventilation and ventilation-perfusion mismatch. • Give respiratory therapy and oxygen, as ordered.
Respiratory alkalosis				
Uncompensated	> 7.45	Decreased	Normal	• Causes include hyperventilation from pain or anxiety, increased respiratory rate on mechanical ventilator, and medullary tumor. • Patient is light-headed and has numbness and tingling of fingers and toes. • Have patient breathe into paper bag. Turn down respiratory rate and volume on ventilator and give sedatives and tranquilizers as needed.
Partially compensated	> 7.45, but moving toward normal	Decreased	Decreasing	• As HCO_3^- begins to decline, give carbon dioxide (CO_2) or have patient breathe into paper bag or take slow, deep breaths. • Turn down respiratory rate on the ventilator.
Compensated	Normal	Decreased, but may start increasing	Decreased	• Not commonly seen in acutely ill patients but, when present, may signal poor prognosis. • Give oxygen therapy. Treatment varies with underlying cause.

ciently. If $Paco_2$ is normal, his acidosis doesn't result from a respiratory problem. So you'll need to look at bicarbonate. If $Paco_2$ is normal and bicarbonate is low, the patient has metabolic acidosis.

If your patient has alkalosis, determine whether it's respiratory or metabolic. If bicarbonate is normal and $Paco_2$ is low, it's a respiratory problem. If bicarbonate is high and $Paco_2$ is normal, then it's metabolic.

The body attempts to correct pH disturbances through a combination of raising and lowering the carbon dioxide and bicarbonate levels. First,

Interpreting arterial blood gas values (continued)

Acid-base imbalance	pH	Arterial carbon dioxide	Bicarbonate	Nursing considerations
Metabolic acidosis				
Uncompensated	< 7.35	Normal	Decreased	• Causes include diabetic ketoacidosis, renal failure, and increased metabolic demand. • Patient may have headache, mental dullness, Kussmaul's respirations. • Treatment varies with underlying cause.
Partial respiratory compensation	< 7.35, but moving toward normal	Decreasing	Decreased	• Body conserves HCO_3^- to increase pH. • Patient may need HCO_3^- I.V. or dialysis. • Respiratory rate increases to blow off CO_2.
Compensated	Normal	Decreased	Decreased, but may start increasing	• Occurs most commonly in patients with chronic renal failure. • Respiratory compensation is minimal. Patient may need HCO_3^- I.V. or dialysis.
Metabolic alkalosis				
Uncompensated	> 7.45	Normal	Increased	• Causes include excessive vomiting, diarrhea, antacid use, and diuretic therapy. • Patient may have confusion, dizziness, numbness, tingling in limbs. • Treatment varies with underlying cause.
Partial respiratory compensation	> 7.45, but moving toward normal	Increasing	Increasing	• Respiratory rate may slow down. • Give sodium chloride, potassium, or diuretic, as ordered.
Compensated	Normal	Increased	Increased, but may start decreasing	• Patient may be asymtpomatic. • Treatment varies with underlying cause.

the body increases or decreases the respiratory rate in an attempt to correct the pH. Next, the internal buffer system raises or lowers bicarbonate levels. Compensation corrects the pH, but it won't correct the cause of the problem. If your patient's body can't compensate, he'll need medical intervention. First correct the pH, and then identify and treat the underlying problem.

Nursing considerations
• Explain the procedure for obtaining ABG measurements to your patient.
• Tell your patient that monitoring his ABGs can help to indicate the effectiveness of his treatment.
• After obtaining an arterial sample, apply pressure to the puncture site for 3 to 5 minutes.
• As you monitor ABG levels, remember that increases in oxygen saturation along with normalization of $Paco_2$ may indicate improved CO.

Coagulation studies
Before beginning any treatments for a cardiac patient, evaluate his blood coagulation studies. If he has an elevated bleeding time, a deficiency in clotting factors, or an abnormal platelet count, some treatments may be temporarily withheld. Com-

mon coagulation studies include bleeding time, platelet count, activated partial thromboplastin time (APTT), prothrombin time (PT), fibrinogen, plasminogen, and activated clotting time.

Bleeding time: This test measures the time it takes for your patient to stop bleeding. Place a blood pressure cuff on the patient's upper arm and inflate it to about 40 mm Hg. Then make a small puncture wound in the forearm. Normally, bleeding stops in 2 to 9 minutes. Prolonged bleeding can result from vascular disorders, deficiencies in clotting factors, and anticoagulation therapy (including aspirin).

Platelet count: This test measures the patient's circulating platelets, or thrombocytes, which have a role in blood clotting. Two-thirds of platelets are found in the circulation and one-third in the spleen. Normally, platelet levels range from 150,000 to 400,000/mm^3. Decreased values prolong the bleeding time and impair clot dissolution. Heparin, antineoplastics, radiation therapy, and disseminated intravascular coagulation (DIC) may cause a low platelet count. Stress or infection may produce thrombocytosis, an elevation in the platelet count.

Activated partial thromboplastin time: This measurement tests the patient's intrinsic clotting system (factors VIII, IX, XI, and XII) as well as the final pathway (factors II, V, and X). It identifies deficiencies of coagulation factors, prothrombin, and fibrinogen and is used to monitor heparin therapy. Normally, APTT ranges from 26 to 45 seconds. The therapeutic range for heparin therapy is 1.5 to 2 times the control value. Prolonged APTT in the absence of heparin therapy indicates a coagulation disorder.

Prothrombin time: This test measures the activity and interaction of factors V, VII, and X; prothrombin; and fibrinogen. It's also used to monitor warfarin therapy. Normal PT is 11 to 12.5 seconds. The therapeutic range for warfarin therapy is 1.3 to 1.5 times the control for deep vein thrombosis, atrial arrhythmias, or pulmonary embolism, and 1.5 to 2.0 times the control for mechanical heart valves. Prolonged PT indicates warfarin therapy or a clotting factor deficiency.

International normalized ratio: Using the international normalized ratio (INR) may be a more accurate way of monitoring warfarin therapy. You can obtain the INR by dividing your patient's PT by the laboratory control value or your patient's own control (baseline) value. Therapeutic guidelines for the INR are 2.0 to 3.0 for deep vein thrombosis, atrial arrhythmias, or pulmonary embolism and 3.0 to 4.5 for mechanical heart valves.

Fibrinogen: This clotting factor converts to fibrin during coagulation, making it an essential element in the process. It's commonly measured by a test called the thrombin time (TT). Normally, TT lasts 25 to 35 seconds. Normal fibrinogen values range from 200 to 400 mg/dl. The TT will be prolonged when fibrinogen levels are below 100 mg/dl. Low levels may indicate liver disease or DIC. High levels may increase the risk of CAD or stroke.

Plasminogen: This protein converts to plasmin, which destroys fibrin and dissolves fibrin clots. Normal plasminogen values range from 2.5 to 4.5 mmol/ml. Decreased values may be seen in fibrinolytic therapy, DIC, or liver disease. Increased values may be seen in pregnancy and inflammatory conditions.

Activated clotting time: This bedside test measures the time blood takes to clot when mixed with an activator. Some facilities use activated clotting time to monitor heparin therapy. Normally, clotting takes 100 seconds. The therapeutic range for heparin is 150 to 190 seconds.

Nursing considerations
- Many cardiac patients begin anticoagulation or thrombolytic therapy during the acute phase of an MI. You'll need to monitor coagulation studies frequently to make the proper dosage adjustments.
- Some cardiac patients with atrial fibrillation, prosthetic valves, or endocarditis have a greater tendency to form clots, which increases their risk of a CVA or pulmonary embolism.
- During and after an MI, coagulation factors may rise, increasing the risk of thrombophlebitis and extension of clots in the coronary artery.
- At high doses, heparin may excessively prolong PT. At therapeutic levels, PT will be prolonged 1.2 to 1.8 seconds.
- Begin bleeding precautions if your patient receives anticoagulation or thrombolytic therapy. Precautions include checking for blood in

urine and stool, having the patient use a soft toothbrush, and avoiding I.M. injections. Watch for bleeding from puncture sites and check for increased bruising, petechiae, and low-back pain.

- If severe bleeding occurs in a patient receiving heparin therapy, give protamine. His APTT will return to normal about 6 hours after you stop giving heparin. If he bleeds while on warfarin, give vitamin K (phytonadione). The PT takes 2 to 3 days to become therapeutic with warfarin therapy.
- If your patient receives heparin, procainamide, or quinidine, be aware that these drugs can lower his platelet count.
- Aspirin and dipyridamole can inhibit platelet aggregation. In fact, taking one aspirin two or three times a week can reduce the risk of an MI or re-infarction. Before beginning aspirin therapy, however, the patient should see his physician.

Electrical and imaging tests

Besides the information available from blood tests, a wealth of diagnostic data can be obtained through electrical and imaging tests.

Electrocardiography

As you know, the events of the cardiac cycle are controlled by waves of electrical impulses that flow from the sinoatrial node to the AV node and then down the interventricular septum and throughout the myocardial tissue. An ECG records the voltage (or strength) of these electrical impulses, the direction of their activity (toward a positive or negative pole), and the types of activity over time. In a person with normal cardiac function, these waveforms show a consistent pattern that includes the P wave, the QRS complex, the T wave, the PR interval, the QT interval, the ST segment, and sometimes the U wave (see *Reading an electrocardiogram,* page 34).

When a patient sustains myocardial ischemia, injury, or infarction, specific changes appear on his ECG tracing. You can use these changes to help identify problems and pinpoint locations. For example, ischemia of the endocardial surface may cause ST-segment depression. Epicardial ischemia may cause ST-segment elevation. Late repolarization of ischemic areas after nonischemic ones have returned to a resting state may cause a large, inverted T wave. And an MI may cause ST-segment el-

evation, T-wave abnormalities, and, in some cases, the development of a Q wave within 1 to 3 days.

Nursing considerations
- Tell your patient that an ECG is safe and painless and that it requires no special preparation.
- Assure him that no electrical current flows to him, but that the machine simply reads the electrical activity coming from his heart.
- Expose only those areas of his body to which you'll attach the electrodes or limb leads.
- Instruct your patient that he must lie still during the ECG. Tell him that leads will be placed on his skin near his upper arms and thighs and across the front of his chest. Mention that the gel, cream, or pads under the leads may feel cool, but not painful.
- When placing electrodes on your patient, make sure you establish good contact with the skin and that you place them in the proper locations (see *Positioning precordial electrodes,* page 35).
- At the time of the test, list any cardiac drugs your patient takes and note whether he has any chest pain.
- Serial ECGs are essential for evaluating the patient's response to many cardiac treatments, including antiarrhythmic drugs, thrombolytic therapy, PTCA, coronary artery bypass graft surgery, and other reperfusion techniques. They also can show an extension or recurrence of an MI.
- After an MI, expect the patient's ST segment to normalize within 6 weeks. The T wave will become larger and more symmetric for 24 hours after an MI, and then, within 1 to 3 days, it will invert for 1 to 2 weeks. Q-wave changes are usually permanent.

Exercise stress test
A valuable tool for evaluating CAD, the stress test combines an ECG with supervised exercise to test the heart's response to increasing oxygen demand. This test helps to diagnose chest pain of cardiac origin, evaluate the effects of cardiac drugs and surgery, and determine the limits of safe exercise during cardiac rehabilitation.

The standard stress test involves increasing the patient's exercise level in increments until he either develops symptoms or reaches a target heart rate that's typically 80% to 85% of the predicted maximum for his age and sex. The duration of the test depends on the type of test being performed and your patient's tolerance.

The two major modes of exercise used during

Reading an electrocardiogram

As an electrical impulse leaves the sinoatrial node, it spreads through the atria, causing them to depolarize and contract. This event produces the P wave on an electrocardiogram (ECG) waveform. The P wave should be rounded and identical to other P waves, and it should occur at regular intervals. You should see one P wave for each QRS complex.

After atrial depolarization, the electrical impulse reaches the atrioventricular node and pauses before proceeding through the bundle of His and down the bundle branches to the Purkinje fibers. The PR interval measures the time from the beginning of atrial depolarization to the beginning of ventricular depolarization. It's measured from the beginning of the P wave to the beginning of the QRS complex.

The QRS complex represents ventricular depolarization. The first downward deflection after the P wave is the Q wave (which doesn't always occur). The first upward deflection of the QRS complex is the R wave, and the next downward deflection is the S wave. If you see no Q wave, measure the QRS interval from the beginning of the R wave.

Between the QRS complex and the T wave is a short segment called the ST segment. It represents the initial phase of ventricular repolarization, the period of returning to the polarized state after an electrical impulse has been conducted. The ST segment should be horizontal and level with the ECG's other baselines. An ST-segment elevation or depression suggests myocardial ischemia or injury or another cardiac disorder.

The T wave follows the QRS complex and represents rapid ventricular repolarization, when the

muscle fibers of the heart begin to relax. The QT interval measures the time from the start of the Q wave to the end of the T wave. In other words, it measures the time from ventricular depolarization to ventricular repolarization. The duration of the QT interval varies with the heart rate; the slower the heart rate, the longer the QT interval.

Sometimes, you may see a U wave after the T wave and before the P wave. This U wave represents the final phase of ventricular repolarization.

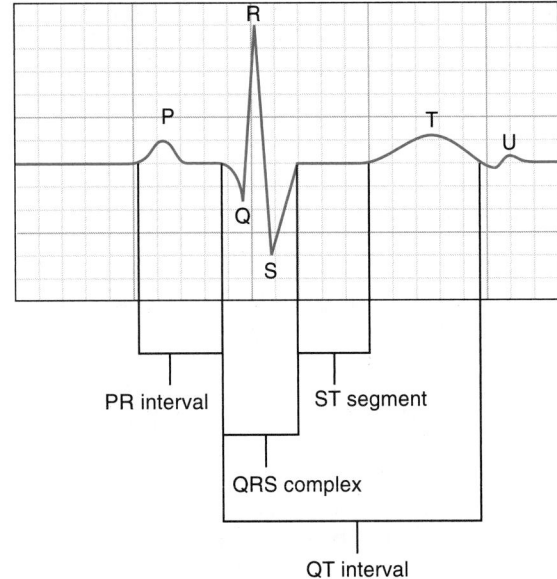

the test are bicycle ergometry and the treadmill. Bicycle ergometry uses a pedal-operated wheel whose resistance can be increased while the patient pedals. The treadmill is a motorized conveyor belt whose speed and incline can be increased while the patient walks on it.

Before undergoing a stress test, your patient must have a baseline physical examination, measurement of vital signs, and an ECG. Contraindications to stress testing include a recent acute MI, unstable angina, life-threatening cardiac arrhythmias, severe heart failure, and severe aortic valvular disease. To take this test, your patient must have a normal baseline ECG, and he must be able to walk or pedal for 20 to 30 minutes.

During the test, a physician or cardiovascular nurse continuously monitors the patient's blood pressure, pulse rate, and ECG. The test takes place in a controlled environment with emergency cardiac drugs and resuscitative equipment nearby. Throughout the test, the patient is monitored for adverse responses, including chest pain, tachycardia, dyspnea, fatigue, cardiac arrhythmias, falling blood pressure, and such ECG changes as a 2-mm ST-segment depression that lasts 0.08 second past the J point.

Nursing considerations
• Determine what your patient knows about stress testing. Use written materials and verbal

instruction to answer any questions he may have.

- Tell the patient not to eat, drink, or smoke for 4 hours before the test.
- Tell the patient to wear comfortable clothes and sneakers or other appropriate exercise shoes.
- Note whether the patient should take his cardiac drugs before or after the test.
- Be aware that benign arrhythmias tend to disappear with exercise but that arrhythmias requiring treatment tend to worsen with exercise.
- Your patient may undergo low-level or alternative stress testing to evaluate treatment of a recent MI.
- If your patient is taking a beta-blocker, his heart rate won't rise enough for an accurate evaluation of his exercise response.
- If the patient develops cardiac signs or symptoms during the exercise stress test, the examiner will stop it.

Signal-averaged electrocardiography

When the myocardium is scarred by an infarct or another cardiac disorder, the damaged tissue may raise the patient's risk of developing sustained ventricular tachycardia—a condition thought to cause most sudden cardiac deaths.

These zones of damaged or infarcted myocardial tissue produce signals at the end of the QRS complex that can be delayed, fractionated, or uneven. Routine ECGs can't pick them up clearly because of their low amplitude and electrical noise. To pick up and record these signals, your patient may need a signal-averaged ECG, in which a computer uses high-gain amplification, signal averaging, and filtering.

Using a low-noise electronic amplifier, the computer greatly amplifies the ECG signal and then converts it to a digital signal. It then averages information from numerous repeating QRS complexes, eliminating random electrical noises in the process. This procedure enables the recording and interpretation of these low-amplitude, high-frequency signals that extend beyond the QRS complex and into the ST segment. Referred to as late potentials, these signals represent late depolarization of the ventricular myocardium (see *Understanding late potentials,* page 36).

This form of ECG helps identify patients at high risk for sustained ventricular tachycardia, such as those who have severe left ventricular dysfunction after an MI.

Positioning precordial electrodes

When conducting 12-lead electrocardiography, place the electrodes for the six precordial leads, V_1 through V_6, as shown.

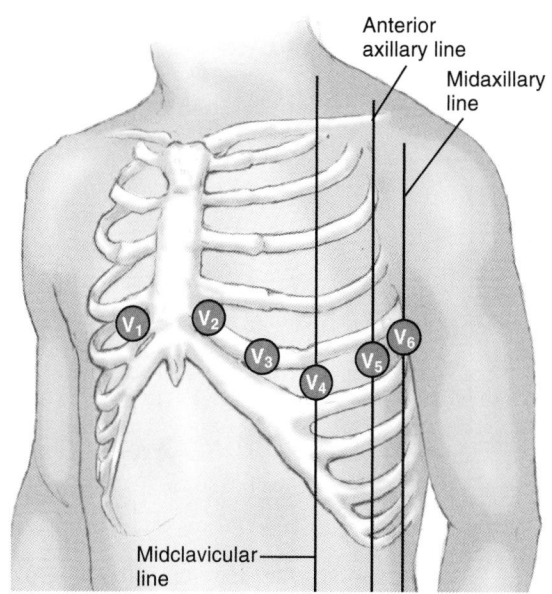

Nursing considerations

- Tell your patient that this is a special kind of ECG used to identify his risk of developing life-threatening arrhythmias. Explain that it's safe and painless, lasts only 10 to 20 minutes, and can be performed at his bedside.
- Tell the patient that he'll need to lie still and avoid talking or moving during the recording period.
- Keep in mind that the results of this test may not be accurate for patients with left bundle-branch block.

Ambulatory cardiac monitoring

For patients who have intermittent cardiac rhythm disturbances, a single ECG may not be sufficient to detect the problem. Ambulatory cardiac monitoring using a Holter monitor and transtelephonic methods can offer ECG recordings over longer periods of time.

Understanding late potentials

A signal-averaged electrocardiogram (ECG) reveals low-amplitude, high-frequency currents in the conduction pathways. Invisible on a standard ECG tracing, these currents are called late potentials. They typically represent myocardial damage and may warn of an increased risk of sustained ventricular tachycardia—a potentially deadly complication.

To produce the waveform, a computer analyzes, filters, and averages many QRS complexes from an extended, perhaps 20-minute, ECG. The result is shown in schematic form below.

Normal signal-averaged ECG

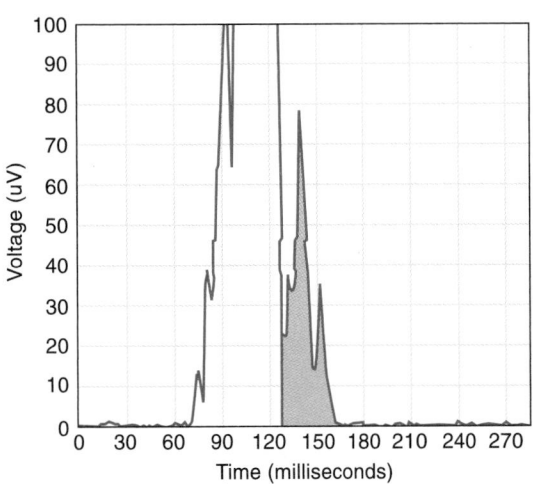

Signal-averaged ECG with late potentials

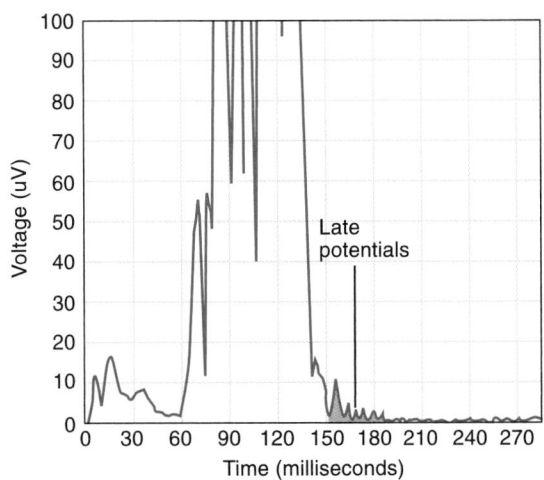

A Holter monitor is a small device worn by the patient during his usual activities of daily living. The device records two or three channels of ECG data onto a cassette tape over 24 to 48 hours. Also, the patient keeps a diary of his activities and his signs and symptoms that can be compared with any changes that show up on the tape. Some Holter monitors have a button the patient can push when he has signs or symptoms; pushing it makes a mark on the tape. A specially equipped computer that can diagnose cardiac abnormalities helps to analyze the information from the Holter monitor.

Unfortunately, the patient's signs and symptoms may not arise even during the extended time available with a Holter monitor. Because continued Holter monitoring may be expensive and the multiple electrodes inconvenient, transtelephonic cardiac event recording offers another option. The patient simply activates a cardiac event recorder when he experiences signs or symptoms. The monitor stores the resulting ECG data in its memory until the patient transmits the data by phone to a receiving center staffed by nurses or other professionals trained in evaluating ECGs.

Two types of cardiac event monitors are available: the looping memory (or presymptom) monitor and the postsymptom monitor. The former monitors cardiac rhythm continuously via two electrodes on the patient's chest. If the patient feels no symptoms and doesn't activate the monitor, it continues to record over itself on its endless loop. However, if the patient does feel symptoms and activates the monitor, it can permanently store up to 5 minutes of his cardiac rhythm, including a few minutes that occurred before activation. Documentation of transient signs and symptoms is one of the system's advantages. When using transtelephonic monitoring, patients can be monitored for several months if necessary.

The postsymptom event monitor may be handheld or resemble a wristwatch. The handheld monitor contains electrode "feet" on the back that conduct impulses from the heart to the monitor's memory system. When the patient experiences signs or symptoms, he simply holds the monitor's feet against his chest while pushing the record button. The device then records his ECG for about 30 seconds using lead II, the lead used most commonly to diagnose cardiac events in ambulatory monitoring. If your patient wears the monitor like a wristwatch on his left arm, it records in lead I. Postsymptom monitors don't record ECG events that occur before activation. When your patient activates the monitor, it stores the resulting data in its memory until the patient transmits it to the receiving center. The postsymptom monitor helps to diagnose arrhythmias that last more than a few seconds, such as atrial fibrillation and supraventricular tachycardias.

Nursing considerations
- Explain that the monitor transmits no electricity and that the machine records electrical events that take place in his heart.
- Stress the importance of maintaining an accurate diary and of pushing the event button during signs and symptoms.
- While the monitor is attached, tell the patient not to bathe and to avoid using electrical appliances, which may cause artifact on the ECG.
- Encourage the patient to pursue his normal activities of daily living so that the monitor can record events that occur during a typical day.
- If the patient has a handheld postsymptom monitor, tell him to keep it in a handy place, such as a pocket, so that it's readily available when signs or symptoms develop.
- Tell him that the electrodes must be firmly attached to the skin for adequate transmission.
- With transtelephonic monitoring, teach your patient to change electrodes every 24 to 48 hours to prevent skin irritation. Show him how to maintain the same lead configuration.
- Tell him to keep the skin under the electrodes clean and free from creams or oils. Before applying the electrodes, he should rub the skin until it's slightly pink to remove dead skin cells.

Then he should clean the area with alcohol and let it air dry.
- Tell the patient that he can use a standard telephone to transmit ECG data to the receiving center; show him how to do it, then ask for a return demonstration.
- Explain that any serious arrhythmias are reported to the physician immediately after arriving at the receiving center.

Chest X-ray
A chest X-ray can reveal cardiac and pericardial calcifications, pulmonary congestion from heart failure, pericardial effusion, and the placement of cardiac catheters as well as show the size, contour, and position of the heart. Typically, a chest X-ray involves three views of the chest: anterior, posterior, and lateral.

Serial chest X-rays can provide valuable information about your patient's response to treatment. For example, they can show whether pulmonary congestion caused by heart failure is improved, worse, or unchanged.

Nursing considerations
Inform your patient that his physician has ordered X-rays of his chest and heart. Assure him that the test requires no special preparation except removal of all metal objects and clothing from the waist up. Explain that he'll be asked to take a deep breath and hold it while the films are being taken.

Radionuclide imaging
By showing blood flow through the coronary arteries (in some cases, after exercise), radionuclide imaging can be used to diagnose impaired cardiac perfusion, evaluate the extent and location of ischemia, and assess the viability of damaged myocardium. Two substances commonly used as imaging agents are thallium-201 and technetium Tc 99m sestamibi. If the patient can't exercise during radionuclide imaging, he may instead receive a drug to dilate his coronary arteries (see *Myocardial perfusion studies without exercise,* page 38).

Thallium-201 is similar to potassium and is easily extracted by cardiac muscle fibers that contain the sodium-potassium active-transport system. However, thallium takes longer than potassium to clear from myocardial cells. Within 5 to 15 minutes after I.V. injection, thallium appears in myocardial

Myocardial perfusion studies without exercise

If your patient has peripheral vascular disease or impaired mobility or if he takes a drug that prevents a maximum exercise response, he may not be able to exercise successfully during myocardial perfusion studies. If he can't, he may benefit from one of two drugs that can dilate his coronary arteries without exercise: dipyridamole or adenosine. Either one can produce exercise-type cardiac effects without actual exercise.

Dipyridamole and adenosine are coronary vasodilators. After an I.V. injection, they increase blood flow to regions of the heart that have normal coronary arteries. Vessels narrowed by coronary artery disease don't dilate normally, so blood flow doesn't increase.

Your patient may not be able to tolerate dipyridamole if he had a myocardial infarction in the past 48 hours or if he has a history of asthma, chronic lung disease, or certain heart conditions. If he has severe airway disease, high-grade atrioventricular block, or hypotension or if he takes a methylxanthine drug, he isn't a good candidate for either dipyridamole or adenosine.

For such patients, dobutamine might provide an acceptable alternative. High doses of dobutamine can increase both the heart rate and the strength of contractions, mimicking the effects of exercise without producing significant peripheral vasoconstriction. Unlike the other two drugs, dobutamine is given by infusion rather than by bolus, a method that more closely parallels the gradual effects of exercise. No matter which drug he'll receive, instruct the patient not to take a calcium channel blocker or beta-blocker for 24 hours before the test.

tissues in proportion to their level of perfusion. Thallium uptake will be decreased or absent in myocardial areas that receive less blood flow and highly concentrated in well-perfused areas.

Technetium Tc 99m sestamibi is a lipophilic cation that enters myocardial cells by passive diffusion in response to changes in electrical potentials. After injection, it doesn't redistribute well in myocardial tissue and can provide only limited information about myocardial viability. However, it produces better images than thallium does, with less scatter and a brighter flash.

Keep in mind that the camera used for imaging can focus clearly at only one distance. For patients who don't fall within the camera's best imaging range, such as those with large chests, technetium Tc 99m sestamibi may provide clearer pictures than thallium-201. Single photon emission computed tomography (CT) cameras may also be used in conjunction with thallium-201 or technetium Tc 99m sestamibi stress testing. Single photon emission computed tomography shows a three-dimensional image of the heart, which will more precisely identify areas of decreased myocardial perfusion.

Nursing considerations

- Find out if your patient has a history of allergy to radioactive isotopes, theophylline, or dipyridamole.
- Usually, thallium-201 and technetium Tc 99m sestamibi produce no adverse effects except a metallic taste during injection.
- Emergency equipment should always be available during stress testing.
- Because the patient is exposed to some radiation, ask a female patient if she could be pregnant.
- Explain that the test involves being attached to an ECG monitor and having the radioisotope injected through an I.V. line.
- Tell the patient to wear comfortable walking shoes or sneakers if the test will involve walking or pedaling.
- If the patient will receive dipyridamole or adenosine, tell him that the injection takes about 4 minutes. After that, the radioisotope will be injected, and images will be taken of his heart.
- Tell the patient not to eat foods or take drugs that contain caffeine or theophylline for 36 to 48 hours before the test. Also, he should avoid beverages that contain caffeine for 2 to 4 hours before the test. The required time intervals vary by facility (see *Thallium scan: Foods and drugs to avoid*).
- As ordered, tell the patient not to eat or drink for 4 to 6 hours before the test to reduce the possibility of nausea or vomiting.
- You don't need to discontinue the patient's oral dipyridamole before the test.
- Tell the patient that he may need to return for more images after 2 to 4 hours.
- Encourage the patient to drink plenty of fluids

after the test to help flush the thallium-201 or technetium Tc 99m sestamibi from his system.
• Monitor his vital signs closely after the test.

Technetium 99m imaging

Testing with technetium Tc 99m pyrophosphate may help to evaluate the presence, extent, and prognosis of an MI, especially for a patient whose cardiac enzyme measurements aren't available or whose ECG results are questionable. It's used less commonly these days because of improved enzyme testing.

Technetium 99m probably combines with the calcium in damaged myocardial cells, causing a hot spot on the scan. This spot shows necrotic myocardial tissue and, in large infarcts, may take a doughnut shape because less of the tracer reaches the center of the necrotic zone. Maximum uptake of technetium 99m takes place 24 to 72 hours after an MI. The myocardium may remain positive for the isotope for up to 6 days.

Nursing considerations
• Explain the purpose of the test and tell the patient how it's done.
• Ask if your patient has a history of allergy to radioactive dyes.
• Because the patient is exposed to some radiation, ask a female patient if she could be pregnant.
• A small MI or subendocardial infarction won't show up on this test.

Radionuclide angiocardiography

Also known as a multiple-gated acquisition scan, radionuclide angiocardiography allows evaluation of the ejection fraction and movements of the left ventricular wall. Damaged areas of the ventricle wall may show decreased (hypokinetic) or absent (akinetic) motion. Likewise, areas made ischemic by narrowed coronary arteries will show decreased wall motion or contractility as well.

Radionuclide angiocardiography offers the opportunity to observe the actual filling and emptying of cardiac chambers by tagging red blood cells (RBCs) with technetium 99m. Then, a scintillation camera records images of blood flow at precise times in the cardiac cycle, cued by signals from the patient's ECG.

During scanning, a computer is synchronized with the ECG to break down the times from one R wave to the next into fractions of a second called gates. Multiple consecutive gates are ob-

---

Thallium scan: Foods and drugs to avoid

Before having a thallium scan, your patient will need to avoid drugs that contain theophylline for at least 36 hours, as instructed. These drugs include the following:
• Aerolate
• Bronkodyl
• Constant-T
• Elixophyllin SR
• Quibron-T/SR Dividose
• Respbid
• Slo-bid Gyrocaps
• Slo-Phyllin Gyrocaps
• Sustaire
• Theo-24
• Theobid Duracaps
• Theochron
• Theoclear L.A.
• Theo-Dur
• Theo-Dur Sprinkle
• Theolair-SR
• Theospan SR
• Theovent Long-Acting
• Uniphyl

The patient will also need to avoid foods and drugs that contain caffeine for at least 4 hours before the test, as instructed. These foods and drugs include the following:
• coffee (including decaffeinated)
• tea (including decaffeinated)
• foods and drinks that contain chocolate
• cola drinks (including sugar-free and decaffeinated)
• other soft drinks (including Dr. Pepper, Ginger ale, Mr. Pibb, Mountain Dew, Mellow Yellow, Orange Crush, Root Beer, Tab)
• Anacin
• Cafergot
• Darvon Compound
• Excedrin
• Fiorinal
• NoDoz
• Synalgos-DC
• Wigraine

---

tained over a period of time to assess ventricular wall motion.

Gated cardiac blood pool imaging can be obtained during stress testing as well. The patient uses a bicycle ergometer with a gamma camera positioned to detect blood pools. If your patient has a normal ejection fraction (58% to 76%), it will increase by 5% with exercise. A patient with ischemic heart disease may show a decrease in ejection fraction with exercise or no increase.

Nursing considerations
- Explain the test to your patient.
- Because the patient is exposed to some radiation, ask a female patient if she could be pregnant.
- As ordered, tell the patient to fast for 3 hours or more before the test.
- Tell the patient to avoid smoking for 8 hours before the test and to avoid caffeinated or carbonated beverages on the day of the test.
- Some cardiac drugs may need to be discontinued before the test, such as beta-blockers and digitalis glycosides.
- If stress testing will be done along with radionuclide angiocardiography, tell the patient to wear comfortable shoes or sneakers.
- Urge the patient to notify the physician if he has any chest pain or other symptoms during the test.
- Encourage plenty of fluids after the test, to help his kidneys clear the radioisotope from his system.
- This study is usually performed in the nuclear medicine department, but it may be performed at the bedside if necessary.

Ultrafast computed tomography
In CT, an X-ray machine sends many narrow X-ray beams, or slices, through a selected area of tissue. A computer then processes this information and converts it to a three-dimensional image of changes in tissue density that can be transferred to X-ray film. Contrast agents may be administered to increase the clarity of the images.

An ultrafast CT (also known as a cine-CT) uses a scanner capable of taking high-resolution, three-dimensional images at speeds fast enough to capture pictures of the beating heart. Ultrafast CT can help in diagnosing many cardiac disorders, including aortic dissection or aneurysm, congenital heart disease, pericardial disease, the location and size of an MI, and ejection fraction. It also may help to assess the patency of coronary artery bypass grafts.

Nursing considerations
Explain the purpose of the procedure to your patient as well as how the equipment works. Ask whether your patient has any allergies to contrast agents because they may be used during the test. Tell the patient that the test usually takes about an hour, during which time he must lie still in a dark, usually enclosed space.

Magnetic resonance imaging
Magnetic resonance imaging (MRI) uses a strong magnetic field and radio waves to detect differences between healthy and diseased tissues. For cardiac patients, it offers valuable information about myocardial chamber size, wall motion, valve function, and blood flow through the great vessels. An MRI scan also can help in diagnosing cardiomyopathies and pericardial disease and in identifying aortic aneurysms, congenital heart disease, and tumors.

Nursing considerations
- Tell your patient that he must remove all metal items, including his watch, jewelry, zippers, and coins, because the test uses a strong magnetic field. Credit cards must also be removed.
- Patients who have implanted metallic objects—such as a cardiac pacemaker, prosthesis, aneurysm clip, or intracoronary stent placed within the previous month—are ineligible for an MRI scan. The magnetic field may move the object within the body, causing internal injury.
- Tell the patient that the test takes 45 minutes to an hour, during which time he must lie still on a table inside an enclosed scanner that makes a loud knocking noise.
- Claustrophobic patients may require sedation.

Positron emission tomography
The positron emission tomogram (PET) is a noninvasive scan that can be used to diagnose cardiac dysfunction. Radioisotopes are administered by I.V. injection. One compound travels through the blood and serves as a tracer for normal physiologic activity. The other compound localizes in the myocardium, revealing metabolic function in the myocardial cells. Uptake of this compound is proportional to glucose metabolism in the myocardial cells, which provides an excellent indication of tissue viability in the myocardium.

The PET camera provides detailed three-dimensional images of these compounds. It can help determine myocardial viability by comparing the level of glucose metabolism in the myocardium with the degree of blood flow. Myocardial tissue that's viable but ischemic shows decreased blood flow and increased metabolism. Coronary artery bypass grafting, PTCA, or other reperfusion procedures may be required to improve coronary circulation in that area.

Also, PET scans can assist in monitoring a patient's response to coronary artery bypass grafting or PTCA. They also reveal the patency of previous coronary artery grafts as well as collateral circulation.

Nursing considerations
- Tell your patient to avoid caffeine, alcohol, and tobacco for 24 hours before the procedure.
- Because the patient is exposed to some radiation, ask a female patient if she could be pregnant.
- Tell the patient that he must lie still on the examining table during the scan.
- Encourage plenty of fluids after the test to help flush the radioisotope from the patient's body.

Echocardiography
An echocardiogram is a noninvasive ultrasonic test used to evaluate structural and functional changes in the heart. High-frequency sound waves are transmitted into the heart from a transducer placed on several areas of the chest wall. As sound waves return to the transducer, they're picked up and recorded as a series of echoes and then converted to electrical signals. These signals are transmitted to the echocardiogram machine, which displays an image on an oscilloscope and records it on a videotape. An ECG is recorded simultaneously so that visual events can be correlated with events of the cardiac cycle.

Echocardiograms help in evaluating many cardiac functions and disorders, including cardiomyopathy, valve problems, pericardial effusion, cardiac shunts, chamber size, left ventricular function, cardiac tumors, and aneurysms. By showing heart valves, chambers, walls, and wall motion, echocardiography also provides valuable evidence of the patient's response to treatment.

Nursing considerations
- Explain that an echocardiogram is a safe, noninvasive test that requires no special preparation.

- Although it may be performed at bedside, echocardiography usually takes place in the imaging laboratory.
- Tell the patient that he'll have ECG leads attached during the test. Also, mention that conduction gel will be applied to his chest to improve the transmission of sound waves to the transducer. Tell him that the examiner will need to press firmly on his chest with the transducer to obtain good images.
- Explain that the procedure usually takes 15 to 45 minutes.
- Tell your patient that he'll be lying on his back or his left side during the test.
- Obesity, chronic obstructive pulmonary disease, and chest-wall abnormalities may alter the display of ultrasonic waves on the recorder.
- The test's unidimensional mode, also known as M-mode, shows heart structures and their movement during a cardiac cycle. The two-dimensional mode shows a sophisticated, spatially correct image that offers more information about the shape of the heart and the spatial relationships of structures during the cardiac cycle.

Stress echocardiography
Two-dimensional echocardiography may be combined with stress testing to detect abnormalities of wall motion caused by inadequate blood flow during exercise. Changes in wall motion can be seen via echocardiography even before they appear on the patient's ECG.

For patients who can't exercise, drugs—such as adenosine, dipyridamole, or dobutamine—may be used to dilate the coronary arteries. A drug-aided stress echocardiogram allows real-time imaging of ischemic events as they occur in the heart. During traditional stress testing, the patient must move quickly from the treadmill to the table for echocardiography imaging.

Stress echocardiography may be indicated for patients who probably have CAD but who show inconclusive results on the standard stress test. It's also helpful for evaluating patients' responses to such treatments as bypass grafting, PTCA, or other reperfusion techniques and for assessing patients at high risk for myocardial ischemia or infarction before they undergo surgery. Stress echocardiography is contraindicated if your patient has unstable angina or severe aortic stenosis.

Nursing considerations
- The stress echocardiogram is noninvasive, has no radiation risk, and is more cost-effective than radionuclide imaging.
- Dobutamine stress echocardiography may be done at the bedside if your patient can't be transferred.
- Tell the patient to fast for 3 to 6 hours before the test, as ordered. Also, tell him to withhold certain drugs before the test, as ordered.
- Before the test, help to obtain the patient's baseline vital signs, pulse oximetry, ECG, and echocardiogram. Throughout the stress echocardiogram, the patient's oxygen saturation may be monitored along with his cardiac rhythm.
- Tell the patient to report chest pain or other symptoms to the physician right away if they arise during the test.
- Resuscitative equipment and emergency drugs must be available during the test, including esmolol to reverse the effects of dobutamine.
- Tell your patient that he will be positioned on his left side for the echocardiogram because this position brings the heart closer to the chest wall and provides a better image.
- Explain that he'll exercise either until he develops signs or symptoms or until his heart rate reaches about 85% of the maximum rate for his age and sex.
- The patient most likely will undergo a post-infusion echocardiogram when his vital signs normalize.

Transesophageal echocardiography
A transesophageal echocardiogram provides a clearer image of the heart than a standard echocardiogram does, especially in obese patients and those with thickened chest walls. To obtain the image, an examiner passes an endoscope with a transducer at its distal end down the patient's esophagus to a position behind his heart (see *A view of transesophageal echocardiography*).

The transducer emits sound waves that echo off the heart's structures and return to the transducer for translation into images on an oscilloscope. Because the transducer is so close to the heart, this test allows for more accurate diagnosis of valvular disorders, aneurysms, and masses. It also allows detailed evaluation of valve repairs or prosthetic valve replacement and may be used during surgery to monitor for the onset of myocardial ischemia or infarction.

Transesophageal echocardiography is contraindicated in patients with esophageal disorders, such as varices or strictures, and patients with a history of dysphagia or chest-wall radiation therapy. High-risk patients include the elderly and those with decreased ventricular function, CAD, and peripheral vascular disease. Complications of the procedure include perforation of the esophagus, arrhythmias, vasovagal reactions, minor pharyngeal bleeding, and transient hypoxemia.

Nursing considerations
- Tell your patient to fast for 6 hours before the test.
- If your patient has valvular heart disease or a mechanical heart valve, administer prophylactic antibiotics as ordered.
- Baseline vital signs will be obtained before the procedure, and then monitored throughout. Skin color, pulse oximetry, and cardiac rhythm are also monitored during the procedure.
- The patient will receive I.V. sedation, probably with meperidine, diazepam, or midazolam, to reduce anxiety.
- Lidocaine will be sprayed on the back of the patient's throat to suppress his gag reflex while the catheter moves down his esophagus.
- Mucosal drying agents and suction help reduce oral secretions during the test.
- Tell your patient that the catheter tip will be lubricated with a water-soluble gel. Then he'll be placed on his left side and asked to swallow while a physician gently advances the transducer.
- The test probably will last about 15 minutes.
- To reduce the risk of aspiration, withhold fluids and food after the procedure until the patient's gag reflex has returned.
- After the procedure, assess your patient for gastrointestinal bleeding or pain—indications of esophageal perforation.

Doppler echocardiography
This test provides information about blood flow through the great vessels, across the valves, and through the heart's chambers. It's used to evaluate the velocity of blood flow and to assess valvular dysfunction, intracardiac pressures and shunts, and CO. Two techniques are available for Doppler echocardiography (pulsed wave and continuous wave), either of which may be used with two-dimensional echocardiography.

A view of transesophageal echocardiography

To perform transesophageal echocardiography, an examiner passes a flexible, transducer-tipped endoscope down the patient's esophagus to the level of his heart, as shown.

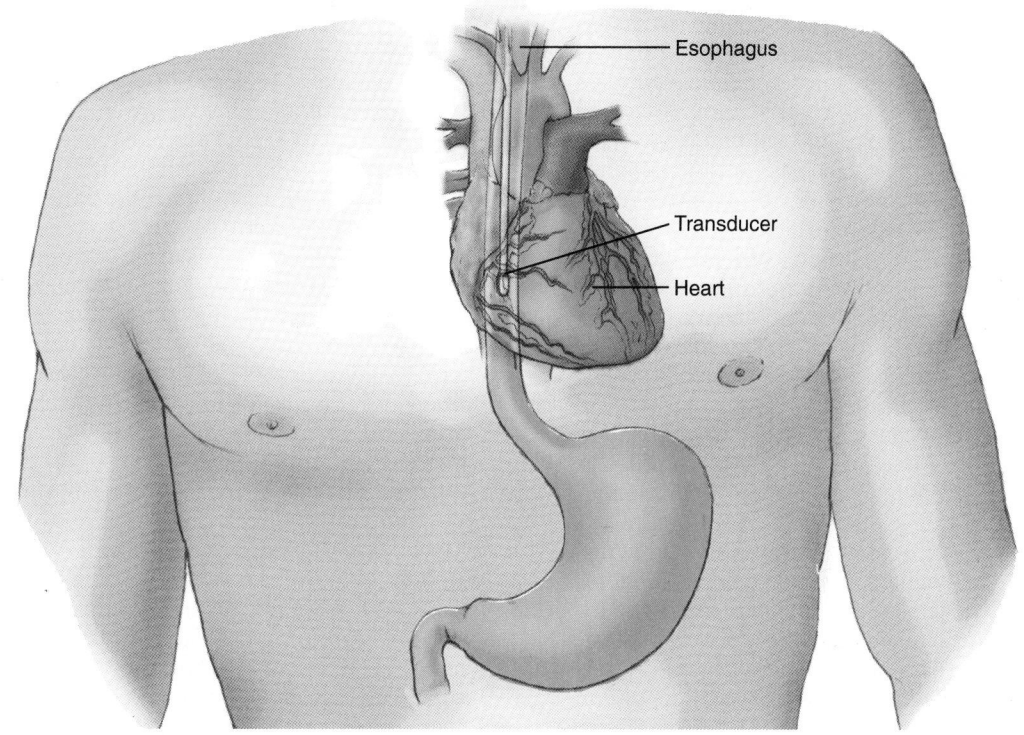

The pulsed wave Doppler emits short bursts of ultrasound from one crystal; they're echoed back by a sample volume of RBCs moving through the heart. Then two-dimensional echocardiography is combined with pulsed wave Doppler to make a visual display of the sample blood volume in the chamber. This display can be used to detect abnormal blood flow through cardiac structures, but it can't be used to quantify high-velocity flow.

Continuous wave Doppler uses two crystals: One continuously emits ultrasound and the other continuously receives the reflected signal. This form of the test allows measurement of high-velocity flow; however, it doesn't specify the origin of the flow. Color added to the Doppler scan identifies the direction, degree, and turbu-lence of flow across stenosed or regurgitant heart valves. The colors blue and red represent the direction of blood flow and improve its visibility through the cardiac chambers during the cardiac cycle. This is especially helpful in diagnosing valvular disorders.

Nursing considerations
Tell your patient that echocardiography is safe and noninvasive and requires no special preparation. The nursing considerations listed for standard echocardiography apply here as well.

Cardiac catheterization
Cardiac catheterization commonly provides the most valuable information about structural and

functional abnormalities in the heart. The procedure can be used to assess pressures and oxygen levels in the heart chambers, measure CO, detect structural problems, collect biopsy specimens, and reveal occlusions in the coronary arteries.

To perform the procedure, a physician inserts a specialized catheter through a puncture or cutdown in the patient's groin or antecubital fossa and advances the catheter to the heart. To assess the right side of the heart, the physician passes the catheter through the inferior or superior vena cava to gain entry to the right atrium. To assess the left side of the heart, a more difficult and risky procedure, the physician passes the catheter against the aortic blood flow, through the aortic valve, and into the left ventricle.

Complications of cardiac catheterization include hematoma formation and infection at the catheter insertion site. Heparin given to prevent clotting during the procedure can increase the risk of retroperitoneal or external bleeding. The arterial puncture needed for catheterization of the left side may cause arterial spasm or thrombus formation. Direct stimulation of cardiac tissues by the catheter may lead to arrhythmias. Some patients develop allergic reactions to the iodine-based contrast medium; signs and symptoms include flushing, nausea, vomiting, tingling, numbness, weakness, and urticaria. Also, the hypertonic contrast medium causes strong osmotic diuresis, which may lead to dehydration. Rarely does a catheter perforate the myocardium or aorta but, if it does, the result can be life threatening.

Nursing considerations

- Have the patient fast for 6 to 18 hours before the test; withhold liquids for at least 4 hours.
- Before the test, reiterate the physician's explanation of the procedure. Tell the patient that he'll need to lie still on a hard, movable X-ray table for about 2 hours, awake but mildly sedated. Explain that he'll receive a local anesthetic to numb the insertion site.
- Tell the patient that the injection of the dye will probably produce a warm, flushed feeling for a minute or less and (with right-sided catheterization) a strong desire to cough.
- Make sure his height and weight are in his chart; these values influence the amount of dye he'll receive.
- Prepare the insertion site according to your facility's policy.
- Assess the patient's vital signs and auscultate his heart and lungs. Record the quality of his pulses.
- Administer a sedative and possibly an antibiotic, as ordered, just before the procedure. If the patient could be allergic to the contrast dye, administer an antihistamine, as ordered.
- Tell the patient to report any chest pain during the procedure.
- During the procedure, monitor the patient's vital signs and ECG continuously.
- If the patient experiences excessive premature ventricular contractions, administer an antiarrhythmic drug, usually lidocaine, as ordered.
- After the procedure, assess his vital signs every 15 minutes for the first hour, every 30 minutes for 2 hours or until his vital signs are stable, and then every 4 hours or in keeping with your facility's policy.
- Keep the limb distal to the insertion site straight for 4 to 6 hours. Check the pressure dressing over the insertion site at regular intervals and watch for hematoma formation. Follow your facility's policy for bed position; depending on the vessel used for catheterization, you may need to keep the patient flat, or you may raise his head up to 30 degrees for several hours.
- Check pulses, color, warmth, and sensation in the distal limb every 30 minutes for the first hour, then less often as ordered. Notify the physician right away if the patient reports numbness or tingling; if the limb becomes cool, pale, or cyanotic; or if you suddenly become unable to palpate his peripheral pulses.
- Monitor the patient continuously for arrhythmias and chest pain; if you detect either, notify the physician.
- Encourage the patient to drink plenty of fluids to help his kidneys rid his body of the contrast medium. Also, continue to check for signs and symptoms of an allergic reaction to the dye, such as nausea, vomiting, and skin rash.

CARDIAC ESSENTIALS

Suggested Readings

Bullock BL. *Pathophysiology: Adaptations and Alterations in Function.* 4th ed. Philadelphia: Lippincott-Raven Pubs; 1996.

Charuvastra EH, Dance DD. *How transtelephonic cardiac event recording helps patients.* Sunnyvale, Calif: Nurseweek Publishing, Inc; 1996: http/www.nurseweek.com. Continuing Education Article for NurseWeek Course #1115A.

Chernecky CC, Berger BJ. *Laboratory Tests and Diagnostic Procedures.* 2nd ed. Philadelphia: WB Saunders Co; 1997.

Dubin DB. *Rapid interpretation of EKG's.* 5th ed. Tampa: Cover Pub Co; 1996.

Fischbach F. *A Manual of Laboratory & Diagnostic Tests.* 5th ed. Philadelphia: Lippincott-Raven Pubs; 1996.

Giger JN, Davidhizar RE. *Transcultural Nursing: Assessment and Intervention.* 2nd ed. St Louis: Mosby, Inc; 1995.

Graceffo MA, O'Rourke RA, Hibner C, Boulet AJ. The time course and relation of positive signal-averaged electrocardiograms by time-domain and spectral temporal mapping analyses after infarction. *Am Heart J* 1995;129(2):238-251.

Guyton AC, Hall JE. *Textbook of Medical Physiology.* 9th ed. Philadelphia: WB Saunders Co; 1995.

Higgins C. Laboratory diagnosis of acute myocardial infarction. *Nurs Times.* 1996;92(3):36-37.

Huether SE, McCance KL. *Understanding Pathophysiology.* St Louis: Mosby, Inc; 1996.

Kim MJ. *Pocket Guide to Nursing Diagnosis.* 6th ed. St Louis: Mosby, Inc; 1997.

Kinney MR, Packa DR. *Andreoli's Comprehensive Cardiac Care.* 8th ed. St Louis: Mosby, Inc; 1995.

Lewis SM, Collier IC, Heitkemper MM. *Medical-Surgical Nursing: Assessment and Management of Clinical Problems.* 4th ed. St Louis: Mosby, Inc; 1996.

Pagana KD, Pagana TJ. *Mosby's Diagnostic and Laboratory Test Reference.* 3rd ed. St Louis: Mosby, Inc; 1996.

Seidel HM. *Mosby's Guide to Physical Examination.* 3rd ed. St Louis: Mosby, Inc; 1995.

Selvester RH. The signal-averaged high-resolution ECG. *J Electrocardiol.* 1995;28 suppl:216-225.

Sherman A. Critical care management of the heart failure patient in the home. *Crit Care Nurs Q.* 1995;18(1):77-87.

Thompson EJ, Detwiler DS, Nelson CM. Dobutamine stress echocardiography: a new, noninvasive method for detecting ischemic heart disease. *Heart Lung.* 1996;25(2):87-97.

Williams PL, Gray HL, Bannister LH. *Gray's Anatomy: The Anatomical Basis for Medicine and Surgery.* 38th ed. New York: Churchill Livingstone, Inc; 1995.

Woods SL, Froelicher ES, Halpenny CJ, Motzer SU. *Cardiac Nursing.* 3rd ed. Philadelphia: Lippincott-Raven Pubs; 1995.

CORONARY ARTERY DISEASE AND ANGINA

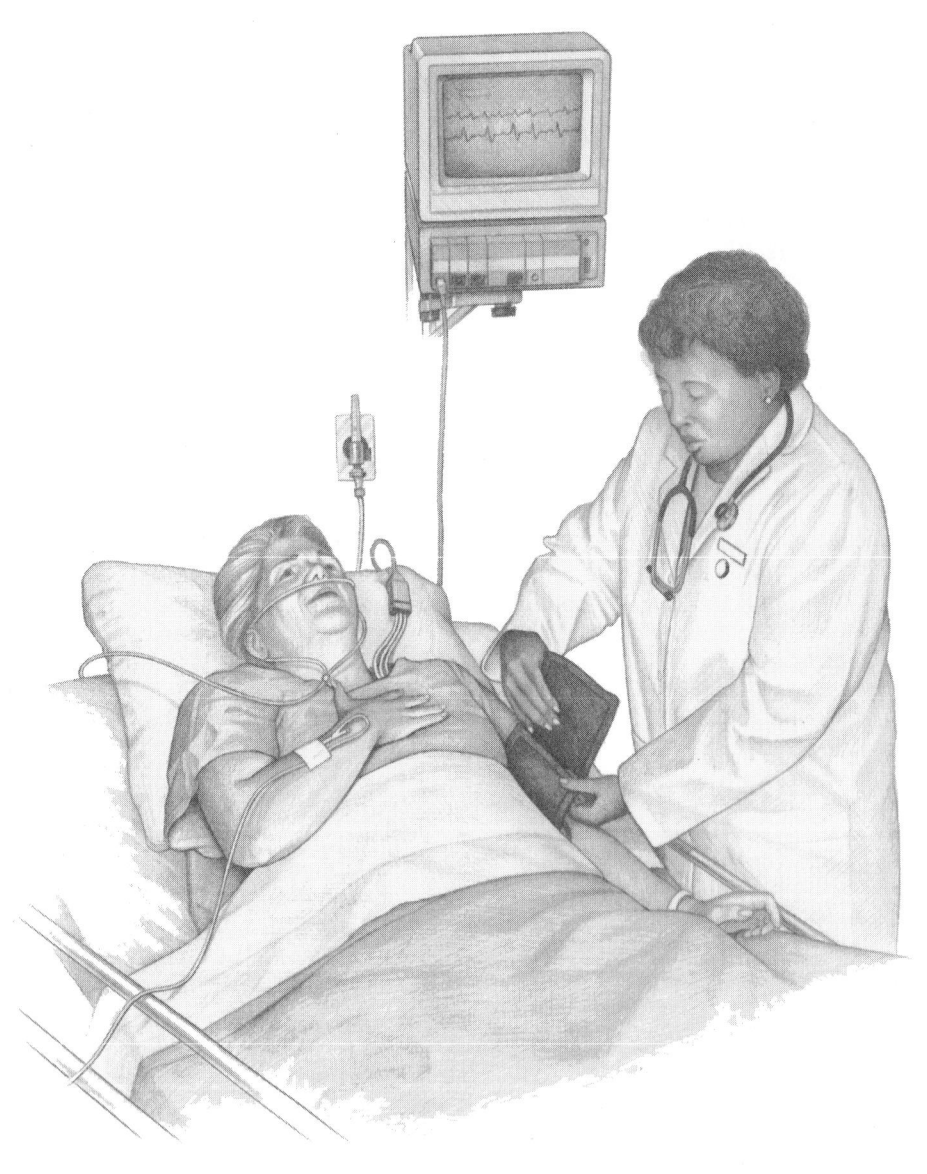

3

CORONARY ARTERY DISEASE AND ANGINA

Overview

Coronary artery disease (CAD) and angina pectoris play leading roles in the onset, signs and symptoms, and outcomes of some of the most serious cardiac disorders. Indeed, disorders resulting from CAD—primarily myocardial infarction (MI)—remain the leading cause of death in the United States today. Nearly 500,000 Americans died of CAD-related illness in 1994 alone, the latest year for which statistics are available.

In this chapter, you'll find an up-to-date review of the pathophysiology of CAD and angina that you can use to help refresh your memory and sharpen your skills.

Coronary artery disease

As you know, the potentially devastating effects of CAD result largely from progressive blockage of the lumens of coronary arteries. That blockage reduces the amount of oxygenated blood available to myocardial tissues, possibly holding it below the level those tissues need to function normally. When that happens, the affected patient develops signs and symptoms of myocardial ischemia (angina) or MI. Unfortunately, however, by the time the patient develops these signs and symptoms, her coronary arteries already have undergone dramatic internal changes.

How coronary artery disease develops

Like all arteries, the coronary arteries are made up of three tissue layers:

- the adventitia, or outer layer
- the media, or middle layer
- the intima, or inner layer.

The adventitia is primarily composed of smooth-muscle cells, fibroblasts, and loose connective tissue; the media, almost entirely of smooth-muscle cells; and the intima, of a single layer of cells called the endothelium. Normally, the endothelium is impermeable to proteins and doesn't interact with platelets, leukocytes, or fibrinolytic clotting factors. Instead, it provides a smooth barrier that allows blood to flow freely through the vasculature.

When something damages the endothelium, however—such as the effects of hyperlipidemia, hypertension, or another risk factor—circulating monocytes may stick to adhesive molecules released by the endothelium at the site of injury. The monocytes then invade the intima and accumulate lipids (see *How atherosclerotic lesions develop,* page 48). These lipid-laden cells are called foam cells. Eventually, they form a fatty streak, which is the first stage of CAD. These streaks have been found even in very young children.

Fatty streak

Composed of lipids (mainly cholesterol) and elongated smooth-muscle cells, a fatty streak is yellow and smooth. It protrudes slightly into the lumen of the artery but typically doesn't obstruct blood flowing through the vessel. Fatty streaks may be reversible, and they don't cause clinically observable signs or symptoms. However, they almost certainly contribute significantly to the two later stages of atherosclerotic lesions.

How atherosclerotic lesions develop

Like all arteries, the coronary arteries consist of three layers, as shown in this cross-sectional view.	When the intima, the innermost layer, becomes damaged, lipids may build up into a fatty streak.	Then smooth-muscle cells may begin to proliferate and protrude into the lumen, forming a typical arterial plaque.	As the plaque enlarges and calcifies, it may become a complicated lesion prone to hemorrhage or thrombus formation.

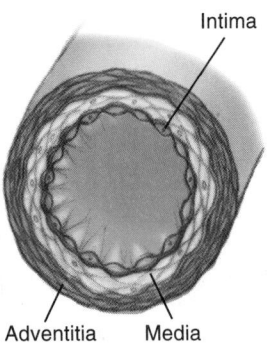
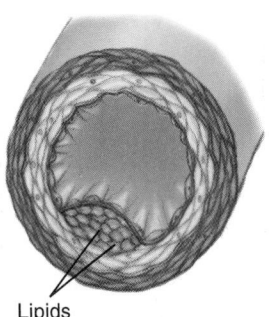
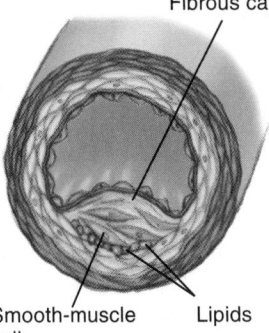
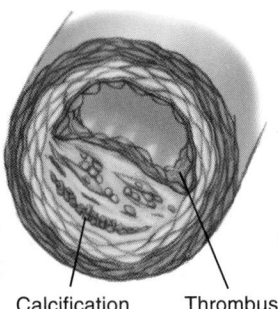

Intima

Adventitia Media

Lipids

Fibrous cap

Smooth-muscle cell Lipids

Calcification Thrombus

Raised plaque

In the second stage of CAD, smooth-muscle cells begin to proliferate at the site of the fatty streak. Connective tissue and lipids, transported through the endothelium on lipoproteins, enter the foam cells and smooth-muscle cells. Over time, the fatty streak becomes a raised plaque that may continue to enlarge and protrude into the arterial lumen. Lipids, fibrin, white blood cells, and calcium are commonly found in these plaques, topped by a fibrous cap that develops over the lesion. This type of raised fibrous plaque is the typical atherosclerotic lesion. It's common in people who are over age 30.

Complicated lesion

As time passes, the plaque may grow and become complicated by additional platelets, calcification, hemorrhage, collagen, and an increasing risk of thrombus formation. Such a complicated lesion—the third stage of CAD—may rupture or block the arterial lumen suddenly and completely. If the lesion completely obstructs blood flow, an MI may result.

Keep in mind that this description of plaque formation is only a theory. Other theories exist as well. However, all include the concepts of endothelial injury, proliferation of smooth-muscle cells, lipid accumulation, fibrosis, thrombus formation, and calcification.

The course of plaque development varies widely from patient to patient. Some patients maintain stable plaques for many years. Others develop serious cardiac signs and symptoms over a relatively short period of time. No one knows precisely why. But everyone acknowledges the profound effect of many important risk factors on the development and progression of CAD.

Recognizing risk factors

Naturally, the best approach to CAD is to prevent it from advancing to the point of danger. To help do that, you'll need to understand the pathophysiology of risk factors that predispose patients to CAD or accelerate its development. The more risk factors a person has, the greater her risk of developing CAD.

But keep in mind that a person without risk factors can develop CAD as well. Consequently, you'll want to help patients identify and reduce their personal risk factors, and you'll want to educate patients who have no apparent risk factors about the dangers of CAD. By doing so, you can help to slow the atherosclerotic process—before it produces dangerous signs and symptoms.

Nonmodifiable factors

Nonmodifiable risk factors are those over which the patient has no influence or control. They include the patient's family background, sex, race, and age.

Family background

If your patient has siblings, parents, or grandparents who have had CAD, she's more likely to develop it herself through heredity, environment, and a learned lifestyle. The risk of developing CAD increases if a patient's family history includes:
- an MI in a first-degree male relative under age 55
- an MI in a first-degree female relative under age 65
- diabetes
- hypertension
- gout
- hyperlipidemia.

Sex and race

Until middle age, men experience more CAD-related problems than women. However, this difference becomes less marked as age increases, probably because of the hormone changes associated with menopause.

Race is also a risk factor for CAD, with African-American patients three times more likely to have severe hypertension than white patients. Also, African-American women are at higher risk for developing heart disease than white women.

Advancing age

Four out of five people who die of CAD-related illness are over age 65. That's largely because without behavior and lifestyle changes, CAD continues to develop over time. The older the patient, the more time CAD has to develop into pronounced plaques with a high risk of rupture, thrombus formation, and arterial blockage.

Modifiable factors

Modifiable factors are those over which the patient does have some influence. They include

Interpreting serum lipid levels

These guidelines from the National Cholesterol Education Program will help you assess your patient's risk of coronary artery disease.

Lipid	Serum level (mg/dl)	Interpretation
Total cholesterol	< 200	low risk
	200–239	borderline high risk
	> 239	high risk
High-density lipoproteins	> 35	low risk
	< 35	increased risk
Low-density lipoproteins	< 129	low risk
	130–159	borderline high risk
	> 159	high risk
Triglycerides	< 200	low risk
	201–399	borderline high risk
	400–1,000	high risk
	> 1,000	very high risk

hyperlipidemia, hypertension, smoking, alcohol consumption, the effects of diabetes, obesity, a sedentary lifestyle, stress, and hormone changes.

Hyperlipidemia

Because of the role lipids play in the formation of atherosclerotic plaque, the level of certain lipids in your patients' blood can make a marked difference in the onset and course of CAD. Specifically, elevated cholesterol and triglyceride levels increase the risk of CAD and its consequences (see *Interpreting serum lipid levels*).

As a group, blood lipids include cholesterol, triglycerides, and phospholipids. Because these lipids can't dissolve in blood, they must be carried to the body's tissues in lipoproteins. The protein portion of a lipoprotein is made of polypeptides called apolipoproteins; they attach to receptor sites on the cells, thus enabling lipids to enter the cells.

Lipoproteins come in three major types: very-low-density lipoproteins (VLDLs), low-density lipoproteins (LDLs), and high-density lipoproteins (HDLs). The VLDLs carry mostly triglycerides.

The LDLs result from the metabolism of VLDLs and transport cholesterol from the blood to the tissues. These LDLs build up within the arterial walls and contribute to the formation of atherosclerotic plaque, thus increasing a person's risk of CAD. Apolipoprotein B (apo B) is the major polypeptide in LDLs. In particular, apo B-100 helps deposit cholesterol in cells and may offer a more specific marker of a person's risk of CAD.

The HDLs are made mostly of protein, which removes cholesterol from the arteries and carries it to the liver for metabolism and excretion. This process prevents lipids from collecting on arterial walls and protects against CAD. Therefore, the higher the HDL level, the lower the person's risk of CAD. Apolipoprotein A (apo A) is the major polypeptide in HDL. Specifically, apo A-I makes up most of the apo A in HDL and may offer a more specific predictor of CAD than total HDL levels.

You may hear LDL called bad cholesterol because it increases the risk of CAD. And you may hear HDL called good cholesterol because high levels of it appear to reduce the risk of CAD. Low HDL levels are more likely to lead to CAD in women, while high LDL levels are more likely to increase the risk in men.

If your patient has high LDL or low HDL levels, especially if she also has other risk factors (such as hypertension), you'll need to teach her about diet, exercise, and other methods of risk modification. Remember that smoking, obesity, a sedentary lifestyle, alcohol use, high triglyceride levels, and the use of corticosteroids or beta-blockers may reduce HDL levels. A patient who exercises regularly, reduces her weight, and stops smoking can raise her HDL levels.

Even if your patient has no evidence of CAD, recommend that she have her total serum cholesterol level measured at least once every 5 years. Remind her what the measurements mean:
• a level below 200 mg/dl indicates a relatively low risk of CAD
• a level of 200 to 239 mg/dl indicates an increased risk of CAD
• a level of 240 mg/dl and above indicates a high risk of CAD.

A patient with a total cholesterol level of 200 mg/dl or above, especially if she also has other risk factors, should have a serum lipid profile that includes total cholesterol, HDL, LDL, and triglyceride levels (see *Lipid profile: Patient teaching tips*).

Afterward, you can determine the ratio of total cholesterol to HDLs by dividing the HDL level into the total cholesterol level. For example, if the patient's total cholesterol level is 250 mg/dl and her HDL level is 25 mg/dl, her ratio would be 10:1—a strong warning of CAD and its related disorders. Tell the patient that the ratio of total cholesterol to HDL cholesterol should remain below 5:1, preferably below 3.5:1.

Hypertension
Defined as a repeated systolic blood pressure of 140 mm Hg or above or a repeated diastolic pressure of 90 mm Hg or above, *hypertension* is a major modifiable risk factor for CAD and its effects.

Probably by damaging the intimal arterial layer, hypertension increases the rate of atherosclerosis development, causing the arteries to thicken and narrow. As a result, the arteries lose their elasticity and the heart must work harder to pump blood. At the same time, hypertension raises the myocardial oxygen demand by requiring the heart to contract more forcefully to circulate blood against increased arterial resistance. Over time, untreated hypertension results in a hypertrophied left ventricle, which also requires more oxygen. Eventually, arteries narrowed by atherosclerosis may not be able to deliver enough oxygenated blood to meet the myocardial demand, resulting in angina or an MI.

Hypertension is more common among African-American, Puerto Rican, Cuban, and Mexican-American people than among white people. African-Americans tend to develop a more severe level of hypertension.

Hypertension also is more common among older people. What's more, patients over age 65 may have *isolated systolic hypertension,* which is a systolic blood pressure of 160 mm Hg or above coupled with a diastolic reading below 90 mm Hg. Isolated systolic hypertension results from a loss of elasticity in the aorta and its larger branches. Among the elderly, it represents the most important risk factor for cardiovascular disease other than age itself.

Keep in mind that some risk factors for CAD are also risk factors for hypertension. For example, women who have taken oral contraceptives for more than 5 years have two to three times the risk of developing hypertension compared to demographically similar women who haven't taken oral contraceptives. Smoking, obesity, and diabetes also raise the risk of hypertension.

Smoking

People who smoke have more than twice the risk of an MI. Also, they're more likely to die of an MI if they have one, and they're more apt to die suddenly, within 60 minutes after the infarction.

We don't know exactly how smoking increases the risk of CAD-related disorders. However, we do know a number of facts that, when combined, create a compelling picture of the harmful effects of smoking.

For example, we know that cigarette smoke contains nicotine and carbon monoxide. Nicotine prompts the sympathetic nervous system to release epinephrine and norepinephrine—two hormones that increase heart rate, blood pressure, stroke volume, cardiac output, and contractility. These responses make the heart work harder, thereby increasing its need for oxygen. If the smoker already has some amount of CAD, her arterial system may not be able to meet that increased need.

Carbon monoxide only aggravates the situation by decreasing the oxygen-carrying capacity of the blood. The problem is that carbon monoxide attaches more readily to hemoglobin than oxygen does. Consequently, the more carbon monoxide in the patient's system, the less hemoglobin will be available to bond with oxygen. As a result, the patient may become hypoxic.

Carbon monoxide also contributes to the development of CAD by damaging the endothelial lining of arteries.

Clearly, the combined effects of arterial constriction, increased myocardial oxygen demand, and the decreased oxygen-carrying capacity of blood sets the smoker up for trouble. What's more, smokers have an increased tendency to form blood clots because smoking increases the adhesiveness of platelets and raises fibrinogen levels. Smoking also lowers HDL levels and raises LDL and triglyceride levels.

All of these factors combined yield a measurable—sometimes dramatic—increase in CAD risk for smokers, especially for people who have other risk factors as well, such as a positive family history, oral contraceptive use, antihypertensive use, and an overindulgence in alcohol.

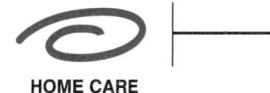

HOME CARE

Lipid profile: Patient teaching tips

Explain to your patient that her physician will delay a lipid profile by at least 8 weeks if she has had a myocardial infarction, surgery, a traumatic injury, or an acute infection because these conditions can falsely decrease lipid levels. Also, a physician will delay the test by at least 2 weeks after changing the patient's drug regimen. When your patient is scheduled for a lipid profile, urge her to follow these instructions to ensure the most accurate test results.
- Don't make any changes in your diet or activity level for at least 2 weeks before the test.
- Don't have anything to eat or drink for at least 12 hours before the test.
- Don't exercise just before the test because doing so can increase triglyceride levels.
- If you're undergoing repeated lipid profile tests, have them done at the same time of day because cholesterol and triglyceride levels tend to rise as the day progresses.
- Sit quietly for at least 5 minutes before having blood drawn for the test.
- Make sure you're in the same position every time you have blood drawn. Changing positions can change your cholesterol level.

Even environmental tobacco smoke, also known as secondhand smoke or passive smoking, increases the risk of CAD in nonsmokers. That's because in an enclosed space, cigarette smoke increases the level of carbon monoxide in the air. Anyone who inhales it will experience some increase in heart rate and blood pressure, some decrease in exercise capacity, and some increase in the risk of endothelial damage and CAD.

Excessive alcohol consumption

Heavy consumption of alcohol can increase VLDL and triglyceride levels in the blood and can increase the risk of arrhythmias that cause alcoholic cardiomyopathy. Heavy alcohol consumption is also a risk factor for hypertension. Plus, alcohol and cigarettes commonly go hand in hand.

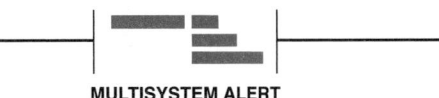

MULTISYSTEM ALERT

Understanding syndrome X

Some people have a constellation of several disorders that raise their risk of coronary artery disease and Type 2 diabetes. This constellation is known as syndrome X (or insulin resistance syndrome). The disorders include the following:
- hyperglycemia
- hyperinsulinemia
- hyperlipidemia (especially increased triglyceride levels and decreased high-density lipoprotein levels)
- hypertension
- insulin resistance
- upper-body obesity.

You may be able to help a patient with syndrome X to reduce her risk of developing heart disease *and* control her diabetes by following guidelines from the American Heart Association. Urge such a patient to schedule regular appointments with her physician and teach her the importance of doing the following:
- monitoring and controlling blood glucose levels
- monitoring and treating hyperlipidemia
- exercising regularly and monitoring the effects of exercise
- achieving and maintaining ideal body weight
- monitoring blood pressure and treating hypertension.

People who smoke and consume too much alcohol raise their risk of CAD even more.

Diabetes

In people who have diabetes, CAD tends to develop at an earlier age; in people with Type 2 diabetes, it's the most common cause of death. Diabetic people tend to have high triglyceride, cholesterol, and LDL levels but low HDL levels, a combination that may accelerate the atherosclerotic process.

Plus, people with diabetes also have an increased risk of atherosclerosis in the large and medium-sized arteries (called macrovascular disease), which results in CAD, peripheral vascular disease, and cerebrovascular disease. This increased risk may stem from the fact that high blood glucose levels increase platelet adhesiveness and cause a proliferation of smooth-muscle cells in arteries.

What's more, factors that normally protect a person from CAD, such as being female, don't offer such protection in those with diabetes. In fact, women with diabetes have a greater risk of CAD than men; they also have a fivefold to sevenfold risk over women who don't have diabetes. Men with diabetes have twice the risk of men without it.

A person with diabetes may have other risk factors for heart disease as well, such as hypertension and obesity. Naturally, having multiple risk factors increases the diabetic patient's risk of developing CAD. A set of conditions called syndrome X may arise in some diabetic patients. The syndrome includes insulin resistance, hypertension, hyperglycemia, hyperinsulinemia, obesity, and lipoprotein abnormalities—a risk-raising combination (see *Understanding syndrome X*).

Obesity

An obese person probably has high blood cholesterol and triglyceride levels and low HDL levels, which increases her risk of CAD. What's more, obesity also tends to lead to hypertension and diabetes, which also increase the risk.

The pattern of fat distribution on a person's body may have more to do with CAD risk than overall obesity. Specifically, a man may face a greater risk if his waist measurement exceeds his hip measurement. A woman may face a greater risk if her waist measurement exceeds 80% of her hip measurement.

Sedentary lifestyle

People who don't exercise tend to have higher cholesterol and triglyceride levels and lower HDL levels. They're also more likely to be obese and have hypertension, both of which increase the risk of heart disease.

Personality and stress

For many years, people with aggressive, or type A, personalities have been warned of their increased risk of developing CAD or having an MI. Characteristics of a type A personality include competitiveness, ambition, impatience, a preoccupation with time and deadlines, and hostility.

However, it may be that only type A people who display hostility have an increased risk of CAD.

Stress increases the risk of CAD by acting on the sympathetic nervous system, which increases heart rate and myocardial contractility, mobilizes free fatty acids, and increases platelet adhesiveness and aggregation. Stress influences other risk factors as well, including hypertension, smoking, drinking, and poor nutrition.

Hormone changes

Women who take oral contraceptives face an increased risk of developing CAD or having an MI, especially those who are over age 35 and smoke or have other risk factors. The increased risk stems especially from the tendency of high-dose oral contraceptives (which contain estrogen and may contain progestin) to raise LDL levels, lower HDL levels, raise blood pressure, and promote the formation of blood clots. Lower-dose oral contraceptives may produce fewer harmful effects.

After a woman goes through menopause and her estrogen levels fall, her LDL levels will tend to rise. As a result, her risk of CAD may meet—or exceed—that of men who are her age.

This hormone change provides the most likely explanation for the shift in risk: Men have a higher CAD mortality rate than women up to age 55 but, after menopause, women have the greater risk. Women over age 65 have an 11% higher mortality rate from CAD than men.

Clearly, many factors influence the pathophysiology of CAD, most of which can be eased or exacerbated by the patient's lifestyle and behavior. Keep in mind, however, that though many patients have good intentions, only about a third succeed in following risk-reducing strategies over the long term. Consequently, many progress from asymptomatic CAD to the next and more ominous stage of heart disease.

Angina

When the myocardium demands more oxygen than the coronary arteries can deliver, the patient develops certain signs and symptoms. If reversible, they're called angina pectoris. In the United States, more than 7 million people know the feeling of angina, almost 3 million men and

more than 4 million women. About 350,000 new cases of angina are diagnosed each year.

Angina occurs in 5.2% of African-American women, 4.6% of Mexican-American women, and 4.1% of white women. It occurs in 2.6% of African-American men, 3.4% of Mexican-American men, and 3.4% of white men.

A sharply higher percentage of people ages 75 to 84 have angina. According to the Cardiovascular Health Study, angina affects:
- 4.4% of non-black men ages 65 to 74; 5.6% of non-black men ages 75 to 84, and 4.3% of non-black men age 85 and over
- 2.6% of black men ages 65 to 74; 5.2% of black men ages 75 to 84; and 4.4% of black men age 85 and over
- 1.9% of non-black women ages 65 to 74; 3.1% of non-black women ages 75 to 84; and 2% of non-black women age 85 and over
- 2.5% of black women ages 65 to 74; 3.8% of black women ages 75 to 84; and 1.5% of black women age 85 and over.

To maintain and even increase your expertise in responding promptly and accurately to angina, take time to review its underlying pathophysiology.

How angina develops

When CAD progresses to the point where arterial plaques restrict the blood flow to the myocardium, the patient is poised for problems. The next time her heart requires more oxygenated blood than those restricted vessels can provide, her myocardial tissues will become ischemic and painful.

Over time, collateral circulation may develop around the narrowed section of artery. However, this mode of compensation eventually fails in most cases, leaving the patient once again open to myocardial ischemia and its attendant signs and symptoms. Unfortunately, most patients have no signs or symptoms until about 75% of the arterial lumen is blocked.

Depending on the degree of blockage and the length of time the blockage has existed, your patient may go beyond the effects of angina alone and develop a myocardial injury or an MI. Indeed, for some patients, the first sign of CAD may be sudden death.

Recognizing angina

If a patient develops angina while in your care, expect to observe an increase in her heart rate, respiratory rate, and blood pressure. She may look pale and anxious. Her skin may feel clammy, and she may report feeling nauseated. Although complaints of chest discomfort vary from patient to patient, a feeling of heaviness or pressure in the chest is common. Obtain a 12-lead electrocardiogram immediately and look for these changes: a flattened T wave in lead I, a peaked T wave in lead II, an inverted T wave in lead III, a depressed ST segment with an inverted T wave in lead V_1, and a depressed ST segment in leads V_2, V_3, and V_4.

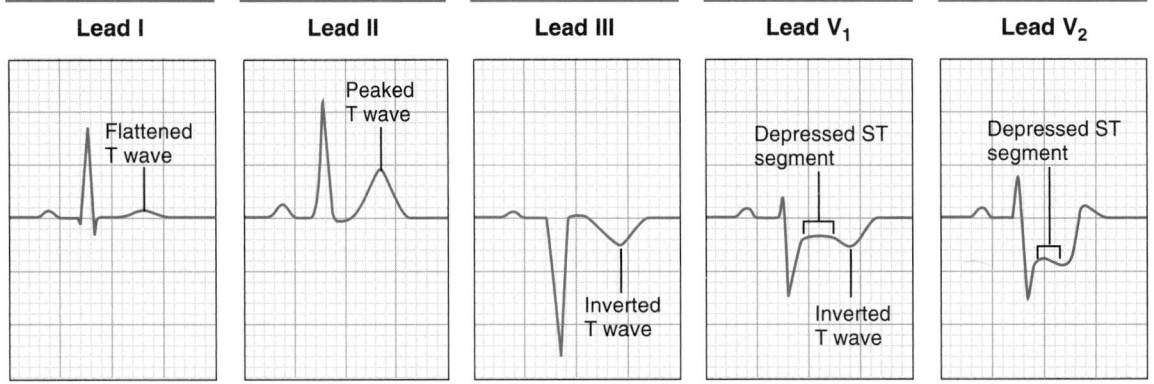

Lead I	Lead II	Lead III	Lead V_1	Lead V_2
Flattened T wave	Peaked T wave	Inverted T wave	Depressed ST segment / Inverted T wave	Depressed ST segment

Recognizing angina

A patient with CAD may develop several types of angina, including:
• stable
• unstable
• variant (also called Prinzmetal's).

Unstable and variant angina are dangerous complications. Stable angina, also called effort or exertional angina, is a syndrome that occurs over several weeks or more in a predictable, repetitive pattern. It arises with exercise or any condition that increases myocardial oxygen demand beyond the capacity of the narrowed arteries. Such conditions include stress, anxiety, a big meal, fever, tachycardia, anemia, hypoglycemia, and hyperthyroidism. By definition, angina resolves with rest or nitroglycerin. It typically lasts 15 minutes or less. Stable angina has a mortality rate of 3% to 4% per year.

Most patients with angina can describe which factors trigger an episode, how long it typically lasts, and how intense the discomfort is. They also can tell you whether the sensation has remained the same over time or evolved. On occasion, you may observe an anginal episode (see *Recognizing angina*).

The most common symptoms of stable angina are substernal chest pain and pressure or heaviness with activity. Keep in mind, however, that the patient may deny having chest pain at all, describing it instead as discomfort or pressure. Your patient may report feeling as though she has an elephant sitting on her chest or a rubber band squeezing her chest. She may place her clenched fist over her sternum while describing the sensation, a gesture known as the *Levine sign*. When your patient describes her chest signs and symptoms, listen for such words as:
• heaviness
• crushing
• burning
• indigestion
• nausea or vomiting
• shortness of breath
• fatigue or weakness
• sweating
• anxiety or restlessness.

Because the patient may ignore signs or symptoms that don't involve her chest, thinking that they're unrelated, you should make sure to ask her specific questions. Have her point to any other areas where she has felt pain or discomfort, and ask her if the sensation radiates to another area (see *Using PQRST to assess chest pain*).

Angina may radiate to the left shoulder, down the left arm, or into the neck, shoulders, or epigastrium. Rarely, it may radiate down the right arm. The patient may have shortness of breath or pain between the scapulae, typically toward the left side. Ask whether the patient has numbness or tingling in her arm and hand. To objectively measure the patient's pain level, have her rate it on a scale of 0 to 10, in which 0 is no pain and 10 is the worst pain imaginable. Also, ask how long the pain typically lasts.

Classification systems

In the earliest stages of angina, the patient may experience no decline in her ability to carry out normal activities of daily living. As CAD progresses, however, the degree of arterial blockage increases, and the patient's ability to function without chest pain decreases—altering her lifestyle and activities.

To help express these changes in a consistent manner, several systems have been developed to classify cardiovascular disability. You can use these systems to establish a functional baseline for your patient and then to follow changes in her activity level over time.

In general, these classification systems grade activities into four classes. A patient with no limitation in activity would be assigned to Class I. As less strenuous activities provoke angina, however, the patient moves up the classification system. By the time she reaches Class IV, her activities are severely limited by angina.

The New York Heart Association has published such a classification system. The Canadian Cardiovascular Society Classification (CCSC) is another system that relates angina to specific activities for each class or level of disability. For instance, if your patient experiences angina after walking from her car to her office, a distance of about one block, her physician may classify her condition as CCSC Class III. Over time, if this same patient reports having angina while dressing and occasionally at rest, her CCSC status may pro-

---

Using PQRST to assess chest pain

The PQRST method allows you to collect data from your patient using an organized approach. Just ask the following questions to obtain a complete understanding of your patient's chest pain.

P *Provocation and palliation.* What provoked your angina? When it began, were you engaged in a physical activity? Resting? Sleeping? What did you do to relieve the pain?

Q *Quality.* What did the pain feel like? Was it accompanied by other problems, such as sweating, nausea, shortness of breath, light-headedness, or palpitations?

R *Region and radiation.* Where did the discomfort arise? Did it seem to radiate to any other locations?

S *Severity.* On a scale of 0 to 10, with 0 being no pain and 10 being the worst pain possible, how severe was the pain you felt?

T *Timing.* How long did the pain last? Did you take nitroglycerin to make it go away?

---

gress to Class IV. After her physician makes adjustments in her therapy, and the patient can once again carry out her daily activities without experiencing angina, she can be reassigned to Class III.

The Goldman system is based on the amount of energy needed to perform specific activities. It uses metabolic equivalents as a way to measure the oxygen uptake required to perform a specific activity. Specifically, 1 metabolic equivalent equals an oxygen uptake of 3.5 ml/kg of body weight per minute. For example, sitting quietly in a chair requires 1 metabolic equivalent. So, if your patient weighs 60 kg, she'll have an oxygen uptake of 210 ml of oxygen per minute (60×3.5) while sitting in a chair. This same patient walking down the hall at a slow pace may require 3 metabolic equivalents, or 630 ml of oxygen per minute. By using metabolic equivalents, Goldman's specific activity scale allows you to objectively classify your patient's activity level.

Whichever classification system you use, you'll need to follow the progress of your patient's angina using the same set of measurements each time. Keep in mind that many patients move up and down the classification system as CAD progresses, therapies change, and invasive procedures (such as angioplasty) are performed. Also, keep in mind that an increase in the frequency, severity, and duration of angina may signal the development of unstable angina or an increased risk of having an MI. This is especially true if the patient's angina becomes less responsive to rest and nitroglycerin—a sign that she may need immediate treatment.

4

CORONARY ARTERY DISEASE AND ANGINA

Treatment

The good news about coronary artery disease (CAD) and angina is that they need not cause permanent myocardial damage. Indeed, lifestyle changes, drugs, and, if necessary, a range of invasive procedures can help reverse a person's course toward myocardial infarction (MI) and lead her instead toward increasing health. This chapter reviews the options available for treating patients who have CAD or angina as well as your role in attaining a successful outcome.

Coronary artery disease

Several drugs can help patients lower their lipid levels and control hypertension. As you know, however, pharmacologic and even surgical treatments for CAD produce only limited benefits if the patient isn't willing to modify her lifestyle to reduce her level of cardiac risk.

Lifestyle changes

Most people know that their lifestyle choices can raise or lower their risk of heart disease. However, that knowledge alone commonly does little to precipitate lifestyle changes—until CAD creates a threat the person simply can't ignore.

In fact, a frightening diagnosis or anginal episode may provide just the impetus a patient needs to commit to difficult lifestyle changes. In general, people are most receptive to change just after experiencing a life-threatening event or confirming an ominous diagnosis. They realize that lack of action could cause permanent disability

or even hasten their death. Clearly, this is an ideal time for you to teach and promote lifestyle changes designed to reduce the odds of a life-threatening event in the future.

When doing so, keep in mind that change itself—even positive change—can create dangerous stress levels for the cardiac patient. Especially for a patient with marked CAD who needs to modify several lifestyle areas, you'll want to remain sensitive to her level of anxiety over the needed changes, her success in accomplishing them, and her ability to tackle more than one topic at once.

By adopting a lifetime commitment to a new and healthier lifestyle, the patient not only can prevent progressive cardiac damage but also can improve the quality of nearly every aspect of her daily life.

Your influence and teaching can do much to convince her to stop smoking, follow healthy dietary guidelines, adopt an exercise program, and adhere to other important elements of a heart-healthy life. As a result, she'll begin to reduce her lipid levels and control her hypertension—two keys to keeping angina and an MI at bay.

Smoking cessation
Avoiding cigarettes and other products containing nicotine is the single most important step your patient can take to reduce her risk of CAD-related adverse events (see *Risks of smoking, strategies for quitting,* page 58).

If your patient smokes, especially if she smokes heavily, tell her about the increased cardiac risk, encourage her to stop smoking, and let her know about the numerous resources avail-

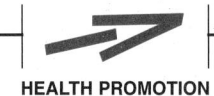

HEALTH PROMOTION

Risks of smoking, strategies for quitting

To help motivate your patient to stop smoking, explain some of the risks:

- Using nicotine doubles the risk of death from coronary artery disease and cerebrovascular accident (CVA).
- Inhaling or chewing nicotine increases the risk of mouth, larynx, and lung cancer by 6 to 12 times.
- Cigarette smoke carries carbon monoxide, a substance that lowers the ability of blood to carry oxygen.
- Nicotine increases the body's tendency to form clots on the inside of blood-vessel walls. Taking a daily aspirin tablet won't reduce this risk.
- If a woman uses birth-control pills and smokes, her risk of having a CVA increases by 10 times.
- Smoking during pregnancy raises the risk of miscarriage, premature birth, low birth weight, and stillbirth.
- Children exposed to cigarette smoke in their homes have an increased number of upper respiratory and inner ear infections.
- A person with diabetes who smokes further impairs circulation to the hands and feet, which can result in the development of wounds that won't heal.

Helping your patient quit

If your patient wants to quit smoking, be honest about withdrawal signs and symptoms. Tell her that she may have periods of fatigue, restlessness, headache, dizziness, coughing, constipation, hunger, and poor concentration for 2 to 4 weeks. Stress that these signs and symptoms result from the body's process of freeing itself from the effects of smoking.

Also, help her to identify her most tempting situations and to find ways to avoid succumbing to the desire to smoke. Suggest that she try avoiding tempting situations altogether for the time being. Or she can try distracting herself by sipping water poured over lots of cracked ice, chewing sugarless gum, or using a toothpick. Remind her that the urge to smoke won't disappear, but it will fade.

Using nicotine replacement therapy

If your patient is pregnant, urge her to try to quit without using nicotine replacement therapy. If she isn't pregnant, discuss the use of nicotine patches and chewing gum.

Tell her that most patients find nicotine patches easier to use than gum and explain that each morning she simply needs to place a new patch on a fairly hairless spot between her neck and waist. Some patients develop a mild skin reaction to the patches; if she does, she should use hydrocortisone cream 2.5% to treat it.

If she wants to use nicotine gum, tell her not to eat or drink anything for 15 minutes before and after chewing it. Also, tell her to chew the gum on a fixed schedule each day, at least one piece every 1 to 2 hours.

Explain that she should chew the gum until it begins to taste peppery. Then she should place it between her cheek and gums for 30 minutes to allow the nicotine to be absorbed through the lining of her mouth. In some people, the chewing gum causes a sore mouth, aching jaw, hiccups, and stomach upset. Usually, these problems are mild and resolve with the proper chewing technique.

---

able to help her. Many support groups and therapies are available to help your patient quit. For example, she can use nicotine-laced chewing gum or one of several types of transdermal patches to gradually lower the level of nicotine in her body. Doing so will also reverse the additional multisystem dangers created by smoking or chewing tobacco. These therapies are available without a prescription.

A prescription drug called bupropion helps reduce withdrawal symptoms and the urge to

smoke without delivering nicotine. The patient probably will start bupropion therapy by taking one 150-mg tablet each morning for 3 days. On the fourth day, she'll take one pill in the morning and another in the evening, at least 8 hours later. Most patients continue this regimen for 7 to 12 weeks. She should stop smoking at the end of the first week, when the drug has reached therapeutic levels. Caution the patient to avoid taking extra doses and to drink little or no alcohol while taking the drug. Warn her not to chew or crush the tablets, but rather to swallow them whole. Mention that the drug may have a distinctive odor. The drug's adverse effects include a dry mouth and insomnia, both of which typically resolve in a few weeks. A few patients may face an increased risk of having a seizure. Contraindications to bupropion include a history of seizures, a current or previous eating disorder, recent use of a monoamine oxidase inhibitor, or current use of any drug that contains bupropion. Tell the patient to contact her physician if she develops a rash.

Which method the patient chooses to help herself quit isn't as important as simply choosing one and getting started. If the first attempt isn't successful, urge her to try a different method. Acknowledge to your patient that quitting is hard, and that it may take a few attempts. But emphasize that an unsuccessful past attempt to quit will not reduce her odds of success now.

Whichever method the patient chooses to help herself quit smoking, take time to review with her the guidelines for using it safely and correctly. For example, if the patient choose a nicotine patch, warn her that smoking while wearing the patch can actually increase her risk of developing angina or having an MI by raising her nicotine level above that created by smoking alone. Also, urge her to check with her physician before taking new drugs or undergoing treatments or diagnostic tests.

Within a year after your patient quits smoking, the myocardial risk raised by nicotine will decline by about half, although hematologic alterations caused by tobacco can take up to 5 years to normalize. Explain to your patient that reduced risk translates into longer life—an average of 5 years longer for a man who quits between ages 35 and 39 and 3 years for a woman in the same age-group.

Alcohol moderation
If your patient drinks alcohol, tell her that she can reduce her risk of developing angina and having an MI by limiting intake to 1 ounce of pure alcohol daily. That translates to one of the following options:
• 24 ounces of beer
• 2 ounces of 100-proof liquor
• 3 ounces of 80-proof liquor
• 8 ounces of wine.
Remind patients that a can of beer contains 12 ounces, a typical shot glass holds 1.5 ounces, and most wine glasses hold 6 to 8 ounces.

Sound nutrition
As you know, nutrition and weight are related but not inseparable. That's why, no matter what your patient weighs, you'll want to take time to explain the principles of basic nutrition and the importance of consuming a diet that includes the proper balance of carbohydrates, proteins, minerals, vitamins, water, fiber, and fats. Let your patient know that a low-fat diet that contains plenty of fruits and vegetables forms a cornerstone of a heart-healthy lifestyle.

You may want to start your discussion of nutritional health by explaining the roles of cholesterol and fats. Although most people know that high cholesterol levels lead to heart disease, far fewer understand the relationship of fats to blood cholesterol levels, and the influence of different types of fats on the progress of CAD. Explain to your patient that cholesterol is essential to the nervous system and brain. It also contributes to the manufacture of certain hormones, aids digestion, and helps to maintain bone integrity. Mention that the body burns fats to produce energy. From these descriptions, the patient will correctly conclude that cholesterol and fats aren't all bad.

However, too much cholesterol and too high a percentage of fats in the diet do contribute to the growth of arterial plaques that eventually convert CAD into a symptomatic problem: angina and possibly an MI. Consequently, dietary guidelines are one of the first and most important recommendations for people with heart disease.

Specific dietary recommendations may vary with the results of the patient's lipid profile test. In general, however, a healthy diet should derive at least 55% of its calories from carbohydrates, 15% from protein, and a maximum of 30% from fats. Of that 30%, saturated fats should constitute no more than a third; unsaturated and monounsaturated fats, each about a third. Urge the patient not to consume more than 300 mg of cholesterol daily. The patient's body size and her level of physical activity will determine the total daily calories she needs to maintain a desired weight.

Remind the patient that saturated fats are found primarily in animal products, such as meats, butter, cheese, and eggs. Polyunsaturated and monounsaturated fats, on the other hand, generally come from plant and vegetable sources. Examples include corn oil, safflower oil, sunflower oil, and peanut oil. Commonly, saturated fats remain hard at room temperature; polyunsaturated and monounsaturated fats turn liquid at room temperature. Warn the patient to avoid polyunsaturated and monounsaturated fats that have been hardened by hydrogenation.

Today, few people take time to calculate the percentage of calories they consume from each important food category. For the patient with CAD, however, doing so can make all the difference between a healthy diet and one that worsens her cardiac health. Remind your patient that when calculating calories, she should assume that 1 gram of carbohydrate or protein contains about 4.5 calories and that 1 gram of fat contains about 9 calories. By lowering her fat intake, your patient can reduce her cholesterol level by up to 30% while increasing her beneficial, high-density lipoprotein (HDL) level.

Impress upon your patient that so-called health foods may not be healthy for her. For example, a food labeled *no cholesterol* may still contain plenty of fat. That's why the patient should learn to read and understand food labels. Tell your patient that food labels have become standardized in the past few years and contain all the information she'll need to make wise diet choices. Over time, reading labels should—and will—become an integral part of her grocery shopping routine.

Finally, make sure the patient's family understands the importance of a well-balanced diet as well. Family members may be your most important allies in helping the patient stick to her commitment to follow a heart-healthy diet.

Sodium restriction
Not all cardiac patients need tight sodium restriction, but most receive a prescription for some degree of restriction to help prevent fluid overload, which can lead to dyspnea, edema, and increased anxiety—all of which increase the possibility of myocardial ischemia. Many physicians prescribe a sodium ceiling of 4 to 6 grams daily.

To help your patient reduce her sodium intake, remind her that prepackaged, frozen, and some ethnic foods contain high sodium levels, as do fast foods and convenience meals, such as TV dinners. Fresh foods, including plenty of fruits and vegetables, will provide many nutritional benefits and a reduced sodium level. Also, remind the patient that many nonfood products contain sodium as well, including antacids, toothpaste, even chewing tobacco.

Most people find sodium restriction to be a difficult dietary change because their foods taste bland and thus become unappealing. You can help your patient to maintain her prescribed sodium restriction by suggesting that she try one or more of the many salt substitutes readily available at grocery stores. She also can try various combinations of herbs and seasonings to add flavor to her food. Emphasize, however, that even the use of salt substitutes will require a period of taste adjustment.

As you know, sodium and potassium are crucial, interrelated elements in the regulation of fluids and electrolytes. Consequently, when the patient reduces her sodium intake, her potassium level may fall as well. You'll need to take steps to make sure it doesn't dip too far. For example, you could suggest that she use a salt substitute that contains potassium. You might want to give her a list of potassium-containing foods. Her physician may want to prescribe a potassium sparing diuretic rather than a potassium-wasting one. If necessary, she may need to take an oral potassium supplement.

Your salt-restricted patient also may need to restrict her fluid intake. In keeping with her physician's orders, she'll probably need to consume about 75% of her daily fluids with meals and about 2% with drugs. She can drink the remaining volume at will throughout the day.

Weight reduction
If your patient is overweight (10% to 19% over her ideal weight) or obese (20% or more over her ideal weight), she'll need to adopt a reduced-calorie version of a heart-healthy diet. By achieving a healthy weight, she'll accomplish a number of goals, including the following:
• decreasing her heart's workload
• raising her HDL levels
• reducing hypertension
• controlling her blood glucose levels.

Aiming for a healthy weight
Various institutions have published tables of ideal weights. Clearly, achieving such an ideal confers multisystem benefits. From a cardiac—and a practical—standpoint, however, you may attain better results by having your patient concentrate on reaching a healthy weight rather than struggling in frustration while trying to meet an unnecessary ideal.

She can progress toward that healthy goal by following a sensible diet designed to suit her age, metabolism, general health, disabilities, activity level, and so on. In other words, when it comes to creating dietary plans, a one-size-fits-all mentality rarely yields long-term success.

Planning a suitable diet

To design a diet suitable to your patient's individual needs, start by determining the physician's goals for reducing her risk of CAD-related events. Then begin to construct a collaborative plan of care that involves you, the patient, the physician, a dietitian if necessary, and appropriate members of the patient's family.

Start with a dietary history. Note any foods the patient especially likes or dislikes. Assess her ability and willingness to read food labels. Question her about any oral, dental, or throat problems that could hinder her ability to chew or swallow. Find out if she battles shortness of breath; if so, she may benefit from eating small meals more frequently. Note any physical disabilities, such as arthritis, paralysis, or muscle tremors, that might prevent her from preparing meals or shopping for food.

Inquire about any digestive problems, such as diarrhea or constipation, that may be affected by a change in diet. Determine whether the patient takes any drugs, either prescription or over-the-counter (OTC), that could alter her taste sensation. And investigate the patient's living situation and her ability to cook and store food. If necessary, consider consulting a social worker for a referral to Meals on Wheels.

Talk with your patient and her family about the possible influence of ethnic and cultural factors (including language barriers) on her health beliefs, her food choices, and any special preparations her foods must undergo.

As necessary and if possible, consider referring the patient to a dietitian for a thorough nutritional evaluation. An active member of the health care team, the dietitian's main role involves working with your patient to assess her nutritional status and needs, formulating a nutritional plan, and evaluating her progress. The dietitian also can help with patient teaching in the realm of diet and nutrition.

Changing habits

Typically, a patient who's trying to lose weight will require substantial teaching and support. That's partly because the patient's food choices and her responses to food involve complex psychological reactions and habits that must be ad-

dressed before she can successfully change them. She also must adapt to the uncomfortable physical sensation of hunger. And she must minimize her expectations that weight will drop quickly.

Patients trying to lose weight typically want to do so rapidly. Not only is rapid loss an unrealistic goal, however, it may be a dangerous goal for a cardiac patient. Tell your patient that a weight loss of 1 to 2 pounds weekly is plenty. Over the course of a year, she could lose 50 pounds or more. A slow and steady loss will allow your patient to become accustomed to a new way of eating without creating high levels of frustration based on feelings of hunger and deprivation.

Becoming accustomed to a new way of eating holds the key to long-term success with dietary therapy. That's because it allows the patient to recognize and replace food habits that obstruct her progress. For example, she may have a habit of eating potato chips while watching television. After helping her recognize that habit, you can also help her convert it to a better habit. You might suggest that she eat plain popcorn or fresh fruit instead of potato chips, for instance.

Even as she works at building new habits, the patient's resolve may flag as time takes her further from the frightening event that prompted her to begin her weight-reduction program. If your patient departs from the principles of her diet, try to minimize the likelihood that she'll abandon it altogether. Tell her that virtually everyone lapses from time to time, but that she should try to make any lapses as brief as possible.

When she reaches her healthy weight, urge her to continue counting calories and to maintain a healthy proportion of carbohydrates, proteins, and fats. Emphasize that a diet is a lifelong eating pattern, not a short-term endeavor to drop pounds.

Exercise

Diet and exercise go hand in hand, especially for a patient trying to reverse the effects of CAD. Regular exercise can benefit your patient's cardiovascular status in the following ways:
• raising HDL levels
• decreasing platelet adhesiveness and improving fibrinolytic activity
• improving glucose tolerance
• decreasing blood pressure
• decreasing resting heart rate
• reducing weight.
Regular exercise offers many other multisystem benefits as well. For example, it can help improve

stamina and muscle strength, control the joint pain and swelling associated with arthritis, and increase feelings of well-being.

However, despite the unequivocal benefits of exercise, a patient with compromised coronary vasculature will need to begin and carry out her exercise program with considerable care. In fact, you'll want to recommend that she discuss her plans with her physician before beginning to exercise. Depending on her age, her risk factors, and her level of CAD, the physician may have her undergo an exercise electrocardiogram (ECG) before beginning her exercise program.

Constructing a plan

As with her dietary plan, you'll want to construct your patient's exercise routine with her specific needs and capabilities in mind. If possible, have her aim to achieve the U.S. Surgeon General's recommendation for moderately intense physical activity that lasts 30 minutes or more on most days of the week. Examples of such aerobic exercise include brisk walking, swimming, or biking, all of which increase the patient's heart rate through continuous rhythmic use of large muscle groups in her arms and legs.

However, keep in mind that physical exercise doesn't have to be strenuous to produce health benefits. If CAD or other disabilities prevent your patient from engaging in aerobic exercise, she'll still benefit from low-intensity activity. Even some moderate exercise—such as walking, performing range-of-motion exercises while sitting, wheeling about in a wheelchair, and simple stretching—can increase cardiorespiratory function in the disabled, acutely ill, or elderly cardiac patient.

For a patient with cardiac disease, a physician may prescribe exercises based on her metabolic equivalents (see *Activities and metabolic equivalents*).

Avoiding injury

The most common problems caused by exercise are musculoskeletal. They typically arise when the patient does too much or begins exercising without an adequate warm-up. Of special note for cardiac patients, however, is the distinct possibility of cardiopulmonary complications after overly aggressive exercise. These complications are especially likely if the patient has excess body weight and an otherwise sedentary lifestyle. For this patient, abrupt strenuous exercise could be disastrous.

That's because any physical or psychological stress on the body results in the release of catecholamines, such as epinephrine and norepinephrine. As a result, the heart rate rises, systolic blood pressure rises, and respirations increase. The duration and intensity of exercise affect the level of catecholamine release and the resulting physiologic response. Massive catecholamine release could lead to myocardial ischemia and an MI in a patient whose coronary arteries are already compromised by CAD.

When working with a CAD patient who's about to begin an exercise program, you'll need to provide detailed patient teaching to help keep her safe. You may even want her to start her exercise program in a monitored inpatient or outpatient environment. Provide her with exercise goals and signs of potential problems. Also, instruct her on activity limits to prevent overexercise, cardiac pain, or a worsening of CAD. And teach her to measure her own heart and respiratory rates and to determine the metabolic equivalent levels of her activities.

Hormone therapy

Because estrogen replacement therapy reduces low-density lipoprotein (LDL) levels and raises HDL levels in postmenopausal women, it may decrease the risk of CAD-related events, especially in high-risk patients.

Specifically, the risk of having an MI is reduced by up to half among women who take estrogen replacement therapy. Other positive effects of this therapy include the following:
- arterial vasodilation, which improves blood flow and decreases blood pressure
- improvement in endothelial function, which decreases platelet adhesiveness and atherosclerotic plaque formation
- protection against osteoporosis
- improvement in carbohydrate metabolism, which decreases glucose levels.

A woman taking unopposed estrogen faces an increased risk of endometrial cancer. However, adding progestin, a synthetic form of the female hormone progesterone, reduces this risk and may even protect against endometrial cancer. Progestin can increase LDL levels and decrease HDL levels, but it nevertheless doesn't seem to cancel out estrogen's beneficial effects.

Activities and metabolic equivalents

You can determine a patient's daily activity level by categorizing each activity using metabolic equivalents of her tasks. Keep in mind, however, that a patient's general fitness level can alter metabolic equivalent levels, as can fatigue, excitement, or emotional stress.

Metabolic equivalents	Home activities	Occupational activities	Exercise or sports activities
1	• Resting in bed • Sitting • Sewing • Watching television	• None	• None
1–2	• Dressing • Brushing teeth • Making bed • Driving a car	• Typing (electric typewriter or computer)	• Walking 1 mph (1.6 km/hr) on level ground
2–3	• Bathing in tub • Cooking • Waxing floor • Riding a lawn mower	• Driving a small truck • Using hand tools • Typing (manual typewriter)	• Walking 2 mph (3.2 km/hr) on level ground • Fishing • Golfing (with a riding cart)
3–4	• Doing general housework • Doing light gardening • Pushing a light power mower • Having sexual intercourse	• Working on an assembly line • Driving a large truck • Plastering	• Walking 3 mph (4.8 km/hr) • Bicycling 6 mph (9.7 km/hr) • Golfing (pulling a hand cart) • Fly-fishing
4–5	• Doing heavy housework • Doing heavy gardening • Doing home repairs, including painting and light carpentry	• Painting • Doing masonry work • Paperhanging	• Performing calisthenics • Playing table tennis • Golfing (carrying a bag) • Playing tennis (doubles) • Swimming slowly
5–6	• Sawing soft wood • Digging in a garden • Shoveling light loads	• Using heavy tools • Lifting 50 lb	• Walking 4 mph (6.4 km/hr) • Bicycling 10 mph (16.1 km/hr) • Skating • Fishing with waders • Hiking
6–7	• Shoveling snow • Splitting wood • Mowing lawn with a hand mower	• Shoveling 10 lb for 10 min	• Walking or jogging 5 mph (8 km/hr) • Bicycling 11 mph (17.7 km/hr) • Playing tennis (singles) • Waterskiing
7–8	• Sawing hard wood	• Digging ditches • Lifting 80 lb • Moving heavy furniture	• Playing paddleball • Swimming (backstroke) • Playing basketball
8–9		• Lifting 100 lb	• Running 5 mph (8 km/hr) • Bicycling 13 mph (20.9 km/hr) • Swimming (breast stroke) • Cross-country skiing
10 or more		• Shoveling 16 lb for 10 min	• Running 6 mph (9.7 km/hr) • Playing handball (competitive) • Performing gymnastics

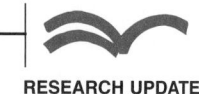

RESEARCH UPDATE

Does anger raise the risk of a myocardial infarction?

After interviewing more than 1,600 patients within days after they'd had myocardial infarctions (MIs), researchers discovered that many had been intensely angry a few hours before the event. Specifically, the researchers determined that fierce anger more than doubled the risk of having an MI during the subsequent 2-hour time span. They suspect that strong anger somehow precipitates thrombus formation and resulting coronary artery occlusion.

The good news? Their data show that regular aspirin use reduced by half the increased risk of an MI created by anger.

Stress reduction

Nontraditional, or so-called alternative, therapies may play a role in the treatment of CAD-related disorders as well. Many of these therapies aim to reduce stress; they include meditation, distraction, use of coping skills, progressive relaxation, biofeedback, and various forms of massage. While many of these techniques have not undergone rigorous scientific study, common sense suggests that benefits accrue to CAD patients who experience relaxation and stress reduction in the same way that benefits accrue to all patients.

Keep in mind that the daily stresses of modern society affect different people in different ways. For most people, however, continuous or overwhelming stress raises the risk of angina and having an MI. This stress may involve concerns about work, money, health, love, death, and any other aspect of life that raises the patient's anxiety level. Of all the strong emotions felt by people under stress and those with aggressive, type A personalities, strong anger is most closely tied to an increased risk of CAD-related symptoms (see *Does anger raise the risk of a myocardial infarction?*). Engaging various methods of stress reduction just might help ease your patient's anger and anxiety.

When counseling patients about alternative or unproven therapies, emphasize the universal benefits of those listed here. Also, emphasize that products or remedies that sound too good to be true probably are.

Using meditation

A form of quiet concentration that can be used for stress reduction, meditation has been practiced since ancient times by people of various religions. Meditation decreases mental stress and lowers the heart rate. It also reduces levels of cortisol, a hormone released in response to stress.

Advise your patient about resources that can help her understand the purpose and procedures involved in meditation. Explain that meditation involves an intentional emptying of stress and that many of its practices can be self-taught. It can be performed anywhere and has sometimes been described as a spiritual experience. Refer your patient to self-help books, videos, and audiotapes available at local bookstores and libraries.

Using distraction

Like meditation, distraction can reduce the effects of pain, anxiety, or other types of stress by changing the focus of awareness from one subject to another. Distraction techniques include imagery, focusing, and centering.

Imagery: This technique involves bringing positive experiences or pleasant scenes into focus to replace negative thoughts.

Focusing: In this technique, the patient uses another activity or object—such as watching television, reading, or playing cards—to redirect physical pain and stressful thoughts.

Centering: This ancient skill focuses awareness into a single point that gathers energy, thus helping the patient to channel that energy more easily into another chosen activity.

Explore these and other distraction techniques with your patient, and then help her select and learn to use the one that appeals to her most. Provide the necessary environment for your patient to practice, and then follow up with her. Ask her how she felt before, during, and after the activity. Help her to evaluate the experience and modify her approach as needed. Reinforce her successes, and remind her that these techniques are all skills that improve with practice.

Building coping skills

In general, people deal with stress using some combination of coping skills and defense mechanisms. Coping skills are positive, healthy methods for dealing with stress. Defense mechanisms are unhealthy methods that don't address the real reasons behind the stress. Examples of defense mechanisms include denial, displacement, and conversion.

Denial allows your patient to cope by minimizing or ignoring a problem. Common just after a cardiac diagnosis, denial is the mind's unconscious refusal to accept the anxiety-causing circumstances. Denial is considered a normal reaction if it lasts for a reasonable period of time. It becomes maladaptive, even lethal, if the patient refuses to seek needed treatment or medical advice.

Displacement allows the patient to cope with stress by unconsciously shifting emotions to other objects or things. For example, your patient may believe that her MI resulted from a fight with her husband rather than from her refusal to quit smoking, improve her diet, and get more exercise.

Conversion is an unconscious coping mechanism that shifts the stress into physical signs and symptoms that have no physical basis. For example, the patient may develop a nervous twitch, paralysis, or dyspnea for no identifiable reason.

Some people possess powerful, healthy coping skills; others don't or must work to understand and use healthy coping skills instead of these unhealthy, negative mechanisms. You can help your patient build her coping skills by helping her to identify the strategies she uses to cope with stress. Then help her to determine which of these strategies are helpful and which are hurtful, and encourage her to practice the helpful strategies whenever she encounters a stressful situation. Refer her for professional counseling, if necessary, to help her address her use of defense mechanisms.

Performing progressive relaxation

Your patient can use progressive relaxation to purposefully relax her entire body. To perform it, have her begin by sitting or lying in a comfortable position in an area that promotes relaxation—a darkened room, for example. Then have her concentrate on relaxing the muscles of her scalp and forehead, followed by the muscles of her face, her neck, her shoulders, and so on in a systemic, step-by-step fashion until she reaches the soles of her feet. She may find it helpful to first contract each set of muscles before relaxing it.

If she prefers, the patient can use audiotapes to guide her through this process of relaxation. Typically, such tapes provide music and a soft monotone script that systematically talks her through a series of contraction-relaxation activities that cover her entire body.

Although the technique of progressive relaxation may not produce complete relaxation every time, it does provide a simple, nondrug method for managing stress and encouraging sleep. Emphasize to your patient that progressive relaxation is a skill; the more she practices, the more skilled she'll become.

Using biofeedback

In conjunction with other relaxation methods, biofeedback (a behavior-modification method) reduces a variety of symptoms caused by psychological and physiologic disorders. In biofeedback, a patient observes monitoring devices while willfully attempting to control her blood pressure, heart rate, and other physiologic responses.

Using massage therapy

Shiatsu, Swedish massage, reflexology, and effleurage are forms of massage therapy that can be used as nondrug relaxation techniques.

Shiatsu is a form of physical therapy that involves using finger pressure on acupuncture points.

In Swedish massage, the practitioner concentrates on deep manipulation of the patient's muscle groups.

Based on the principle that certain points or zones correspond to certain glands or organs, reflexology involves massaging those points to reduce pain and stress. Commonly, it's performed on the patient's feet.

Effleurage is the only form of massage that doesn't exert pressure. Instead, it employs a light touch that slides over the skin. The practitioner uses fingertips to create rhythmic circles or lines in a fashion similar to lightly petting a cat or dog.

Lipid level reduction

If your patient has elevated LDL or triglyceride levels, she may require lipid-lowering drug therapy as well as lifestyle modifications. Specifically, she may need drug therapy if she has one or more of the following:

- an LDL level above 160 mg/dl with more than two risk factors for CAD
- an LDL level above 190 mg/dl, regardless of risk factors
- a triglyceride level between 400 and 1,000 mg/dl if her LDL level is elevated and HDL level is reduced
- a triglyceride level above 1,000 mg/dl.

For an LDL level below 160 mg/dl, the patient may start with dietary changes alone. The Step I diet for reducing the LDL level mirrors the standard heart-healthy diet by limiting the intake of saturated fats to less than 10% of total calories, total fat to less than 30% of calories, and cholesterol to less than 300 mg daily. If this diet fails to reduce the patient's LDL level, her physician may prescribe a Step II diet. It places more stringent limits on fat intake: Saturated fats should constitute less than 7% of her total calories, and she should consume less than 200 mg of cholesterol daily.

If after 6 months on the Step I diet and 6 months on the Step II diet, the patient still has abnormal LDL levels, drug therapy may begin with a cholesterol synthesis inhibitor, a bile acid–binding resin, nicotinic acid, a fibric acid derivative, or probucol (see *Reviewing antilipemic drugs*).

These antilipemic drugs prevent the formation of, slow the progression of, and cause the regression of atherosclerotic lesions. To varying degrees, they do so by altering total cholesterol, triglyceride, and lipoprotein levels. Adverse reactions to these drugs commonly limit a patient's compliance and may influence the selection of one drug over another.

If your patient's physician prescribes an antilipemic drug for her, make sure you reiterate the continued need for faithful adherence to her prescribed diet. Impress upon her that the drug will not cure her CAD. Indeed, its effectiveness may depend on her compliance with both her drug therapy and her dietary plan. Without constant attention, her serum lipid levels will return to their pretreatment levels.

Cholesterol synthesis inhibitors

Commonly known as statins, cholesterol synthesis inhibitors are most appropriate for patients with elevations in total cholesterol, triglyceride, LDL, and very-low-density lipoprotein (VLDL) levels. All of the drugs in this class decrease cholesterol production by inhibiting HMG-CoA reduc-

tase, an enzyme essential to cholesterol synthesis. A decrease in cholesterol leads to a decreased risk of an MI and death.

Therapy with a cholesterol synthesis inhibitor can result in a 25% to 60% increase in LDL clearance. Inhibited cholesterol synthesis causes LDL and VLDL levels to decrease. Triglyceride levels can decrease by 10% to 37%. Plus, cholesterol synthesis inhibitors may increase HDL levels by up to 14%. You'll observe an initial response to the therapy about 2 weeks after it begins; most patients achieve their maximum response in about 4 to 6 weeks.

Your patient will take her cholesterol synthesis inhibitor once or twice daily. If she has once-daily dosing, tell her that taking the drug at bedtime will yield the best results because more cholesterol is synthesized at night. Most cholesterol synthesis inhibitors can be taken without regard to meals. Lovastatin, the exception, should be taken with food to increase its effectiveness.

As with all antilipemics, cholesterol synthesis inhibitors cause considerable gastrointestinal (GI) effects for many patients, including gas, abdominal pain, diarrhea, constipation, nausea, and upset stomach. Simvastatin, atorvastatin, and cerivastatin cause fewer such problems than others in this class.

About 1 patient in 100 may show elevated liver enzyme function tests within 6 weeks after starting therapy, but this finding rarely requires discontinuation of the drug. An elevation that exceeds three times the normal level indicates toxicity and typically warrants stopping the drug.

Cholesterol synthesis inhibitors should be used with caution in patients who have liver dysfunction and in alcoholics because of the possible effects on their liver enzymes. Some patients may need blood testing every 4 to 6 weeks for the first 15 months of therapy to monitor elevations in their liver enzymes.

Urge any woman taking a cholesterol synthesis inhibitor to notify her physician right away if she thinks she could be pregnant. These drugs may cause birth defects and should never be used during pregnancy. Also, urge patients to report muscle cramps and weakness to their physician and to have an annual vision examination to detect changes in visual acuity.

Bile acid–binding resins

These drugs work by binding with bile acid, the precursor of cholesterol, in the intestine and ex-

Reviewing antilipemic drugs

Drug	Dose	Adverse effects
Cholesterol synthesis inhibitors		
fluvastatin	20–40 mg once daily	• gas, abdominal pain, diarrhea, constipation, nausea
lovastatin	20–80 mg once daily or divided into two doses	• elevated liver enzyme and creatine kinase levels
pravastatin	10–40 mg once daily	• myalgia, muscle cramps • changes in visual acuity
simvastatin	5–40 mg once daily	• birth defects
atorvastatin	10–80 mg once daily	
cerivastatin	0.3 mg once daily or 0.2 mg once daily in patients with moderate to severe renal impairment	
Bile acid–binding resins		
cholestyramine tablets	8–24 g once daily or divided into two doses	• constipation, gas, bloating, diarrhea
cholestyramine powder	16–24 g once daily	
cholestyramine chewable bar	initial dosage: 4 g (one bar) once daily; maintenance dosage: 8–16 g divided into two doses	
colestipol tablets	2–16 g once daily or divided into two doses	
colestipol granules	20–25 g once daily or divided into two doses	
Fibric acid derivatives		
gemfibrozil capsules	600 mg twice daily	• with long-term use, liver disease, gallbladder disease, risk of liver cancer
gemfibrozil tablets	600 mg twice daily	• dyspepsia, abdominal pain, diarrhea, nausea, vomiting, constipation, appendicitis, cholecystitis
clofibrate	500–1,000 mg twice daily	• skin rash • fatigue, dizziness, headache
Other antilipemics		
nicotinic acid	1–2 g three times daily	• at start of therapy, light-headedness, dizziness • within 30 minutes of ingestion, flushing, warmth in face and upper body, itching, burning or tingling, headache • nausea, vomiting, diarrhea, aggravation of gastric ulcers, abdominal pain
probucol tablets	500 mg twice daily	• diarrhea, gas, bloating, nausea, abdominal pain, vomiting • arrhythmias

creting the resulting compound in feces. As a result, the liver must synthesize new bile acid from cholesterol, thereby reducing LDL levels. These actions render this class of drugs most effective in patients with hypercholesterolemia secondary to increased LDL levels, rather than in patients with elevated VLDL or triglyceride levels.

Therapy with cholestyramine or colestipol, the two bile acid–binding resins, can reduce serum LDL levels by 20% within the first 4 to 7 days. They reach their maximum effect in 2 to 4 weeks. However, the patient's cholesterol levels typically return to pretreatment levels after she stops taking the drug.

Cholestyramine may increase or have no effect on triglyceride, VLDL, and HDL levels. Colestipol may increase or have no effect on triglyceride and HDL levels, but it usually increases VLDL levels.

These resins are taken 2 to 4 times daily, with meals and at bedtime. If your patient receives a prescription for a powdered form, instruct her to mix the powder with at least 4 ounces of fluid or pulpy fruit (such as applesauce or crushed pineapple) before taking it. Warn her to avoid accidentally inhaling or choking on the powder as she's mixing the drug. Cholestyramine is also available as a chewable bar.

Because these drugs are binding resins, they may interfere with absorption of other drugs, such as fat-soluble vitamins, folic acid, anticoagulants, digoxin, thiazide diuretics, penicillins, beta-blockers, tetracyclines, and thyroid hormones. Instruct your patient to take all other drugs at least 1 hour before or 4 to 6 hours after taking a bile acid–binding resin.

As with cholesterol synthesis inhibitors, the most common adverse effects of the bile acid–binding resins involve the GI tract. This is especially true with high doses and in patients over age 60. About 1 patient in 5 becomes constipated; to help your patient avoid this effect, recommend using stool softeners, drinking plenty of liquids, getting regular cardiovascular exercise, and taking doses either before meals or with bran cereal or another source of soluble dietary fiber. Some adverse effects may resolve with continued therapy. Bile acid–binding resins are contraindicated in patients with biliary obstruction.

Nicotinic acid

Also known as niacin (a B-complex vitamin), nicotinic acid reduces cholesterol, triglyceride,

LDL, and VLDL levels while increasing HDL levels. It's effective for all types of hyperlipidemias.

Nicotinic acid works by inhibiting secretion of VLDLs by the liver, an action that directly decreases LDL production and triglyceride levels. The decrease in LDL production results in a decrease in total serum cholesterol. Within the first 4 days of therapy, the patient's triglyceride and VLDL levels will most likely drop 20% to 40%. It takes 5 to 7 days for LDL levels to drop, and 3 to 5 weeks to achieve the maximum response. A patient's HDL levels may rise by 20%.

Because most patients have transient lightheadedness and dizziness for the first week or two of therapy, instruct your patient to stand slowly during that time to avoid fainting. Nicotinic acid can also cause a reaction called a niacin flush (see *Recognizing a niacin flush*).

Bothersome GI effects may include nausea, vomiting, diarrhea, aggravation of gastric ulcers, and abdominal pain. These reactions may worsen if the patient takes nicotinic acid with hot drinks or alcoholic beverages. They may abate somewhat if she takes it with food, milk, or antacids. Extremely high doses (more than 8 g/day) can induce hyperglycemia in both diabetic and nondiabetic patients.

Nicotinic acid is available both by prescription and OTC. However, encourage your patient to talk with her physician about the proper dosage before she buys any OTC product. Most patients take nicotinic acid three times daily.

If possible, discourage your patient from taking a sustained-release form of nicotinic acid. Only rarely will it decrease the incidence of adverse reactions, and it may significantly increase the patient's risk of hepatotoxicity. If your patient uses a sustained-release form, warn her not to crush the tablets or capsules. If she wishes, she can mix the capsule beads with soft foods, but she shouldn't chew them. Extended-release niacin may be less hepatotoxic and produce less severe and frequent flushing episodes than typical sustained-release forms.

Bear in mind that bile acid-binding resins, cholesterol synthesis inhibitors, and nicotinic acid may be prescribed in dual or triple combinations to help maximize their effect. Because each drug has a slightly different effect on cholesterol, triglycerides, and lipoproteins, combination therapy may create beneficial synergistic effects. Many physicians reserve these combination therapies for patients with hyperlipidemias that haven't responded to the typical combination of diet, exercise, and maximum dosages of single-drug therapy.

Fibric acid derivatives
Largely because of their dangerous adverse effects, drug interactions, and lack of advantages over other antilipemics, the fibric acid derivatives typically are not used as first-line therapy. In fact, they're usually reserved for patients whose hypertriglyceridemia hasn't responded to diet, exercise, and maximum dosages of other drugs. Fibric acid derivatives are ineffective against hypercholesterolemia.

Gemfibrozil and clofibrate both work by activating lipoprotein lipase, an enzyme responsible for catabolism and increased clearance of VLDL. A reduction in VLDLs then leads to a reduction in triglycerides. Gemfibrozil also inhibits the secretion of VLDLs by the liver. Clofibrate may increase HDL levels slightly; gemfibrozil may raise them by 10% to 20% in some patients. Clofibrate can reduce triglyceride levels by 30% to 40%; gemfibrozil can reduce them by 50% to 60%.

Unfortunately, however, long-term therapy at maximum doses may lead to liver disease, gallbladder disease, and an increased risk of cancer. These drugs also commonly cause GI reactions, including dyspepsia, abdominal pain, diarrhea, nausea and vomiting, constipation, and acute appendicitis. Combination therapy with gemfibrozil and lovastatin may destroy muscle tissues and cause acute renal failure; don't give these two drugs in combination.

Because gemfibrozil also may enhance the effects of oral anticoagulants, monitor your patient's prothrombin time (PT) and adjust her anticoagulant dosages as needed at the start of therapy.

Probucol
Also reserved for patients who haven't responded to other therapies, probucol is prescribed for those with elevated cholesterol and LDL levels. It has little or no effect on triglycerides and causes a decrease in HDL levels. The drug has a very slow onset, requiring 1 to 3 months of therapy before reaching its maximum cholesterol-lowering effects. It may lower total cholesterol and LDL levels by 10% to 15%. Instruct your patient to take it in two divided doses with morning and evening meals because food increases its effectiveness.

On the plus side, probucol has few adverse ef-

Recognizing a niacin flush

Niacin, also known as vitamin B_3, contributes to the smooth functioning of more than 50 of the body's vital processes and fights hyperlipidemia. Within about 30 minutes after taking niacin, however, your patient may develop a harmless but mildly uncomfortable reaction called a niacin flush.

She'll most likely describe a prickling or tingling sensation in her face and upper body, possibly accompanied by a patchy rash and a headache. The sensations typically fade within 30 to 60 minutes.

You may be able to minimize the niacin flush by recommending that your patient take 325 mg of buffered aspirin 30 minutes before each dose of niacin. You also can try gradually increasing the niacin dosage so that the patient takes just enough to achieve an antilipemic effect.

---

fects. About 1 patient in 10 develops diarrhea, gas, bloating, nausea, abdominal pain, indigestion, or vomiting—reactions that seldom require a discontinuation of therapy. Because probucol occasionally causes cardiac arrhythmias and a prolonged QT interval, your patient probably will need a baseline and twice-yearly ECGs.

Hypertension control

Because chronic increases in blood pressure can damage the intimal layer of arteries and encourage formation of arterial plaques, hypertension control forms another important facet of CAD treatment. Without doubt, reducing your patient's blood pressure will reduce her risk of CAD-related complications.

Hypertension control involves many of the lifestyle alterations already discussed. For example:
• The patient should stop smoking. A hypertensive person who continues to smoke raises her risk of MI to a level three to five times higher than a hypertensive person who doesn't smoke.
• She should moderate her alcohol intake. People who consume more than 2 ounces of alcohol each day significantly increase their risk of hypertension.

- She should lose weight, if necessary, and exercise regularly. By itself, being overweight can lead to hypertension.
- She may need to follow a sodium-restricted diet. Especially in patients with isolated systolic hypertension, limiting sodium intake may help lower blood pressure.

If your patient's hypertension hasn't responded after 3 to 6 months of lifestyle adjustments, her physician may prescribe drugs to help accomplish the goal. They may include diuretics, beta-adrenergic blockers, vasodilators, angiotensin-converting enzyme (ACE) inhibitors, or calcium channel blockers, based on your patient's individual situation.

For many patients with CAD, combining faithful adherence to lifestyle adjustments and, if necessary, the use of antilipemic or antihypertensive drugs can prevent this disorder from progressing to its next and more symptomatic stage, a stage that commonly requires invasive testing and interventions.

Stable angina

In a general sense, the treatment of angina involves three related goals:
- to identify and respond to anginal attacks rapidly and effectively
- to establish a prophylactic drug regimen that minimizes the likelihood of recurrent attacks
- to widen or circumvent blocked arteries, if necessary, to restore adequate blood flow to the myocardium.

Accomplishing all these goals may require a combination of treatment approaches that includes drugs and procedures for easing acute episodes, maintenance drugs, invasive procedures, patient and family teaching, and possibly extensive rehabilitation and follow-up care. If your patient's angina results from an identifiable medical condition, such as arrhythmia, hypoxia, anemia, acute blood loss, dehydration, or shock, you'll need to administer treatment for that condition as well.

Initial response

If a patient previously undiagnosed with angina develops what you believe to be an acute anginal attack, you'll need to respond promptly to confirm the condition, restore blood flow to the ischemic myocardium, reduce the cardiac workload, stabilize the patient's vital signs, prevent life-threatening arrhythmias, and ease the patient's symptoms (see *Caring for a patient with angina,* pages 72 and 73).

History
Naturally, you'll want to obtain pertinent medical and family history information as soon as possible and in as much detail as possible to corroborate your suspicion of angina. Such information includes the patient's risk factors for CAD, her lifestyle characteristics, her ability to cope with stress, her family history, previous treatments and surgeries, and any other data that could shed light on her current situation.

However, you'll need to balance the importance of obtaining appropriate information with the importance of restoring myocardial perfusion. Use your powers of observation and judgment to determine how long and in what detail you should question the patient, based on her signs and symptoms, her level of discomfort, and her vital signs. Obtain only enough information to justify treating acute angina; you can gather the rest later, after her condition has been stabilized.

Signs and symptoms
Have the patient lie in bed while you assess her blood pressure, heart rate, respirations, and pattern of signs and symptoms. If she's having an anginal attack, her blood pressure will be significantly elevated. Her heart rate and respirations also may increase slightly from the discomfort and anxiety.

Ask her to describe what she's feeling in her own words. If she doesn't give you enough information, ask a few pertinent questions to pinpoint the location of her discomfort. Ask how it started, what it feels like, and whether it radiates to another location. Ask her to rate her level of pain on a scale of 0 to 10, and then have her continue to rate it as you administer drugs and other treatments. Remember that some patients don't experience the substernal pain and pressure typical of most anginal attacks. She may have pain in her jaw, her shoulder, or her arm, for instance. If she complains of epigastric discomfort but her vital signs are normal, consider the possibility that she isn't having an anginal attack at all.

Also, quickly check for signs and symptoms associated with angina, such as diaphoresis, a cough, fatigue, palpitations, nausea, or dyspnea. If the patient's constellation of signs and symptoms convinces you that she's having an anginal attack, notify her physician right away.

Oxygen

If you have an order for nasal oxygen to be given as needed, begin administering it at 2 to 4 L/minute, as prescribed or according to your unit's protocol. If the patient has pulmonary disease, set a lower flow rate, perhaps 1 to 1.5 L/minute, until you can confirm the rate preferred by the patient's physician. Some facility policies specify that you titrate the flow rate based on the patient's oxygen saturation levels, as measured by pulse oximetry. In any case, do not administer oxygen without an order to do so.

Nitroglycerin

The cornerstone of treatment for acute angina, nitroglycerin produces rapid and pronounced vasodilation of the coronary arteries, improving blood supply to the myocardium. The drug also acts as a systemic vasodilator, reducing preload by relaxing the venous system and, consequently, reducing the pressure and amount of blood returning to the heart. To a lesser extent, it reduces afterload as well. Overall, it acts to reduce myocardial workload and oxygen demand while providing increased coronary blood flow, a combination that typically eases the symptoms of angina within about 15 minutes.

Nitroglycerin is available in many forms. Most likely, the patient will already have taken sublingual nitroglycerin before arriving at the hospital. If not, you may need to administer it sublingually after she arrives. If the first dose doesn't ease her chest pain, give another dose after 5 minutes has passed and, if necessary, a third dose after 5 more minutes (see *Nitroglycerin administration tips,* page 74). Before and after administering each dose, watch the patient's blood pressure closely because it may drop sharply from the drug's systemic effects. If it does, you may need to hold subsequent doses, as ordered.

Nitroglycerin commonly causes headache and facial flushing; stay alert for these reactions. As ordered, give acetaminophen to relieve the headache.

Morphine

If sublingual nitroglycerin doesn't relieve your patient's angina, you'll probably need to switch to I.V. nitroglycerin along with morphine. Besides being a narcotic pain reliever, morphine reduces anxiety and venous return to the heart, thereby reducing the heart's workload. Usually, you'll give 2 to 4 mg of morphine by I.V. push as often as every 20 minutes until the patient's discomfort subsides.

Like nitroglycerin, morphine causes hypotension; however, giving small amounts at frequent intervals should create less hypotension than nitroglycerin does. Because morphine tends to decrease blood pressure and respiratory rate, you'll need to monitor the patient's vital signs often.

If rest, oxygen, nitroglycerin, and morphine fail to resolve your patient's signs and symptoms, she most likely is having an MI. At this point, more potent treatment is necessary, and you'll need to transfer the patient to an intensive care or coronary care unit, where she has access to continuous telemetry monitoring.

If, on the other hand, the anginal attack does subside, you'll need to institute and maintain a regimen of prophylactic drugs designed to minimize the chance of additional attacks. As ordered, you'll also obtain serial ECGs and serial tests of the patient's cardiac enzymes and isoenzymes. The patient also may undergo diagnostic tests, to determine the cause of her angina and any needed interventions.

Make sure to document as many details of the patient's anginal attack as possible, including the signs you observe, the symptoms she reports, her vital signs, and any drugs or other treatments you administer.

Prophylactic drugs

A patient with compromised coronary arteries and a tendency to develop angina needs prophylactic drug therapy to minimize the chance of recurrent angina or the development of an MI. Drugs used for that purpose include beta-blockers, calcium channel blockers, and nitrates. They improve coronary artery perfusion, keep the pa-

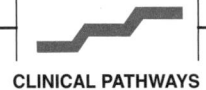

CLINICAL PATHWAYS

Caring for a patient with angina

	History and physical examination	Diagnostic tests	Discharge planning	
Day 1	• activities that precipitated chest pain • characteristics of chest pain • patient's pain rating (scale of 0 to 10) • other signs and symptoms, such as epigastric burning, back pain, nausea, dyspnea • patient's and family's knowledge of disorder • risk factors for CAD • assessment of intake and output every 8 hours • assessment of analgesic effectiveness • assessment of activity tolerance every shift	• 12-lead electrocardiogram (ECG) • blood screening, including complete blood count, electrolyte levels, thyroid function test, lipid profile, and coagulation studies • cardiac enzyme, isoenzyme, and protein levels • chest X-ray	• Arrange a dietary consultation. • Arrange a cardiac rehabilitation consultation. • Arrange a social services consultation. • Arrange a home care consultation.	
Day 2	• characteristics of chest pain • patient's pain rating (scale of 0 to 10) • other signs and symptoms, such as epigastric burning, back pain, nausea, dyspnea • assessment of intake and output every 8 hours • assessment of analgesic effectiveness • assessment of activity tolerance every shift	• 12-lead ECG • cardiac enzyme, isoenzyme, and protein levels • stress ECG test (exercise or pharmacologic) • nuclear imaging with radioisotope • echocardiogram • cardiac catheterization • ambulatory ECG monitoring	• Arrange for ambulatory ECG monitoring.	

tient's heart rate and blood pressure under control, and reduce myocardial energy expenditure. Most patients take a beta-blocker, calcium channel blocker, or both for long-term treatment of stable angina. The patient may need an anticoagulant as well, to reduce the risk of thrombotic complications.

Beta-blockers
Beta-blockers can be used in combination with calcium channel blockers, nitrates, or both in the prophylactic management of chronic stable angina.

The patients who benefit most from beta-blockers include those whose major problem is a myocardial oxygen demand that exceeds supply. Patients with exercise-induced angina are primary candidates for beta-blocker therapy.

How beta-blockers work
As you may recall, the body contains two main subgroups of adrenergic receptors: alpha and beta. Both are stimulated by neurotransmitters, primarily norepinephrine. Stimulation of small numbers of alpha receptors in the heart and smooth muscle of arterioles causes increased myocardial contractility and vasoconstriction.

Drugs	Interventions	Patient teaching
• antianginal drugs, such as sublingual nitroglycerin up to three doses 5 minutes apart • if pain doesn't subside, 2–4 mg of morphine by I.V. push every 20 minutes • antianxiety drugs, as prescribed • stool softener and laxative, as prescribed	• vital signs every 15 minutes until pain subsides; then every 2 to 4 hours • oxygen at 2–4 L/min via nasal cannula • cardiac monitoring or telemetry • pulse oximetry continuously during angina, then every 4 hours • breath sounds every 4 hours • bed rest with bathroom privileges • low-cholesterol, low-fat, sodium-restricted diet • ECG, as ordered, with chest pain	• Instruct patient to report chest pain and related symptoms immediately. • Teach use of pain scale. • Review drug regimen. • Instruct patient to avoid straining.
• prophylactic drugs, such as beta-blocker, calcium channel blocker, nitrate, anticoagulant • stool softener and laxative, as prescribed • sublingual nitroglycerin to stop acute anginal attack	• vital signs every 15 minutes until pain subsides, then every 2 to 4 hours • oxygen as necessary • direct-current cardiac monitor or telemetry • pulse oximetry reading every 4 hours • breath sounds every shift • low-cholesterol, low-fat, sodium-restricted diet • ECG, as ordered, with chest pain	• Explain underlying mechanism of disorder. • Teach lifestyle modifications, such as smoking cessation and exercise. • Outline treatment options. • Review correct use of drugs and any food or drug interactions. • Expain use and storage of nitroglycerin. • List signs and symptoms to report to physician. • Emphasize importance of seeking emergency help for chest pain that's unrelieved by nitroglycerin and rest. • Review importance of returning for follow-up medical appointments.

Although no one knows exactly what role these receptors play in regulating coronary blood flow, they may lead to vasoconstriction that complicates CAD, angina, and coronary artery spasm.

Beta$_1$ receptors are located in the heart. Stimulating them causes an increase in heart rate, contractility, and conduction velocity. Beta$_2$ receptors are located in arterioles, primarily in the skeletal muscles and lungs. Stimulating them causes arterial dilation and increased blood flow in skeletal muscles.

Beta-blockers inhibit the stimulation of both beta$_1$ and beta$_2$ receptors. Thus, these drugs reduce myocardial oxygen demand by decreasing heart rate, electrical impulse conduction, and contractility. They may also indirectly increase oxygen supply because the decreased heart rate results in a prolonged filling time, which enhances coronary artery perfusion.

However, beta-blockers typically don't enhance the heart's oxygen supply, which limits their usefulness in patients with an oxygen supply compromised by atherosclerosis. Instead, they're most effective for patients with stable, exercise-induced angina or angina provoked by an increase in heart rate. Beta-blockers shouldn't be used for

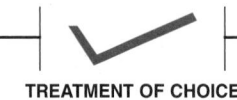

Nitroglycerin administration tips

After more than 100 years, nitroglycerin is still considered the first-line treatment for anginal attacks among patients with chronic stable angina. As you know, the drug is available in many forms. To manage an attack, most patients use either buccal tablets, sublingual tablets, or translingual spray. For prophylaxis and long-term control, most use ointment, transdermal patches, translingual spray, transmucosal tablets, or sustained-release tablets. Usually, you'll administer the I.V. form only in a hospital setting with cardiac and hemodynamic monitoring in use.

Sublingual tablets
Tell your patient to place a tablet under her tongue when chest pain begins. If the pain doesn't subside, she can place another tablet under her tongue 5 minutes after the first and, if necessary, a third tablet 5 minutes after the second. If the pain doesn't subside 5 minutes after she takes the third tablet, the patient needs emergency attention and more powerful drugs.

Explain that sublingual tablets should sting slightly when first placed under the tongue. If they don't sting, the patient should assume they're not working and discard them.

Buccal tablets
Explain the same procedure as for sublingual tablets, but have the patient place buccal tablets between her gum line and lip.

Sustained-release tablets
Have the patient swallow a whole tablet with 8 ounces of water on an empty stomach. Warn her not to crush or chew the tablet.

Translingual spray
Advise the patient to spray once or twice under her tongue when chest pain begins. Warn her not to inhale or swallow the spray and not to shake the canister before use. As needed, she can repeat the sprays every 5 minutes for a total

of three doses. If her chest pain persists, she should obtain emergency care.

Topical ointment
Instruct your patient to clean old ointment thoroughly from her skin. Then have her measure the correct amount of fresh ointment using the applicator papers packaged with the drug. Remind her that 1 inch of ointment contains 15 mg of the drug.

After she measures the correct amount, she should use the applicator to spread the ointment on an area of her chest or back. Stress that she should avoid rubbing or massaging the drug into the skin. Also, advise her to rotate application sites and avoid placing fresh ointment in an area just used. Warn her not to use her fingers to apply the ointment because excess drug will be absorbed through her skin. Tell men to avoid placing the drug on hairy areas. Instruct the patient to remove the ointment after 12 to 14 hours to establish a nitrate-free period that will prevent her from developing a tolerance to the drug.

Transdermal patch
Explain that she should apply a fresh patch to a site on her upper arm or body at the same time each day. The site should be clean, dry, not hairy, and free from cuts, scars, and irritation. Urge her to remove the patch after 12 to 14 hours to establish a nitrate-free period that will prevent her from developing a tolerance for the drug. Rotate application sites to avoid skin irritation.

I.V. injection
Administer I.V. nitroglycerin from a glass bottle through tubing not made of polyvinyl. Because the drug binds with polyvinyl, using this type of tubing reduces the amount of drug delivered to the patient. Remember that nitroglycerin isn't compatible with any other I.V. drug, either in a syringe or in solution. Titrate the infusion to achieve the desired response.

---

patients with vasospastic angina because they may worsen the condition by leaving stimulation of coronary alpha receptors unopposed.

Selecting a beta-blocker
When choosing a beta-blocker for a patient with stable angina, a physician considers receptor se-

Reviewing beta-blockers

Drug	Lipid solubility	Usual dose for angina
Cardioselective drugs		
acebutolol	low	• 100–600 mg twice daily
atenolol	low	• initially 25 mg once daily; in elderly patient, 12.5–25 mg • maximum 200 mg once daily • in renal dysfunction with creatinine clearance of 15–35 ml/min, 50 mg once daily • with creatinine clearance under 15 ml/min, 25 mg once daily
bisoprolol	low	• 2.5–20 mg once daily • in renal dysfunction with creatinine clearance under 40 ml/min, start with 2.5 mg and titrate to desired response
metoprolol	moderate	• 25–200 mg twice daily; in elderly patient, 6.25–12.5 mg • maximum 400 mg once daily
Nonselective drugs		
carteolol	low	• 2.5–10 mg once daily • in renal dysfunction with creatinine clearance above 60 ml/min, give every 24 hr • with creatinine clearance of 20–60 ml/min, give every 48 hr • with creatinine clearance under 20 ml/min, give every 72 hr
labetalol	moderate	• 200–400 mg twice daily; in elderly patient, 100–200 mg twice daily
nadolol	low	• initially 40 mg once daily; in elderly patient, 20–40 mg once daily • maintenance 40–80 mg once daily • maximum 240 mg once daily • in renal dysfunction with creatinine clearance above 50 ml/min, give every 24 hr • with creatinine clearance of 31–50 ml/min, give every 24–36 hr • with creatinine clearance of 10–30 ml/min, give every 24–48 hr • with creatinine clearance under 10 ml/min, give every 40–60 hr
pindolol	moderate	• 5–30 mg twice daily; in elderly patient, 2.5 mg twice daily
propranolol	high	• immediate-release: 80–160 mg twice daily; in elderly patient, 20–40 mg twice daily • extended-release: 80–320 mg once daily
timolol	low to moderate	• 10–30 mg twice daily; in elderly patient, 5–10 mg twice daily

lectivity and lipid solubility (see *Reviewing beta-blockers*).

Receptor selectivity: Beta-blockers that inhibit beta$_1$ receptors and have little effect on beta$_2$ receptors are called *cardioselective.* Those that inhibit beta$_1$ and beta$_2$ receptors equally are called *nonselective.*

Because the heart's oxygen demand decreases primarily through blockade of that organ's beta$_1$ receptors, cardioselective drugs yield the best antianginal effect with the fewest adverse effects. Examples of cardioselective beta-blockers include atenolol and metoprolol.

Beta$_2$-receptor inhibition in the bronchioles and vessels leaves alpha-adrenergic bronchocon-

MULTISYSTEM ALERT

Beta-blockers for angina: Effects on other disorders

Beta-blockers may affect more than just myocardial oxygen demand. In fact, they may complicate several other major disorders.

Bronchospastic disease
Nonselective beta-blockers leave alpha-induced bronchoconstriction unopposed, which may worsen acute bronchospasm in a patient with asthma or chronic obstructive pulmonary disease. If such a patient needs a beta-blocker, the physician may prescribe a cardioselective one.

Diabetes mellitus
Nonselective beta-blockers may inhibit beta-stimulated insulin release from the pancreas, leading to hyperglycemia. These drugs also may mask signs and symptoms of hypoglycemia. If your diabetic patient needs a beta-blocker, the physician may prescribe a cardioselective one.

Hyperlipidemia
Beta-blockers may increase serum levels of low-density lipoproteins and decrease serum levels of high-density lipoproteins. That's why a physician may prescribe a calcium channel blocker for a patient with hyperlipidemia.

Peripheral vascular disease
Nonselective beta-blockers leave alpha-induced peripheral vasoconstriction unopposed, which may worsen tingling, numbness, pain, and coldness in the hands and feet. If a patient with peripheral vascular disease needs a beta-blocker, the physician may prescribe a cardioselective one.

striction and vasoconstriction unopposed. As a result, nonselective beta-blockers may worsen bronchospasm or peripheral vascular disease, making cardioselective agents a better choice for patients with these conditions (see *Beta-blockers for angina: Effects on other disorders*). Because bronchoconstriction and vasoconstriction may still occur even with cardioselective drugs, patients with these disorders should take the lowest possible dose.

Lipid solubility: Drugs that are highly lipid soluble are easily absorbed into the central nervous system (CNS); therefore, they increase the risk of CNS-associated adverse effects, including dizziness, lethargy, fatigue, sedation, insomnia, headache, depression, and an altered mental status.

Propranolol has the highest level of lipid solubility among the beta-blockers, and it produces the most CNS adverse effects. Metoprolol is moderately lipid soluble; atenolol and nadolol are the least lipid soluble. A less lipid-soluble drug, such as atenolol, can be helpful in elderly patients and those prone to CNS adverse effects.

Nursing considerations
During the start of beta-blocker therapy, many patients feel lethargic and tired. These effects usually resolve after a few weeks. Your patient also may complain of cold hands and feet; this reaction stems from arterial constriction in the extremities.

Elderly patients are most likely to experience adverse reactions to beta-blockers, possibly including bradycardia and hypotension as well as lethargy. Hypotension can be more pronounced if the patient takes a nitrate, a calcium channel blocker, or certain other drugs besides the beta-blocker (see *Beta-blockers and the elderly: Avoiding the dangers*).

Check your patient's blood pressure regularly if she's receiving combination antianginal therapy to make sure her systolic pressure stays above 90 mm Hg. Also, check to be sure her heart rate stays at or above 60 beats per minute (bpm). Severe bradycardia (a heart rate less than 40 bpm) and hypotension (systolic pressure less than 80 mm Hg) can be treated with 0.6 mg of I.V. atropine as ordered. This dose can be repeated every 3 minutes until you've given a maximum of 2 to 3 mg.

Instruct the patient to check her own blood pressure after discharge. Give her specific blood pressure levels prescribed by her physician and tell her what to do if her pressure goes above or below the recommended level.

Also, instruct her to avoid skipping doses of her beta-blocker or abruptly stopping her therapy. If she needs to stop taking her beta-blocker, the drug should be tapered over 1 to 3 weeks. One guideline recommends reducing the dosage in 10-mg increments every 4 days. Another suggests decreasing the dose by 50% every 3 to 7 days.

Patients with severe heart failure make poor candidates for beta-blocker therapy because the drug may worsen the oxygen deficit that already exists. Likewise, beta-blockers shouldn't be used by any patient whose condition could be worsened by decreases in heart rate, conduction, or contractility. This includes patients with sinus bradycardia, some forms of heart failure, cardiogenic shock, and atrioventricular (AV) block greater than first degree (in the absence of a functioning pacemaker).

Calcium channel blockers

Calcium channel blockers decrease myocardial oxygen demand and increase oxygen supply. The result is improved exercise tolerance and decreased anginal symptoms. These drugs can be used alone or in combination with nitrates, beta-blockers, or both. They also may be used in combination with other calcium channel blockers to take advantage of their varied effects.

Of the five categories of calcium channel blockers, three are commonly used as antianginals: diphenylalkylamines, dihydropyridines, and benzothiazepines. You also may administer bepridil. These drugs differ somewhat in their effects on the myocardium, coronary vessels, and peripheral vessels.

Diphenylalkylamines

Verapamil, which represents this category of calcium channel blockers, exerts potent depressant effects on myocardial contractility and the conduction of electrical impulses through the AV node. As a result, the patient's heart rate and myocardial wall tension decline, which in turn decreases the heart's demand for oxygen. Verapamil also moderately dilates coronary and peripheral vessels, which improves oxygen supply to ischemic areas of the heart.

Dihydropyridines

Nifedipine, an example of the drugs in this category, occupies the other end of the calcium channel blocker spectrum. It exerts minimal effects on myocardial contractility and doesn't slow conduction through the AV node. The antianginal benefits stem from its potent dilatory effects on peripheral and coronary vessels.

In contrast to other calcium channel blockers that slow the heart rate, this one leads to reflex tachycardia through dilation of peripheral vessels. This effect limits the drug's usefulness when

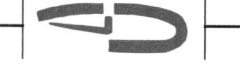

DANGEROUS COMPLICATIONS

Beta-blockers and the elderly: Avoiding the dangers

Many elderly patients take several prescription drugs, plus they have an increased sensitivity to beta-blockers. Before your elderly patient begins taking a beta-blocker, find out which other drugs she takes and when she takes them.

Drugs that could enhance bradycardia and hypotension when used with beta-blockers include:
- angiotensin-converting enzyme inhibitors, such as captopril, enalapril, and lisinopril
- calcium channel blockers, such as verapamil, diltiazem, nifedipine, nicardipine, and amlodipine
- digoxin
- diuretics, such as furosemide, bumetanide, and hydrochlorothiazide
- nitrates, such as nitroglycerin, isosorbide dinitrate, and isosorbide mononitrate
- antidepressants, such as fluoxetine, paroxetine, sertraline, amitriptyline, doxepin, and nortriptyline
- anxiolytics and sedatives, such as temazepam, clonazepam, lorazepam, alprazolam, triazolam, and diazepam.

treating stable angina because reflex tachycardia worsens anginal symptoms in many patients. Two other drugs in this class that are used to treat angina are amlodipine and nicardipine.

Benzothiazepines

Diltiazem, which represents this category, moderately increases coronary and peripheral vasodilation and moderately decreases heart rate and electrical conduction through the AV node. It has minimal depressant effects on myocardial contractility. This results in a smoother decrease in oxygen demand and an increase in oxygen supply.

Bepridil

Bepridil possesses properties of both calcium channel blockers and sodium channel blockers. Despite its approval for use in treating chronic stable angina, most physicians use it only for patients in whom all other antianginal therapies have failed.

Reviewing calcium channel blockers

Drug	Effects	Dose
amlodipine	• peripheral vasodilation strongly increased • myocardial contractility mildly decreased	• initial: 5–10 mg once daily • usual maintenance: 10 mg once daily • elderly: 2.5–5 mg once daily
diltiazem	• peripheral vasodilation moderately increased • conduction of impulses through myocardium moderately decreased • myocardial contractility mildly decreased	*Tablets* • initial: 30 mg once daily • maintenance: 180–360 mg once daily or divided into three or four daily doses *Extended release* • initial: 120 to 180 mg once daily • maximum: 480 mg once daily • elderly: 120 mg once daily
nicardipine	• peripheral vasodilation strongly increased • myocardial contractility mildly decreased	• initial: 20 mg three times daily • maintenance: 20–40 mg three times daily • elderly: 10 mg three times daily
nifedipine	• peripheral vasodilation strongly increased • myocardial contractility mildly decreased	*Capsules* • initial: 10 mg three times daily • maintenance: 10–20 mg three times daily • maximum: 60 mg three times daily *Extended release* • initial: 30–60 mg once daily • maximum: 120 mg once daily • elderly: 30 mg once daily
verapamil	• peripheral vasodilation moderately increased • conduction of impulses through myocardium strongly decreased • myocardial contractility moderately decreased	• initial: 80 mg every 6–8 hr • maintenance: 320–480 mg once daily or divided into three or four daily doses • suggested range: 240–480 mg once daily • elderly: 40 mg every 8 hr or 120 mg once daily

That's because the adverse effects of this drug may include life-threatening ventricular arrhythmias, torsades de pointes, and agranulocytosis.

Nursing considerations

Dosages of calcium channel blockers vary by drug, formulation, and individual patient response (see *Reviewing calcium channel blockers*). Keep in mind that initial and maintenance dosages may be much lower for elderly patients. All antianginal dosages should be adjusted to the minimum required to provide relief of symptoms and adequate exercise tolerance.

When therapy begins, monitor your patient's blood pressure and pulse carefully. If her heart rate drops below 55 bpm or her systolic blood pressure goes below 90 mm Hg, avoid giving her drugs that will further lower heart rate or blood pressure—especially if she's elderly or has mild heart failure or orthostatic hypotension. Also, avoid giving calcium channel blockers to a patient hypersensitive to them or to a patient with sick sinus syndrome, second-degree or third-degree heart block (unless she has a pacemaker), severe aortic stenosis, or cardiogenic shock.

Use caution when giving any drug that affects vasodilation, heart rate, or blood pressure to a patient already taking a calcium channel blocker.

Instruct your patient not to crush or chew extended-release or sustained-release formulations because doing so will alter absorption of the drug and may damage the drug's protective coating, possibly causing mucosal irritation. Inform your patient that some extended-release forms of calcium channel blockers don't dissolve in the body and will be eliminated in the stool. Reassure the patient that the drug will still work. This formulation allows absorption of the active drug and elimination of the undissolved tablet matrix in the stool.

Throughout therapy, monitor your patient for progression of her underlying cardiac disorder. Check for increased pain frequency, anginal attacks of longer duration, and decreased exercise tolerance.

Adverse reactions common to patients taking calcium channel blockers include hypotension and bradycardia. Profound hypotension and reflex tachycardia are more likely to occur with the dihydropyridines. Other reactions to calcium channel blockers may include dizziness, lightheadedness, flushing, headache, weakness, peripheral edema, and nausea. All result from vasodilation and, consequently, are more common with the dihydropyridines.

A cough and constipation are also common. Advise your patient to notify her physician if she develops a persistent cough. Constipation occurs most commonly with verapamil. To help your patient avoid it, recommend a stool softener, such as 50 to 100 mg of docusate sodium at bedtime, or a bulk-forming laxative, such as methylcellulose or psyllium.

Several interactions may arise between calcium channel blockers and other drugs. The most significant ones are enhanced adverse reactions to calcium channel blockers or toxic concentrations of other drugs (see *Drug interactions with calcium channel blockers*).

Nitrates
Nitroglycerin, a nitrate, is the treatment of choice for easing acute anginal attacks, but nitrates typically aren't considered a first-line prophylactic treatment for angina. Even so, depending on a patient's response to beta-blockers and calcium channel blockers, she may take a nitrate alone or in combination with other antianginal drugs.

How nitrates work
When they enter the body, nitrates convert to nitric oxide, a potent vasodilator similar to a sub-

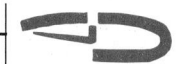

DANGEROUS COMPLICATIONS

Drug interactions with calcium channel blockers

When caring for a patient who's taking a calcium channel blocker, stay alert for drug combinations that could cause trouble. Here are some examples.

Concomitant use of quinidine with verapamil or nifedipine can cause marked decreases in blood pressure and heart rate, ventricular tachycardia, atrioventricular block, and pulmonary edema.

Simultaneous use of a calcium channel blocker and any beta-blocker could worsen hypotension and heart failure.

Diltiazem or verapamil taken with carbamazepine may cause toxic carbamazepine levels. If you must give these drugs together, monitor carbamazepine levels carefully at the start of therapy and adjust the carbamazepine dose, if necessary.

Taking digoxin with diltiazem, verapamil, nifedipine, bepridil, or felodipine may raise digoxin levels by as much as 60%. Because digoxin levels don't peak for at least a week, you'll need to measure your patient's levels at the start of calcium channel blocker therapy, 2 to 3 days after starting therapy, and again at the end of 1 week. Watch for signs and symptoms of digoxin toxicity, including loss of appetite, dizziness, nausea, vomiting, visual disturbances, and tachycardia. If they occur, adjust the digoxin dose.

stance called endothelial-derived relaxing factor that's found naturally in the walls of blood vessels. In intact blood vessels, this factor stimulates smooth-muscle vasodilation. In blood vessels damaged by atherosclerosis or ischemic changes, however, the release of this factor declines, and vasodilation doesn't occur.

Taking a nitrate drug can help to resolve that problem. In fact, nitrates dilate damaged vessels even more effectively than they dilate normal ones. The ability to enhance vasodilation in both normal and damaged endothelial tissues makes nitrates uniquely effective in increasing blood flow to ischemic myocardial areas in patients with advanced CAD.

Also, dilation of peripheral veins decreases venous return to the heart, reducing preload. Dilation of arterial beds decreases systemic vascular resistance and arterial pressure, reducing afterload. The result is decreased myocardial workload and reduced myocardial oxygen demand.

Nitrates also may inhibit the activation and aggregation of platelets, which may reduce potential thrombotic complications.

Types of nitrates

Nitrates other than nitroglycerin that are used to treat chronic stable angina include isosorbide dinitrate and isosorbide mononitrate.

Isosorbide dinitrate is available as sublingual tablets, chewable tablets, immediate-acting tablets, and sustained-release tablets and capsules (see *Reviewing organic nitrates*). Isosorbide mononitrate is supplied in immediate-acting and extended-release tablets. These two forms of nitrates haven't been compared for bioequivalence. Therefore, instruct patients to avoid switching from one form to another.

Because isosorbide mononitrates don't require metabolism by the liver to become active, as the isosorbide dinitrates do, the mononitrates are rapidly becoming the nitrates of choice for long-term oral therapy.

Nursing considerations

Nitrate therapy requires a daily nitrate-free period to avoid drug tolerance, so the physician probably will prescribe it in combination with a beta-blocker or calcium channel blocker to provide 24-hour antianginal coverage. The nitrate-free period lasts 10 to 12 hours and usually takes place at night, the least common time for acute angina to develop. Naturally, patients known to experience angina at night or in the early morning make poor candidates for nitrate monotherapy.

Your patient probably will also receive a prescription for sublingual nitroglycerin to be used if she experiences recurrent anginal attacks. Give her these instructions:

• If you feel chest pain, stop what you're doing, rest, and place a tablet under your tongue. The drug will be absorbed across the moist skin in your mouth.
• If the pain doesn't abate, place a second tablet under your tongue 5 minutes after the first.
• If the pain still doesn't abate, place a third tablet under your tongue 5 minutes after the second.
• If the pain doesn't abate within 5 minutes (15 minutes total), call an emergency medical service or go to the nearest emergency department. You may be having a heart attack.

Instruct your patient not to crush sublingual, transmucosal, or sustained-release nitroglycerin tablets.

Sublingual nitroglycerin tablets may not dissolve fully in patients with decreased levels of saliva—a condition common among elderly patients. An older adult also may have trouble swallowing an intermediate or long-acting preparation, which may make her a good candidate for a translingual spray, transdermal patch, or ointment formulation.

If she uses a translingual spray, tell her not to shake the canister or inhale the drug; either one will interfere with the drug's absorption. To determine when the spray container is empty, have her float it in a bowl of water. The emptier the container is, the more it will float.

Emphasize that nitrates must be stored properly to retain their effectiveness. Urge the patient to keep her nitroglycerin tightly closed in its original container. Have her protect the drug from extremes of heat, cold, and humidity. Also, tell her to protect it from light.

Instruct your patient to write the month and year on the bottle when she first opens her sublingual nitroglycerin tablets. After 6 months, she should discard any unused tablets. Explain that sublingual nitroglycerin should tingle when placed under the tongue. If it doesn't, the tablets should be discarded regardless of their age. Urge her to carry her sublingual nitroglycerin with her at all times in case she develops chest pain.

Adverse effects common with nitrate use include hypotension, headache, and tolerance to the drug's therapeutic effects.

Hypotension results from the drug's vasodilatory effects and becomes most pronounced with large doses, during periods of volume depletion, when making sudden changes in position, or when taking other drugs with hypotensive effects (such as beta-blockers, calcium channel blockers, diuretics, or ACE inhibitors). Tell your patient to avoid sudden changes in position, to drink plenty of fluids, and to avoid taking other hypotensive drugs at the same time she takes her nitrate.

Reviewing organic nitrates

Drug	Dose	Onset (min)	Peak effects	Duration (hr)
Nitroglycerin				
Sublingual tablets	• 0.3–0.6 mg • maximum 1.5 mg within a 15-min period	2–5	up to 15 min	0.5–1
Transmucosal, sustained-release tablets	• 1–3 mg three times daily	2–3	30 min	up to 0.5
Translingual aerosol spray	• 0.4 mg as needed • maximum 2.4 mg	2–5	2–5 min	up to 5
Oral, sustained-release capsules and tablets	• initial: 2.5 or 2.6 mg three or four times daily	20–45	1–2 hr	8–12
Topical ointment	• initial: 7.5 mg (1/2 inch) every 8 hr	20–45	1–2 hr	3–6
Transdermal patch	• 1 patch daily	30–60	2–3 hr	12–24
Isosorbide dinitrate				
Sublingual tablets	• 2.5–10 mg as needed	2–10	30–60 min	1–2
Chewable tablets	• 5–10 mg every 2–3 hr	3	15–45 min	0.5–2
Oral, immediate-release tablets	• 10–100 mg every 3–6 hr	15–60	1–2 hr	4–6
Oral, sustained-release tablets and capsules	• 20–80 mg every 6–12 hr	30–180	1–2 hr	6–12
Isosorbide mononitrate				
Oral, immediate-release tablets	• 20 mg twice daily, 7 hr apart	30–60	1–2 hr	5–12
Oral, sustained-release tablets	• 30–120 mg once daily • rarely, 240 mg once daily	45–60	1–4 hr	8–24

Headaches usually diminish or disappear as nitrate therapy continues. To ease the patient's pain early in therapy, suggest that she take a mild analgesic, such as aspirin or acetaminophen. Starting nitrate therapy with low doses reduces the likelihood of severe headaches.

Over time, a patient taking long-term nitrate therapy may develop tolerance to the drug, resulting in decreased exercise endurance and increased anginal episodes. To help avoid tolerance, suggest that your patient separate nitrate dosages by 6 to 8 hours (7 A.M. and 2 P.M. dosing times, for instance) and maintain a 10-hour to 12-hour nitrate-free period. If she uses a trans-

How ischemia leads to platelet aggregation

Acute ischemia triggers the release of arachidonic acid, a prostaglandin precursor that's derived from platelet membranes. Next, the enzyme cyclooxygenase converts arachidonic acid into prostaglandin G_2 and prostaglandin H_2. Prostaglandin H_2 is converted to thromboxane A_2 by the enzyme thromboxane synthetase. Thromboxane A_2 stimulates vasoconstriction and platelet aggregation, particularly in the coronary arteries.

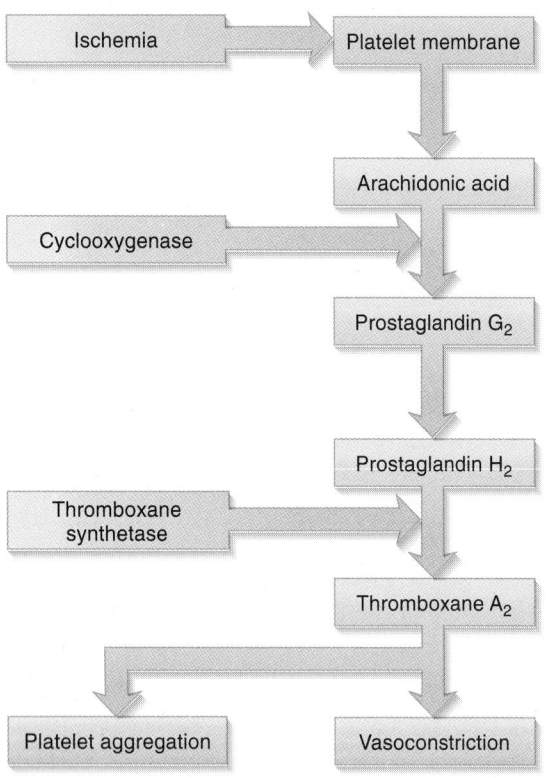

dermal patch, have her remove it each afternoon or evening to allow for a 12-hour nitrate-free period. If she has chest pain during this period, she can take a short-acting sublingual nitrate. Her physician may also add a beta-blocker or calcium channel blocker to her regimen to provide 24-hour prophylactic coverage.

Nitrates are contraindicated in patients with severe anemia, chronic postural hypotension, closed-angle glaucoma, head trauma, cerebral hemorrhage, or hypersensitivity to the drugs or delivery vehicles (such as the adhesive on a transdermal patch).

Anticoagulants

Arterial surfaces roughened and damaged by atherosclerotic plaques provide prime areas for the development of thrombi. By further narrowing an already compromised vessel, the thrombus can lead to ischemia and create symptoms of angina. That's why many patients with angina undergo anticoagulant therapy: It helps avoid the development of artery-blocking thrombi.

The four drugs commonly used to reduce the risk of thrombotic complications include aspirin, ticlopidine, clopidrogel, and warfarin. Aspirin, ticlopidine, and clopidrogel inhibit platelet aggregation; warfarin inhibits formation of certain clotting factors.

Platelets play a pivotal role in the formation not only of atherosclerotic lesions but also of thrombi and tissue hyperplasia. Patients with elevated cholesterol levels and CAD face an increased risk of platelet aggregation. Increases in blood cholesterol levels, specifically LDL levels, raise the cholesterol content of platelet membranes, which causes an increase in arachidonic acid, the substrate for thromboxane A_2 (TXA_2) synthesis. Consequently, production of TXA_2 increases in the vasculature, which activates platelet aggregation and vasoconstriction (see *How ischemia leads to platelet aggregation*).

Hypercholesterolemia also inhibits the release of endothelial-derived relaxing factor, thus reducing its ability to inhibit platelet aggregation and cause vasodilation. The net effect for patients with CAD and hypercholesterolemia is a propensity toward platelet aggregation, atherosclerotic plaque formation, vessel wall hyperplasia, and vasoconstriction.

Direct vascular damage can activate platelets as well, which may ultimately lead to thrombus formation. For all these reasons, patients at risk for angina caused by thrombotic complications of CAD may benefit from platelet-blocking or anticoagulant drugs.

Aspirin

By inhibiting platelet cyclooxygenase, aspirin prevents the formation of TXA_2 and thus prevents platelet aggregation. An irreversible inhibitor of platelet aggregation, aspirin exerts effects that continue through the life of each cell affected.

Patients who benefit most from prophylactic aspirin therapy have chronic stable angina, hypercholesterolemia, hypertension, a strong family history of CAD, or a history of an MI, diabetes, or smoking.

Even these high-risk patients should take only low doses of aspirin: either a baby aspirin (80 mg) or one regular-strength tablet (325 mg) daily. These dosage levels have proven effective in preventing adverse coronary events, especially a second MI. Higher dosages have proven no more effective than lower ones and may increase adverse reactions, notably GI discomfort and bleeding. At high dosages, aspirin actually may heighten the patient's cardiac risk because, in addition to inhibiting TXA_2 production, it also inhibits production of prostacyclin, a natural anti-aggregation chemical.

To minimize GI problems, urge your patient to take her daily aspirin tablet with food. Or ask her physician about switching to an enteric-coated aspirin or a combination of aspirin and antacid to help minimize problems. Stress to your patient that aspirin therapy will not cure her CAD. Rather, it reduces the risk of blood clots that could lead to an MI.

If your patient is at a high risk for thrombus formation—from atrial fibrillation, a history of deep vein thrombosis or pulmonary embolism, hypercoagulability, or heart valve disease or replacement, for example—a stronger drug such as warfarin should be used.

Ticlopidine

An alternative to aspirin therapy, ticlopidine also has an antiplatelet effect; patients may take it as prophylaxis against thrombotic cerebrovascular accident (CVA) after having a transient ischemic attack or first CVA. The disadvantage of ticlopidine is its adverse reaction profile. It can lead to neutropenia and thrombocytopenia within the first 3 months of therapy. It also increases serum total cholesterol and triglyceride levels, giving it limited usefulness among patients with CAD.

If your patient takes ticlopidine, make sure she has a complete blood count at the start of therapy and every 2 weeks during the first 3 months of therapy. Instruct her to report any signs and symptoms of infection or fever because she may be at risk for infection secondary to drug-induced neutropenia.

Clopidrogel

Clopidrogel reduces the risk of an MI, a CVA, or vascular death in patients with peripheral artery disease or a recent MI or CVA. Like ticlopidine, clopidrogel has an antiplatelet effect. However, it causes fewer adverse effects than ticlopidine, and it doesn't require laboratory monitoring.

Warfarin

Warfarin interferes with the liver's ability to synthesize vitamin K–dependent clotting factors, which causes a reduction of clotting factors II, VII, IX, and X and a resultant anticoagulant effect.

The popularity of warfarin has waxed and waned over the years, largely because it can produce pronounced bleeding if dosed or monitored incorrectly. In the last 5 years, however, warfarin has regained popularity based on its effectiveness—at low therapeutic dosages—in preventing and treating many thrombotic cardiovascular disorders. The fact is that warfarin benefits patients with atrial fibrillation, an MI, unstable angina, mural thrombi, and cardiomyopathy. However, effective therapy remains a challenge for a number of reasons.

First, the proper dosage must be meticulously titrated and monitored for each patient. Second, a host of medical conditions and drugs can alter warfarin's effect (see *What alters warfarin's effect?,* page 84). Also, many patients begin warfarin therapy in the hospital while on heparin, which can make accurate dosage adjustments more difficult. Finally, as you know, the consequences of inaccurate warfarin dosing or monitoring can be life threatening.

To track your patient's response to warfarin, you'll need to follow her PT or international normalized ratio (INR). At the start of therapy, the initial increase in her PT will reflect a reduction in clotting factor VII, which has a short, 6-hour half-life. After 3 to 7 days, when other clotting factors are depleted as well, you'll get a better idea of the true anticoagulant effect of the warfarin dosage you're using.

Most patients start with 7.5 to 10 mg of warfarin for 2 to 3 days and then begin maintenance therapy on the third or fourth day. Elderly and female patients, who tend to be more sensitive to warfarin, may start with 5 to 7.5 mg/day. Keep in mind, however, that many patients begin warfarin therapy while still receiving heparin. As you might expect, the combination can result in a falsely elevated PT or INR that drops when the

What alters warfarin's effect?

Many conditions can interact with warfarin to either increase or decrease the patient's international normalized ratio (INR). For example, cancer, heart failure, diarrhea, extended airplane travel, fever, hyperthyroidism, liver disease, noncompliance, prolonged hot weather, and vitamin K deficiency can increase the INR. Edema, hereditary warfarin resistance, hyperlipidemia, hypothyroidism, increased cigarette smoking, and noncompliance can decrease it.

Many drugs can affect the INR.

Drugs that increase INR
- allopurinol
- anabolic steroids
- aspirin
- chloramphenicol
- cholestyramine
- cimetidine
- cyclophosphamide
- dextran
- indomethacin
- kanamycin
- methyldopa
- methylphenidate
- metronidazole
- nalidixic acid
- oxolinic acid
- oxyphenbutazone
- phenylbutazone
- phenytoin
- propylthiouracil
- quinidine
- quinine
- ranitidine
- reserpine
- streptomycin

Drugs that decrease INR
- adrenocortico-steroids
- antacids
- antihistamines
- antipyrine
- barbiturates
- carbamazepine
- chlordiazepoxide
- contraceptives
- digitalis glycosides
- estrogens
- ethchlorvynol
- griseofulvin
- haloperidol
- meprobamate
- phenytoin
- primidone
- rifampin
- thiazide diuretics
- thiopurines
- vitamin K
- xanthines

patient stops receiving heparin. Indeed, the INR may be inaccurate for up to 6 weeks at the start of warfarin therapy, especially in older patients who receive heparin.

Given that it may take several weeks to stabilize the patient's warfarin therapy, you may work with her on an outpatient basis. To maximize anticoagulation rapidly, start a standard warfarin dose and then monitor the patient's response closely. Adjust doses in small increments to achieve the desired degree of anticoagulation and avoid complications. The first PT or INR measurement should be 2 to 5 days after discharge. Document your patient's response to doses and changes on a flowchart kept in her record. In addition to tracking dosage adjustments, the flowchart also will help you identify seasonal changes in her response, document her responses, and note your suspicions of poor compliance with therapy—a common cause of bleeding complications.

If your patient develops excessive bleeding and an INR above 20 that results from overdose, give vitamin K to reverse the effect. Expect to administer 10 mg of vitamin K by subcutaneous injection. Depending on the urgency of the patient's condition, you may also administer fresh frozen plasma or prothrombin complex concentrate.

The amount of information your patient needs to know to maintain her warfarin therapy can be overwhelming. Take several sessions to teach her, and make sure you give her written materials to review between sessions and to use for guidelines at home (see *Teaching your patient about warfarin*).

Invasive interventions

If lifestyle changes and drugs fail to ease your patient's angina, she may need to undergo an invasive procedure to open or circumvent a blocked artery. Many such procedures, commonly called catheter-based interventions, focus on removing plaque and debris from the lumen of the artery. They include angioplasty, atherectomy, and coronary ultrasound. They may be performed in combination if necessary. However, if the patient's CAD is too widespread, she may need a surgical procedure instead, such as coronary artery bypass grafting or a less invasive procedure called minimally invasive direct coronary artery bypass.

Because catheter-based interventions all involve threading a catheter from the patient's groin to her heart, they all create a risk of similar complications, primarily vasovagal syncope and retroperitoneal bleeding. Malignant vasovagal syncope results from stimulation of the vagus nerve by the catheter sheath. It involves bradycardia, vasodilation, low cardiac output (CO), and hypotension. Other possible effects of vagal stimulation include nausea, weakness, yawning, blurred vision, and sweating.

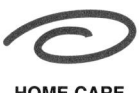

HOME CARE

Teaching your patient about warfarin

Warfarin therapy requires strict patient compliance and careful monitoring. Give your patient these important instructions to help ensure her success.

- Take warfarin at the same time each day, exactly as your physician directs.
- If you miss a dose, take it as soon as possible and then go back to your regular schedule. If you forget to take warfarin for a day, don't take the dose at all. Never take a double dose; doing so may cause bleeding.
- Check with your physician before taking any nonprescription drugs or vitamins. Vitamins K and E can interfere with warfarin. Aspirin and nonsteroidal anti-inflammatory drugs (such as naproxen, indomethacin, ketoprofen, and ibuprofen) can cause bleeding.
- Remember to keep your blood-test appointments. Your physician will use the results to adjust your warfarin dosage.
- Carry medical alert information with you at all times so that emergency personnel will know you're taking warfarin.
- Tell every physician and dentist you see that you're taking warfarin.
- Don't alter your intake of foods high in vitamin K, such as green scallions, dark green leafy vegetables (kale and spinach, for example),

cabbage, fish, mayonnaise, broccoli, cauliflower, and liver.
- If you drink alcohol, limit yourself to one or two drinks a day.
- Check with your physician before starting a weight-loss program or becoming pregnant.
- To reduce the risk of injury, always wear shoes and place a nonskid mat in your bathtub. Shave with an electric razor and use a soft toothbrush.
- Wear gloves when gardening or working outside.
- If you cut yourself, apply direct pressure on the wound with a clean cloth for at least 5 minutes. If it continues to bleed beyond 10 minutes, call your nurse or physician.
- If you get a bruise, apply a cold pack for the first 2 hours afterward and notify your physician. After 48 hours, apply a warm compress to help your body reabsorb the blood.
- Call your physician if your gums bleed when you brush your teeth or if you notice any bruises or purplish marks on your skin. Also, report nosebleeds, heavy bleeding, oozing from cuts or wounds, heavy or unexpected menstrual bleeding, blood in your urine or sputum, bloody or tarry black stools, or vomitus that looks like coffee grounds.

To treat vasovagal syncope, place your patient in Trendelenburg's position to promote blood flow to her brain and heart, and begin volume replacement with I.V. fluids. Give atropine to increase heart rate and blood pressure, as ordered. Anticipate transcutaneous pacing or temporary transvenous pacing if the bradycardia persists.

If the catheter punctures her femoral artery, your patient will develop retroperitoneal bleeding. Look for bruising and hematoma development at the puncture site, in the groin area, and over the flank region. Also, look for an increase in thigh circumference. The patient may complain of low-back pain from pressure caused by the hematoma. Testing the patient's hemoglobin level usually will reveal a drop of 1 g/dl or more.

If you think or know that your patient has retroperitoneal bleeding, evaluate her peripheral

pulses frequently. (If the hematoma enlarges, it could reduce blood flow to the leg and lead to ischemia.) Inspect the groin site frequently for obvious bleeding and hematoma formation. Keep the patient in a recumbent position for 4 to 6 hours and avoid moving or manipulating the cannulated limb for 4 to 6 hours after removal of the sheaths. Carefully regulate anticoagulants according to clotting studies, such as the activated partial thromboplastin time (APTT).

Percutaneous transluminal coronary angioplasty

The most common nonsurgical intervention for angina, percutaneous transluminal coronary angioplasty (PTCA) has a 95% immediate success rate (defined as more than a 20% reduction in stenosis). Not a cure for CAD, it should be ac-

How percutaneous transluminal coronary angioplasty works

In this procedure, a physician positions a balloon catheter in a section of occluded coronary artery and inflates the balloon several times to fracture and compress the plaque, thus widening the arterial lumen.

Balloon catheter in position	Balloon inflated	Arterial lumen widened

companied by lifestyle changes designed to maintain the health of the newly opened vessel.

The procedure involves mechanical dilation of a narrowed or occluded artery using a specially designed balloon-tipped catheter. The examiner directs the balloon catheter to the desired anatomic point using fluoroscopy as a guide, and then dilates the balloon several times. The procedure requires neither general anesthesia nor surgery. However, the patient is typically sedated with diazepam or diphenhydramine before the procedure (see *How percutaneous transluminal coronary angioplasty works*).

Balloon inflation has two effects on plaque in the vessel. First, it creates cracks of various depths from the lumen into the plaque. These cracks may act as additional channels through which blood can flow. Second, it may compress flexible portions of the plaque, leaving a wider lumen for blood to flow through after balloon deflation.

Because balloon inflation results in a temporary occlusion of blood flow, your patient may complain of angina during the procedure. After a successful procedure, she'll experience relief of her anginal symptoms, reperfusion of the coronary arteries, and an improved quality of life.

Patients who are most suitable for PTCA have angina inadequately controlled by drugs and plaque in a single coronary artery. Patients with a calcified occlusion of the left main coronary artery usually make poor candidates because the catheter can't proceed past the calcified blockage.

The most common problem after PTCA remains restenosis. Acute or early restenosis occurs in 4% to 10% of patients who undergo routine PTCA. Possible causes include the following:
• rapid relaxation of the stretched arterial wall opposite an eccentrically shaped plaque
• occlusion from a large intimal flap
• spasm of the coronary artery wall
• thrombus formation with a large, curled intimal flap.

A monoclonal antibody called abciximab can help prevent abrupt restenosis after angioplasty by binding to a platelet receptor, thereby preventing platelets from clumping. Give an I.V. bolus of 0.25 mg/kg 10 minutes or more before the procedure, followed by a continuous infusion of 10 µg/minute for up to 12 hours, along with the usual heparin and aspirin. Monitor the patient closely for bleeding complications.

Chronic or late stenosis affects 25% to 50% of patients after PTCA, usually within 6 months after the procedure. It may relate to the number of balloon inflations used, the inflation pressure, the location of the angioplasty site, or the use of anticoagulants or vasodilators.

Both early and late restenosis may lead to ischemic complications, including chest pain, shortness of breath, ECG changes, an MI, and cardiac arrest. Medical treatment for restenosis includes I.V. heparin, antiplatelet drugs, I.V. nitroglycerin, and thrombolytic therapy. The patient also may need repeat angioplasty, intracoronary stent placement, or coronary artery bypass grafting.

Other complications include coronary artery dissection, malignant vasovagal syncope, and retroperitoneal bleeding. Remember that coronary artery dissection typically causes cardiac arrest; be prepared to perform cardiopulmonary resuscitation.

Nursing considerations

Before PTCA, you'll need to wash your patient's groin with an antibacterial soap and shave or clip the pubic hair. Insert an indwelling urinary catheter to monitor urine output. Make sure she has an I.V. line with fluids running; hydration helps prevent kidney damage from the dye used during the procedure. Locate and mark the patient's pedal pulses so that you can find them more easily later. Also, take a baseline set of vital signs and assess the color, temperature, and sensation in her extremities.

Explain the mechanics of the procedure to the patient and mention that she may feel pressure as the catheter moves along the vessel. Remind her that she'll be awake during the procedure and lying on a hard table. Tell her that it may take 1 to 4 hours to complete the procedure and that she may be asked to take deep breaths from time to time to help the physician position the catheter. Tell her to notify the physician if she feels any anginal pain during the procedure.

Warn her that she'll hear the fluoroscope machine moving and making noise over her chest and that she may feel a flushed sensation and possibly nausea when the dye is injected. Explain that she'll need to stay in bed with her leg straight for several hours after the procedure.

During the procedure, the patient will receive supplemental oxygen to increase the amount of oxygen in her blood and maximize the amount available to cardiac tissue. She'll also receive I.V. nitroglycerin and heparin, and she'll undergo continuous cardiac monitoring. Throughout the procedure, provide support by talking to the patient. Monitor the fluids infusing through the peripheral I.V. line as well as through the sheaths. Monitor urine output at least hourly and report the result to the physician. Be prepared to administer I.V. nitroglycerin, if ordered, for severe angina.

After the procedure, monitor the patient's vital signs every 15 minutes for the first hour and then every 30 to 60 minutes for the next 6 hours. If they're unstable, monitor the patient every 5 minutes and notify the physician. Instruct your patient to stay in bed for 6 hours after the groin sheaths are removed. Monitor the groin site for bleeding or hematoma, and assess circulation in the patient's legs. Monitor her cardiac rhythm continuously and notify the physician of any changes or complaints of chest pain. Maintain the nitroglycerin and heparin infusions, as ordered,

and collect blood samples for APTT measurements as needed. Obtain a 12-lead ECG and compare the tracing to the preprocedure recording.

The physician will remove the sheaths in 6 to 12 hours. Maintain the C-clamp or sandbags over the pressure dressing on the insertion site during that time. Explain to your patient the importance of maintaining pressure on the site to prevent bleeding from the site or within the tissues.

Encourage your patient to drink extra fluids and continue I.V. hydration to promote excretion of the dye. Monitor her urine output closely and assess her for signs and symptoms of fluid overload.

Tell the patient that she can resume her normal activities after discharge. Tell her to report any signs of bleeding or bruising at the arterial puncture site. Stress the importance of keeping follow-up appointments with her physician.

Laser angioplasty

Using laser angioplasty as an adjunct to balloon angioplasty can increase the chances of success and reduce complications, including restenosis. Holmium and excimer lasers have been gaining in popularity for the treatment of total occlusions. In both cases, after inserting the laser through a conventional catheter to the occlusion, a physician rotates and advances it through the occlusion while triggering it to emit rapid bursts of energy. The energy vaporizes the plaque, creating a channel wide enough to admit the balloon catheter, which then widens the channel even more.

Major complications of laser-assisted angioplasty develop in about 3% of patients. They include vessel perforation, dissection, restenosis, and spasm. Perforation and dissection necessitate immediate coronary artery bypass surgery and can result in an MI and death.

Nursing considerations

Care for a patient undergoing laser-assisted angioplasty mirrors that needed for balloon angioplasty alone. In a laser procedure, however, you'll need to pay extra attention to signs and symptoms of possible coronary perforation or dissection. And you'll need to be ready to administer emergency treatment if needed. Urge the patient to report any chest discomfort right away.

You can begin teaching your patient about her drugs as her condition stabilizes and pain at the insertion site is relieved. The most common

Understanding directional coronary atherectomy

In this procedure, a physician positions the atherectomy catheter in a section of occluded coronary artery and inflates a balloon to force a section of plaque into the catheter's cutting chamber. After shaving the plaque with the device's sharp blades, the physician suctions debris through the catheter, deflates the balloon and, if necessary, moves the catheter to a new location to repeat the process.

Atherectomy catheter in place	**Balloon inflated**	**Blade cutting plaque**	**Arterial lumen widened**

postprocedure drugs are antianginal, anticoagulant, and antiplatelet drugs.

Atherectomy

In directional coronary atherectomy, the physician uses a pair of stainless steel blades to excise atherosclerotic material and then aspirate the particles through the catheter's central lumen. Inflation of the catheter's balloon pushes the plaque between the blades for removal (see *Understanding directional coronary atherectomy*).

Benefits and risks are similar to those of PTCA and laser angioplasty. Like laser angioplasty, directional coronary atherectomy has the added benefit of removing some of the plaque rather than simply pressing it out of the way.

In rotational atherectomy, a physician uses a device made of a sheath with a nickel-plated brass or diamond-coated burr. When the foot pedal is depressed, the burr spins at up to 200,000 revolutions per minute, pulverizing plaque into tiny pieces that disappear into your patient's distal coronary artery circulation. When the plaque is attacked by the rotating burr, intense coronary artery vasospasm occasionally occurs. This can be treated with intracoronary nitroglycerin.

Nursing considerations

Care for a patient undergoing atherectomy mirrors that for PTCA or laser-assisted angioplasty. Make sure your patient understands that her faithful adherence to lifestyle adjustments provides the main source of long-term success for this procedure.

Intracoronary stent

An intracoronary stent is a tube of stainless steel mesh that can be positioned at a narrowed portion of coronary artery and expanded against the walls of the vessel to permanently hold it open. It also secures flaps of media and intima against the artery wall.

Stent placement follows a procedure similar to angioplasty. After positioning the closed stent over a deflated balloon, a physician threads the catheter to the area of plaque buildup. With the stent in position, the physician inflates the balloon, which expands the stent to the size of the coronary artery lumen and embeds it in the artery wall. The physician then deflates the balloon and withdraws the catheter, leaving the stent permanently in place (see *Placing a coronary stent*).

Patients who receive stents experience a lower reocclusion rate, a lower risk of having an MI, and a reduced need for emergency coronary artery bypass grafts. They still have a risk of restenosis, but it's much smaller than the risk from angioplasty alone. The incidence of vascular complications is slightly higher because of the larger arterial sheaths needed for the procedure.

Nursing considerations
Besides needing the nursing care typical for all catheter-based interventions, patients who undergo stent placement need special instruction about endocarditis precautions. Your patient will take prophylactic antibiotics for up to 3 months after stent placement. Patient teaching should also focus on the long-term anticoagulation your patient will receive.

Coronary artery bypass grafting
The treatment of choice for multivessel disease or occlusion of the left main coronary artery, coronary artery bypass grafting circumvents the patient's occluded arteries using native or synthetic replacement vessels.

The risks and complications of coronary artery bypass graft (CABG) surgery include an MI, bleeding, infection, CVA, and arrhythmias.

The surgery involves either taking a portion of saphenous vein from the patient's leg or dissecting one of the internal mammary arteries away from the chest wall to use as a graft (see *Two types of coronary artery bypass grafts,* page 90). During the procedure, the patient's blood, diluted and heparinized to prevent clotting, flows through a heart-lung bypass machine. The surgeon immobilizes the heart by injecting a cold cardioplegic solution into the coronary arteries, allowing the bypass machine to circulate oxygenated blood to the body's tissues. The patient's blood (and body) temperature is reduced to conserve oxygen. A moderate degree of hypothermia, 28°C (82.4°F), reduces oxygen consumption by 50%. At 20°C (68°F), oxygen consumption is reduced by about 25%.

After sewing grafts into place around blocked areas of the coronary arteries, the surgeon weans the patient from the bypass machine, brings pacemaker wires through the chest wall into the

Placing a coronary stent

In this procedure, a physician anchors a closed stent over a deflated balloon catheter and then positions the catheter in a section of occluded coronary artery. Inflation of the balloon expands the stent against the arterial walls, widening the lumen.

Closed stent in position	Balloon inflated and stent expanded	Stent in widened arterial lumen

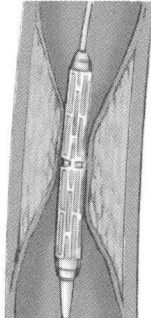 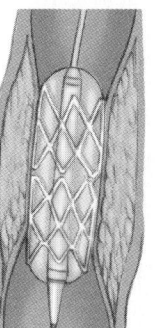 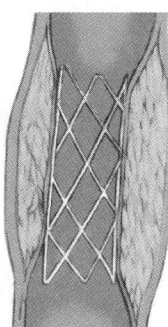

heart muscle, places mediastinal drainage tubes, and closes the sternum with wire. After her chest has been closed, your patient can be moved to the intensive care unit.

Complications of CABG surgery include bleeding, arrhythmias, pneumonia, infection, cardiac tamponade, an MI, and a CVA. Atrial fibrillation may result from swelling caused by stitches used to secure a graft or from hypokalemia, hypomagnesemia, or hypoxemia. Atrial fibrillation can cause a life-threatening CVA if emboli form. If your patient develops atrial fibrillation that fails to respond to initial therapy, she may need atrial overdrive pacing or electrical synchronized cardioversion.

Sinus tachycardia can be corrected by treating the underlying cause: anxiety, pain, or hypovolemia. Sinus bradycardia, junctional rhythm, heart block, or asystole can be treated with epicardial pacing wires. Atrial pacing offers the better option if your patient has a sinus rhythm because it maintains the atrial kick. Second-degree or third-

Two types of coronary artery bypass grafts

A surgeon may restore blood flow to occluded coronary arteries either by using pieces of the patient's saphenous vein or by rerouting the patient's internal mammary artery.

If the surgeon uses saphenous grafts, he'll sew one end into the root of the aorta and the other into a coronary artery on the distal side of the blockage. If the surgeon uses the internal mammary artery, he'll dissect it away from the patient's chest wall and connect it to a coronary artery distal to the blockage. Usually, the proximal end of the artery stays attached to the subclavian artery at its normal point of origin.

Saphenous vein grafts

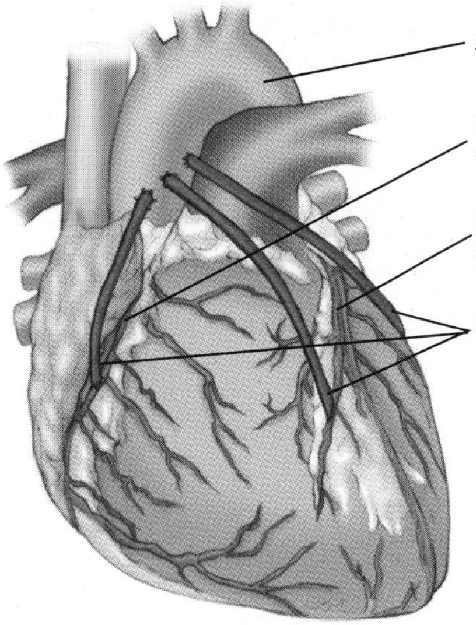

Aorta

Right coronary artery

Left coronary artery

Grafts

Internal mammary artery graft

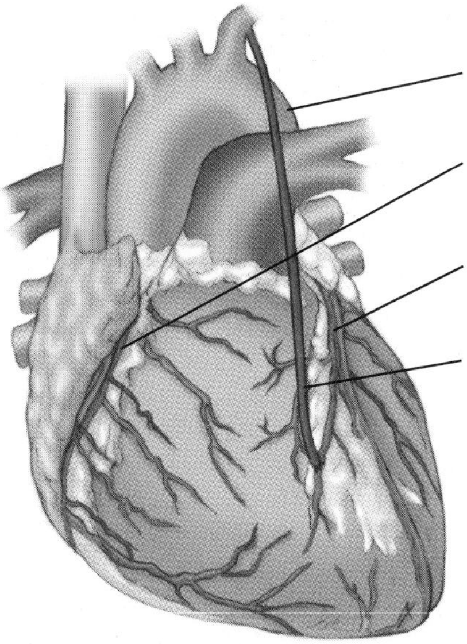

Aorta

Right coronary artery

Left coronary artery

Graft

degree AV block also suggests the need for temporary pacing via the epicardial pacing wires. Sequential pacing (in which the pacemaker first triggers the atria and then the ventricles) works for patients with AV block. Ventricular ectopic activity usually indicates hypokalemia, hypoxemia, or ischemic heart muscle.

An MI or a CVA may result from hypotension, hypoperfusion, or both during the procedure. Afterward, surgical insult and residual anticoagulation from the bypass machine may result in bleeding problems. Poor lung expansion, from pain or immobility, may lead to pneumonia. And nosocomial infections may result from transmission of resident bacteria, possibly from poor hand washing or other poor infection-control technique.

Nursing considerations

After surgery, your patient will be hypovolemic, hypertensive, hypothermic, and tachycardic. An atrial pacer may be required to synchronize atrial contraction and increase CO. You'll need to focus on maintaining hemodynamic stability, monitoring for complications, and rewarming your patient.

Use warmed blankets and warming lights to gradually increase your patient's temperature. Give antihypertensive drugs if necessary; morphine helps to relieve pain, relax vascular smooth muscle, and sedate the anxious patient. Morphine also eases pain as the patient awakens from anesthesia. If the patient had hypertension before surgery, you may need to give her vasopressors, such as sodium nitroprusside.

Monitor your patient's urine output because low urine output warns of low CO. Other signs include hypotension and tachycardia. Low CO usually stems from blood loss during surgery, rewarming, third-space losses, or intraoperative myocardial ischemia. It also may result from myocardial stunning, a temporary dysfunction of the myocardium that usually persists for up to 8 hours after CABG. Treat hypovolemia promptly by giving crystalloids, colloids, albumin, autotransfusion material, or packed red blood cells in sufficient quantities to raise the cardiac index to at least 2 L/minute/m^2.

Assess chest-tube output every 15 minutes for the first 1 to 2 hours to monitor for excessive postoperative bleeding. Low chest-tube output may indicate cardiac tamponade. To remove clots from the tubes, gently milk them by folding and squeezing the tubing, section by section. Observe for other signs of tamponade as well, including hypotension, narrowing of the pulse pressure, tachycardia, and weak pulses.

Continuously monitor the patient's cardiac rhythm. Atrial arrhythmias are common postoperatively and may be treated with atrial pacing to synchronize atrial contraction and increase CO. Monitor electrolyte levels, especially potassium levels. Administer potassium replacement as necessary. Titrate vasoactive drugs to maintain hemodynamic stability and optimize CO.

Assess the patient's breath sounds and watch for signs and symptoms of fluid overload. After 24 hours, most patients experience a fluid shift that can result in pulmonary edema. Monitor arterial blood gases and assess your patient's readiness to be weaned from the ventilator. After the endotracheal tube has been removed, encourage coughing and deep breathing.

Be aware that your patient may experience mild neurologic dysfunction, including a transient inability to focus her eyes, maintain concentration, or pay attention for short periods of time. She may experience mild confusion and mild hallucinations. Possible causes include the circulation of large volumes of fluid during bypass surgery and fibrin and platelet microemboli. The symptoms usually clear in a few days.

Most patients will be discharged in 5 to 7 days, still weak and vulnerable to complications. Teach your patient about signs and symptoms of possible problems, including infection. Include her family in postoperative teaching as much as pos-sible. Emphasize the importance of her keeping follow-up appointments.

Minimally invasive direct coronary artery bypass

Minimally invasive direct coronary artery bypass allows bypass grafting of the left anterior descending artery without the need for a thoracotomy. Instead, a physician operates through a 3-inch incision between the patient's left nipple and sternum after removing a 2-inch section of rib to gain access. The patient's heart continues to beat during the procedure, eliminating the need for a heart-lung bypass machine. Because of the reduced amount of trauma, hospitalization lasts only 2 to 3 days rather than the 5 to 7 days needed after traditional bypass surgery.

Some surgeons prefer to use a bypass machine even when using this approach. The procedure is then called port-access minimally invasive bypass surgery. Benefits of using a bypass machine include increased patient safety and the ease of working on a heart that's still.

Nursing considerations

Nursing care is similar to that required for traditional bypass surgery, although your patient will progress through the stages of recovery much more quickly.

Patient teaching and follow-up

You'll need to use your teaching skills to emphasize the crucial role that lifestyle choices play in the treatment of CAD and angina. Information obtained and behaviors observed during your admission interview, physical assessment, and ongoing interactions with the patient will help you focus your teaching. Obviously, you'll want to start teaching immediately after admission, continue throughout your patient's stay, and hopefully, follow up after discharge.

Start by determining what your patient already knows about CAD and angina. Then get an idea of how your patient prefers to learn. As you know, some people prefer to learn by doing, others by reading, and still others by hearing information spoken aloud. Some, perhaps most, patients learn best when they receive information through several routes: verbal explanation backed by written instructions, for example.

Using the methods you believe best suited to your patient, encourage her to learn as much as possible about CAD, angina, and the influence of lifestyle choices on their development. Give the patient the following information:

- basic myocardial physiology
- development of CAD
- modifiable risk factors for CAD and angina
- basics of a heart-healthy diet, including specifics about fats, sodium, potassium, calorie counting, and label reading
- guidelines for safe exercise
- drugs to take, including their names, intended effects, dosages, and adverse effects
- local groups and agencies to contact for support or additional information
- developments that warrant contacting the physi-

cian or activating the emergency medical system.

Try to involve the patient's family members as much as possible in your teaching.

Make use of whatever resources can help you in the teaching process. For example, solicit help from a dietitian when devising a nutritional plan for your patient. Use videotapes, handouts, and other reading material whenever possible. Remember that a lifetime of habits won't change after one teaching encounter. Provide the patient with positive reinforcement and ongoing evaluation to help her follow through on her resolve to adopt heart-healthy habits. But understand that only she can make real changes in her life.

Document all information provided to your patient, her responses, and the elements included in your plan of care. All this information will prove necessary in monitoring the patient's progress and providing continuity of care.

5

CORONARY ARTERY DISEASE AND ANGINA

Complications

Coronary artery disease (CAD) and stable angina can develop into unstable angina, a complication that may reflect an imminent danger of a myocardial infarction (MI). Also, a patient with CAD or angina may experience a cardiac arrest, a complication that requires immediate lifesaving measures. This chapter refreshes your knowledge of these complications and their treatments so that you can maximize your patient's outcome in each case.

Unstable angina

For most patients with CAD, angina creates a predictable set of signs and symptoms that arise in response to a certain amount of physical exertion. Chest pain typically lasts less than 5 minutes, and it abates readily with rest or nitroglycerin. Many patients become almost comfortable in their knowledge of what produces chest pain, what that pain will feel like, and how long it will last. Each episode reflects the course of previous ones, and each responds to similar therapy.

For many patients, however, this picture of stable angina doesn't fit. Instead, their angina becomes unstable. In fact, according to the National Center for Health Statistics, the number of patients hospitalized for unstable angina in the United States rose from 130,000 in 1983 to 570,000 in 1991. More than half of those patients were over age 65; slightly less than half were women.

Clearly, your ability to differentiate between unstable and stable angina has become more important than ever.

Defining the problem

Commonly, a patient who develops unstable angina will report a change in her pattern of chest pain. She may say that the pain arises in response to diminishing levels of activity, such as when she's sitting still or sleeping soundly. And it doesn't respond readily to repeated doses of sublingual nitroglycerin (see *Characteristics of unstable angina,* page 94).

Even patients with no history of CAD may report symptoms of unstable angina. Whether a patient has a history of CAD or not, however, you should consider any new angina to be unstable until proven otherwise.

Unstable angina represents a medical emergency. In response to it, you'll first help to confirm a diagnosis, if necessary. Then you'll administer treatments designed to reduce the symptoms by increasing myocardial perfusion. Sometimes, you'll need to perform diagnostic and treatment measures simultaneously to stabilize the patient's condition and reduce her risk of having an MI. About 1 in 10 patients with unstable angina eventually has an MI, usually after prolonged episodes of severe chest pain.

Pathophysiology

In most cases, unstable angina probably results from a change in existing atherosclerotic lesions that leads to impaired myocardial perfusion even without an increase in myocardial oxygen demand. For example, a plaque that ruptures may lead to clot formation and coronary artery

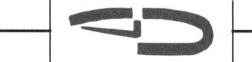

DANGEROUS COMPLICATIONS

Characteristics of unstable angina

A patient with stable angina or coronary artery disease may develop unstable angina, a dangerous complication that may signal an impending myocardial infarction. To help your patient avoid this life-threatening event, stay alert for these telltale signs and symptoms of unstable angina:
- angina that lasts longer than 20 minutes and doesn't abate with rest or sublingual nitroglycerin
- recent increases in the frequency, intensity, or duration of chest-pain episodes
- radiation of pain to a new location
- new signs and symptoms accompanying chest pain, such as diaphoresis, nausea, and palpitations.

spasm, further reducing—even blocking—the myocardial blood supply.

Likewise, a change in the topography of an atherosclerotic lesion could lead to obstruction. Ulcers may form on the plaque's roughened, irregular surface, or a thrombus (commonly a piece of hardened plaque or a fibrin clot created by hemorrhage) may become lodged in the narrowed coronary artery lumen. In either case, platelets migrate to the area and interact with platelets in the thrombus or damaged plaque, possibly triggering vasospasm. These mechanisms cause your patient to experience pain at rest.

For many patients with unstable angina, thrombus-induced vasospasm plays an important role in myocardial ischemia. Thrombosis induces formation of platelet plugs inside the vessel, release of thromboplastin, and subsequent activation of the clotting cascade. As the vessel becomes more and more occluded, the components of the thrombus—platelets, fibrin, erythrocytes, and leukocytes—prompt the release of vasoconstricting substances that cause the surrounding vessel to spasm, thus depleting or blocking the supply of circulating oxygenated blood.

Assessment

If your patient has no history of CAD, you'll first need to determine that her discomfort stems from angina rather than from one of the many other conditions that can cause chest pain and related symptoms. You'll need to confirm that she has unstable angina (rather than stable angina) and determine her risk of having an MI. You'll also need to verify that she hasn't already had an MI. Throughout your assessment, be prepared to administer treatments as needed and ordered to stabilize the patient's condition and ensure myocardial perfusion.

Start by having your patient describe her signs and symptoms. As with patients who have stable angina, a patient with unstable angina probably will describe crushing or squeezing chest pain. She may say it feels as though someone is sitting on her chest. Or she may have trouble describing the pain in specific terms, portraying it instead as a funny feeling, a sensation of fullness in her chest, or a numbness or tingling in her arms or neck.

As your patient describes her symptoms, listen for reports of increasing levels of pain in recent days or weeks or pain that now begins without exertional provocation—both keys to a diagnosis of unstable as opposed to stable angina. Make special note of evidence that the pain no longer subsides with rest or nitroglycerin and that it lasts longer than 20 minutes. Also, stay alert for reports of other symptoms, such as dizziness, weakness, shortness of breath, and nausea, all of which may indicate unstable angina.

If the patient hasn't been diagnosed with CAD, quickly evaluate her risk factors to help rule out other possible causes of chest discomfort (see *Conditions that mimic unstable angina*). Obtain her temperature, blood pressure, and blood samples to test hemoglobin levels, hematocrit, and thyroid function.

Especially if the patient still feels chest pain, obtain an electrocardiogram (EGG) right away. If you can obtain it during an episode of unstable angina, you'll see ST-segment depression of 1 mm or more—a sign of myocardial ischemia. You also may see T waves that are abnormally tall and peaked or deeply inverted. When you examine the patient, you may detect a transient third or fourth heart sound (S_3 or S_4), a murmur of mitral regurgitation, or a precordial lift.

Other tests commonly ordered for a patient who may have unstable angina include the following:

- electrolyte levels, liver function, and kidney function to ensure safe and effective drug action
- cardiac enzyme levels to rule out an MI
- serial ECGs to look for signs of an MI, such as ST-segment elevation, T-wave changes, and Q-wave formation
- cardiac catheterization and coronary angiography to confirm a diagnosis of CAD
- pulse oximetry or arterial blood gas (ABG) analysis to identify problems with myocardial oxygen supply.

Treatment

The treatment for unstable angina depends almost entirely on the severity of the patient's symptoms and the speed with which they've progressed from stable to unstable angina. Naturally, your first priority is to deliver any treatments needed to stabilize your patient's condition. For example, if the patient shows cyanosis and respiratory distress, begin giving her supplemental oxygen, as ordered. Monitor her oxygen saturation levels via pulse oximetry or ABG analysis. And confine her to complete bed rest for as long as her symptoms linger.

Determine as soon as possible whether the patient has just experienced or is still experiencing an MI. If so, her physician may want to begin thrombolytic therapy right away. If not, you'll most likely administer a series of drugs to restore her myocardial perfusion (see *Drug therapy for unstable angina,* page 96). A few patients may need balloon counterpulsation as well.

Drug therapy

Except in cases of hypersensitivity or active bleeding, the first and most basic drug ordered for patients with unstable angina is aspirin. Start by giving the patient a 325-mg aspirin tablet. In all likelihood, unless she receives a stronger anticoagulant, she'll continue this aspirin therapy indefinitely after discharge, as prescribed.

If the patient's symptoms and ECG changes continue, prepare to administer a nitrate sublingually or I.V., morphine I.V., or a beta-blocker I.V. If the patient has hypertension or continued symptoms despite beta-blocker therapy, antici-

Conditions that mimic unstable angina

When you're assessing a patient for unstable angina, remember that several other serious health problems can cause similar signs and symptoms. Consider the possibility that your patient has one of these conditions instead:

- aortic dissection
- aortic valve disease
- esophageal rupture
- gastroesophageal reflux disease
- hiatal hernia
- hypertrophic cardiomyopathy
- leaking or ruptured thoracic aneurysm
- myocardial infarction
- pericarditis with tamponade
- pneumothorax
- pulmonary embolism
- rupture or ischemia of abdominal organs.

pate giving a calcium channel blocker. For patients at high risk for having an MI, expect to give heparin I.V. and titrate the dosage to achieve an activated partial thromboplastin time of 1.5 to 2.5 times the control.

Keep in mind that patients who don't respond to single-drug therapy may benefit from therapy with a beta-blocker, nitrate, and calcium channel blocker. In fact, many physicians begin multiple-drug therapy right away for patients who have unstable angina. Doing so can quickly increase the myocardial oxygen supply while simultaneously decreasing oxygen demand.

Another combination involves tirofiban, which is a platelet aggregate inhibitor, given with aspirin and heparin. Within 30 minutes, tirofiban inhibits platelet aggregation by 90% and continues to do so throughout therapy. As ordered, give your patient a loading dose of tirofiban I.V. over 30 minutes. Then infuse a maintenance dose for up to 48 hours.

Balloon counterpulsation

Usually, unstable angina doesn't respond as well to drug therapy as stable angina does. What's more, patients with unstable angina tend to have poorer heart function. That's why, if your patient's unstable angina fails to respond to

Drug therapy for unstable angina

Drug	Indications	Contraindications	Usual dose
aspirin	• unstable angina with electrocardiogram changes	• bleeding or high risk of bleeding	• 325 mg oral dose or 80 mg chewable dose daily
heparin	• high-risk unstable angina	• bleeding or high risk of bleeding • history of thrombocytopenia caused by heparin • recent cerebrovascular accident (CVA)	• 80 units (U)/kg by I.V. bolus • continuous infusion of 18 U/kg/hr titrated to keep activated partial thromboplastin time at 1.5 to 2.5 times control • if continuous infusion not possible, 5,000 U by I.V. bolus every 4 hours
tirofiban	• unstable angina	• active internal bleeding • bleeding within previous 30 days • history of arteriovenous malformation, CVA, intracranial bleeding, tumor, or aneurysm • major surgery or traumatic injury within previous 30 days • severe hypertension • signs or symptoms of aortic dissection • acute pericarditis	• initial dose, 0.4 µg/kg/min by I.V. infusion over 30 minutes • maintenance dose, 0.1 µg/kg/min by continuous I.V. infusion
nitrates	• unremitting pain or ischemia	• hypotension	• up to three sublingual tablets, one every 5 minutes • 5 to 10 µg/min I.V. • oral or topical therapy after 24 hours symptom-free
morphine	• unremitting pain after administration of nitrate and beta-blocker	• hypotension • respiratory depression • confusion • obtundation	• 2 to 5 mg I.V. • repeated every 5 to 30 minutes, as needed
beta-blockers	• unstable angina	• PR interval < 0.24 seconds • second-degree or third-degree atrioventricular heart block • heart rate > 60 beats per minute • systolic blood pressure < 90 mm Hg • shock • left ventricular heart failure • severe reactive airway disease	• for metoprolol I.V., 1 to 5 mg every 5 minutes by slow (1-minute to 2-minute) infusion to a total of 15 mg; after 1 to 2 hours, 25 to 50 mg orally every 6 hours. • for esmolol I.V., optional loading dose of 0.5 mg/kg over 2 to 5 minutes; then, 0.1 mg/kg/min increased in increments of 0.05 mg/kg/min every 10 to 15 minutes until desired effect achieved or 0.2 mg/kg/min reached. • for propranolol I.V., 0.5 to 1.0 mg. • for atenolol I.V., 5 mg followed 5 minutes later by another 5 mg; after 1 to 2 hours, 50 to 100 mg orally each day.

drug therapy, you should anticipate the possibility of therapy with intra-aortic balloon pump counterpulsation. To begin this therapy, a physician threads a balloon catheter through a femoral puncture or cutdown and up the patient's abdominal aorta almost to the subclavian artery. There the balloon deflates with each systole and inflates with each diastole. As a result, coronary artery perfusion increases, and preload and afterload decrease. A physician sutures the catheter in place until the source of the patient's angina can be identified and corrected. Although patients awaiting heart transplantation have lived for several months on this therapy, it typically lasts from a few hours to a few days.

When the balloon inflates during diastole, it forces blood toward the openings of the coronary arteries located at the base of the aorta. It also forces blood toward the brain and backward toward the renal arteries, increasing perfusion in all three areas. As the balloon deflates just before systole, pressure in the aorta drops, which reduces afterload and some preload.

The reduction in afterload reduces myocardial workload and oxygen demand, which usually causes a rapid and complete resolution of angina. If it doesn't, consider the possibility that the patient may have other problems such as aortic dissection, esophageal rupture, perforated peptic ulcer, or pneumothorax.

As you would expect, successful therapy requires precise timing of balloon inflation and deflation. Indeed, improper timing can harm the patient. That's why the balloon function typically is linked to continuous arterial pressure monitoring; when the balloon inflates in sync with the dicrotic notch, proper timing is virtually guaranteed. To wean the patient from this therapy, a physician may adjust the inflation to take place with every other heartbeat for a prescribed period of time.

In everyday practice, few patients undergo balloon counterpulsation therapy. Other options for those whose symptoms can't be controlled adequately with drugs include angioplasty, atherectomy, and surgical revascularization. The treatment of choice depends on the degree to which the patient's angina affects her lifestyle, the amount of atherosclerosis she has, the risk she faces of having an MI, and her overall health status.

Nursing considerations

In the emergency phase of unstable angina, all members of the health care team must work together efficiently and effectively. Assessing and documenting the patient's pain—and helping to ease her anxiety—probably will fall largely to you.

When asking your patient about her pain, document her description in her own words. Don't interpret what your patient tells you; instead, record what she says. Have her rate the severity of her pain on a scale of 0 to 10. Ask whether her pain is worse than anginal pain she has felt before; if it is, ask how much worse. Then have her continue to rate her pain level as she undergoes treatment.

Be prepared to start at least three I.V. lines to deliver nitroglycerin, heparin, an analgesic, and possibly an antiarrhythmic and a thrombolytic.

Assess your patient's cardiopulmonary status continuously. Palpate her anterior chest wall for thrills or heaves. Auscultate over the pericardium to detect an irregular heart rhythm or a new S_3 or S_4. While you auscultate, palpate your patient's radial pulse to confirm that she has adequate peripheral perfusion. Record her vital signs every 10 to 15 minutes while she continues to feel pain.

Also, make note of your patient's breathing. Assess the amount of effort it requires, and watch for the use of accessory muscles along her chest wall. Auscultate her anterior and posterior lung fields for adventitious breath sounds. Report any abnormal findings to the physician.

Make sure you take time to translate your findings into appropriate nursing interventions. For example, if you auscultate crackles in the patient's lung fields, elevate the head of her bed to ease her work of breathing and, consequently, her myocardial workload.

Patient teaching

Before discharge, help your patient understand the influence of modifiable and nonmodifiable risk factors on her current condition and her risk of future cardiac problems. If she already has been diagnosed with CAD or stable angina, she probably has heard this information before. Perhaps after an even closer brush with death, however, she'll be more ready to listen and respond.

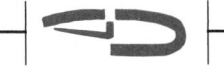

DANGEROUS COMPLICATIONS

Imminent myocardial infarction: Assessing your patient's risk

Identifying your patient's risk of an imminent myocardial infarction (MI) from unstable angina could be the key to saving her life. Use this list to help identify her risk level; remember that she faces the highest risk of having an MI when the signs and symptoms of unstable angina first appear.

High risk
Your patient has a high risk of an imminent MI if she has one or more of the following characteristics:
• angina that lasts more than 20 minutes and that doesn't resolve with rest or nitroglycerin
• angina that occurs at rest and produces ST-segment changes greater than 1 mm on the patient's electrocardiogram (ECG)
• angina accompanied by pulmonary edema, a new or worsening murmur of mitral regurgitation, a third heart sound, new or worsening crackles, or hypotension.

Intermediate risk
Your patient has an intermediate risk of an imminent MI if she has no high-risk factors but one or more of the following characteristics:
• an episode of angina that occurs at rest, lasts 20 minutes or more, and resolves with rest or nitroglycerin
• angina that occurs during sleep
• angina with pathologic Q waves or a resting ST-segment depression of less than 1 mm in the anterior, inferior, and lateral leads on the patient's ECG.
• age 65 or older.

Low risk
Your patient has a low risk of an imminent MI if she has no high-risk or intermediate-risk factors but one or more of the following:
• an increase in the frequency, severity, or duration of angina
• angina caused by lower levels of activity than usual
• anginal episodes beginning within the last 2 months
• no ECG changes.

Whether or not you sense her willingness to change, carefully review the tenets of a heart-healthy life, including diet, exercise, cholesterol reduction, and smoking cessation.

Also, review with her the signs and symptoms of unstable angina. Explain that certain signs and symptoms indicate a relatively low risk of an imminent MI and that others warn of an immediate danger (see *Imminent myocardial infarction: Assessing your patient's risk*). Remind her that her ability and her family's ability to recognize these signs and symptoms can literally save her life.

Finally, make sure the patient knows how to activate the emergency medical system in her area, and describe the circumstances under which she should do so.

Cardiac arrest

Despite all the medical and nursing interventions used to treat CAD and angina, some patients experience cardiac arrest. In rare cases, cardiac arrest is the patient's first sign of CAD.

Obviously, a cardiac arrest requires immediate assessment and a prompt, coordinated response to make sure the patient receives the treatment that can save her life. To function effectively, each member of the responding code team must understand and adhere to assigned roles. Knowing your role in a cardiac arrest situation—and knowing how to perform that role with skill—will set you up to participate fully and successfully in this lifesaving intervention.

Pathophysiology

Many factors contribute to cardiac arrest, but none is more important than arrhythmias. As you know, an arrhythmia can begin for a number of reasons; when the patient has CAD, however, the reason typically relates to myocardial irritability caused by hypoxia. When coronary arteries become occluded, lack of oxygen weakens and injures the heart muscle. This diseased, fatigued myocardium can't contract properly and may eventually stop contracting altogether.

If it continues contracting, it may do so weakly or unevenly. Electrical conduction through the damaged area can become abnormal, slow, or uncoordinated. The amount of electrical energy needed to stimulate a contraction (the action potential or threshold) may be altered as well. What's more, this damaged area of myocardium may generate its electrical impulses at a different rate and rhythm than the rest of the heart. Clearly, any myocardial challenge could spell disaster.

Treatment

Managing a cardiac arrest involves taking a series of steps outlined in the American Heart Association's (AHA's) cardiac life-support protocols. These protocols contain general instructions for handling a cardiac arrest, known as basic cardiac life-support guidelines. The protocols also contain specific instructions for responding to such arrhythmias as ventricular fibrillation (VF), pulseless ventricular tachycardia (VT), pulseless electrical activity, and asystole. These specific instructions are known as advanced cardiac life-support (ACLS) guidelines.

If you discover that your patient is unresponsive, pulseless, and not breathing, you'll need to call a code. Each health care facility defines specific procedures for doing so; make sure you know the proper procedures in your facility.

Also, make sure you know your patient's code status. Each facility has a policy for identifying code status. For example, your patient may have a code number in her chart and next to her name above her bed. Or she may have a colored sticker instead. Your patient's code status could place her anywhere in this range:
• do not resuscitate (also called a no code)
• partial (or chemical) code
• full code.

If you don't know the patient's code status, you must respond to a cardiac arrest with a full code. After following the procedures specified by your facility to initiate the code, begin cardiopulmonary resuscitation (CPR) and continue performing it until someone arrives to help you.

Cardiopulmonary resuscitation

The cornerstone of basic cardiac life support, CPR involves confirming a cardiac arrest; checking the patient's airway, breathing, and circulation; and providing cardiopulmonary support. This response must begin within 4 to 6 minutes after the arrest, or the patient will die (see *When your patient is unresponsive,* page 100).

If the patient isn't breathing and you observe that she's cyanotic and has dilated pupils, open her airway using the head-tilt, chin-lift maneuver. If she doesn't start breathing, begin breathing artificially for her. Use a bag-valve mask whenever possible rather than performing mouth-to-mouth resuscitation. If you can't feel the patient's carotid pulse, begin administering external cardiac compressions as well.

Give 15 compressions at a rate of 80 to 100 beats per minute (bpm), then give two ventilations. After delivering four cycles of this pattern, check for a carotid pulse. If you can't feel one, give two more ventilations and continue the cycle. Check for a carotid pulse every 60 seconds.

Basic and advanced life support both begin with CPR. In fact, once a code begins, CPR continues unbroken throughout the code except for these reasons:
• The patient needs to be assessed (every few minutes but not for more than 7 seconds at a time).
• The patient needs defibrillation.
• The patient's pulse and breathing have returned.
• Other procedures, such as a thoracotomy or drug delivery down an endotracheal tube, must be performed.
• The team leader has pronounced that the patient is dead.

Keep in mind that if you're doing CPR correctly, you'll be able to palpate a carotid pulse and see a QRS complex on the patient's ECG during chest compressions. Also, the patient's chest will rise and fall with artificial ventilations. However, even if done correctly, CPR may still leave the patient at risk for brain damage, aspiration of vomitus, and fractured ribs that may puncture a lung or lacerate her liver.

When possible, have someone else perform CPR when the code team arrives. That leaves you free to assess the situation, identify members of the team, and clear the room of other patients, personnel, and clutter to give team members enough room to work effectively. Immediately give the team leader a brief report of what happened, any drugs the patient takes, any allergies the patient has, and her recent vital signs and cardiac status. Your report will help the team leader make adjustments to the standard resuscitation protocol, as needed.

Keep in mind that intubation offers the best method for managing your patient's airway during a cardiac arrest. An anesthesiologist, a certified nurse anesthetist, or a physician will intubate the patient when the code team arrives. Be-

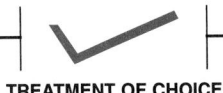

TREATMENT OF CHOICE

When your patient is unresponsive

If you think your patient is in cardiac arrest, respond with these basic cardiac life-support measures:

- Call a code.
- Assess breathing.

Patient is breathing.

Patient is not breathing.

Unless contraindicated, place patient in recovery position.

- Give two slow breaths.
- Assess circulation.

Patient has a pulse.

Patient has no pulse.

- Perform rescue breathing.
- Give oxygen as ordered.
- Establish I.V. access.
- Take vital signs.
- Assist with endotracheal intubation.
- Obtain a 12-lead electrocardiogram.
- Consider history and examination findings to determine cause.

- Start cardiopulmonary resuscitation.
- Watch for pulseless ventricular tachycardia (VT) or fibrillation (VF) on monitor.

Patient has VT or VF.

Patient doesn't have VT or VF.

- Follow steps for treating pulseless VT and VF.

- Assist with endotracheal intubation.
- Confirm tube placement using end-tidal carbon dioxide levels.
- Confirm adequate ventilations.
- Determine the cardiac rhythm and the underlying cause.

Electrical activity is present.

Electrical activity isn't present.

- Follow steps for treating pulseless electrical activity.

- Follow steps for treating asystole.

sides providing a patent airway, the tube allows for administration of drugs to treat the arrest. The AHA lists four drugs that can be administered into an endotracheal tube: lidocaine, atropine, naloxone, and epinephrine. Remember to stop giving chest compressions while drugs are being administered down an endotracheal tube.

Also, remember to monitor your patient's endotracheal tube carefully so that you can quickly determine if it slips into one of her bronchi. Watch carefully for bilateral chest expansion, assess periodically for breath sounds, and track the patient's ABG levels, pulse oximetry readings, and carbon dioxide levels to assess for effective ventilation and oxygenation.

Defibrillation

Although CPR is widely recognized and accepted as a lifesaving procedure for patients in cardiac arrest, patients who undergo defibrillation right away rather than receiving continued CPR are more likely to survive. Consequently, hospitals require that you follow ACLS standards, which include defibrillation, when responding to a cardiac arrest.

As you know, defibrillation involves delivering one or more brief electrical shocks to the patient's heart. The procedure must be performed by a person trained to operate the defibrillator.

To perform defibrillation, the staff member places two paddles on the patient's chest in the specified positions (see *Defibrillation: Placing the paddles correctly*). Then the patient receives a shock of 200 joules. If that fails to convert her heart to a sinus rhythm, she'll receive another shock at 300 joules, possibly followed by another at 360 joules.

To prevent the current from arcing through the air outside the patient's body—or possibly through the operator's body, causing an arrhythmia instead of curing one—the operator must place pads or conduction gel between the paddles and the patient's skin to ensure complete contact.

Oxygen

By giving supplemental oxygen during a cardiac arrest, you can help to ensure delivery of sufficient oxygen to the patient's tissues, especially her brain. Hyperventilation with a bag-valve mask delivers 100% oxygen and helps to reverse the process of metabolic and respiratory acidosis that begins immediately after cardiac arrest.

Defibrillation: Placing the paddles correctly

Place one paddle on the right midclavicular line over the third intercostal space. Place the other on the left midclavicular line at the fifth or sixth intercostal space. With the paddles in these positions, the ventricles lie in the path of the electrical current. Incorrect placement of the paddles can leave the ventricles outside this path.

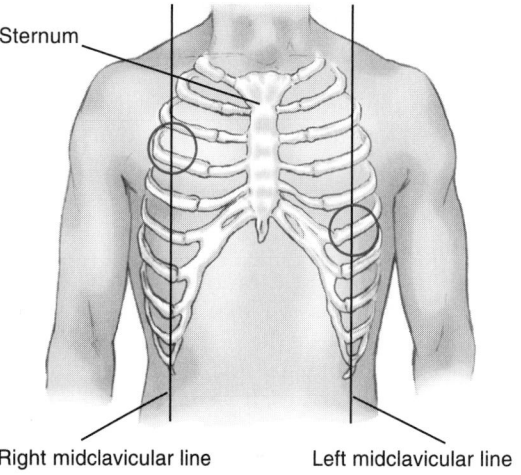

Sternum

Right midclavicular line   Left midclavicular line

Drug therapy

Depending on your patient's rhythm at the start of the cardiac arrest, you may be asked to administer a number of drugs, including atropine, epinephrine, lidocaine, procainamide, bretylium, magnesium sulfate, and sodium bicarbonate.

Atropine

A parasympathetic inhibitor, atropine stops the effects of certain chemicals that create bradycardia and blocks the atrioventricular (AV) node by stimulating the vagus nerve. Thus, atropine raises the heart rate and increases conduction through the AV node.

Epinephrine

This beta-agonist stimulates the heart, constricts blood vessels, and increases heart rate and irritability. You'll use it to treat a cardiac arrest (mainly asystole) because it exerts strong cardiac stimulation, makes the waves of VF more coarse, and may help to convert pulseless VT into a normal sinus rhythm. It also increases coronary artery perfusion pressure and increases the heart rate in patients unresponsive to atropine.

Lidocaine
Used to increase the electrical stimulation threshold (action potential) of the myocardium, lidocaine depresses spontaneous depolarization and automaticity in the ventricles. It's highly effective for treating ventricular arrhythmias.

Procainamide
Typically, you'll use procainamide (also an antiarrhythmic) if your patient doesn't respond to or can't tolerate lidocaine. Procainamide has properties similar to those of lidocaine; it slows conduction and prolongs the refractory period for repolarization, making it useful for treating both atrial and ventricular arrhythmias.

Bretylium
Another antiarrhythmic, bretylium can be used to treat VF or pulseless VT that resists lidocaine or procainamide. It raises the VF threshold and lengthens the action potential and effective refractory period of the ventricles. It also interferes with release of norepinephrine, a neurotransmitter that speeds the heart rate, increases atrial and ventricular conduction and contractility, and boosts catecholamine uptake by the nerve endings.

Magnesium sulfate
Magnesium sulfate helps to counteract the excitability of irritable myocardial tissue that occurs with VF and VT. A low serum magnesium level leads to increased neuromuscular irritability by diminishing the excitation threshold of the motor nerves and enhancing myofibril contraction.

Sodium bicarbonate
Used on occasion to correct metabolic or respiratory acidosis, sodium bicarbonate is a pH buffer produced by the body that binds with free hydrogen ions. It's no longer given routinely, but you may be asked to administer it to a patient who responds poorly to other treatments. Many drugs have a reduced effect when the patient develops acidosis.

Responding to arrhythmias
The most common rhythms of cardiac arrest include VF, pulseless VT, pulseless electrical activity, and asystole. Each requires immediate intervention, including CPR to generate temporary oxygenation and circulation. Even with prompt CPR, however, only 20% to 30% of patients survive these arrhythmias without receiving ACLS. Indeed, unless effective treatment begins within 4 to 6 minutes of the arrest, the patient may sustain permanent brain damage or may die.

Pulseless ventricular tachycardia and ventricular fibrillation
Any factor that greatly increases the body's metabolic demands—such as burns, drug toxicity, electrolyte imbalance, hemorrhage, shock, or traumatic injury—could cause VT, VF, or cardiac arrest. Most likely VT results from a reentry mechanism, in which an electrical impulse fires during a vulnerable portion of the cardiac cycle, usually ventricular repolarization. Initially, a patient with VT may have a pulse. The ventricle contracts rapidly, commonly at 150 bpm or faster. Eventually, the shortened ventricular filling time causes a rapid drop in blood pressure, resulting in hypoxia and hypoperfusion of the brain, heart, and vital organs. Carbon dioxide accumulates in the bloodstream, and the body enters an acidotic state, causing further myocardial irritability. The myocardium becomes hypoxic and fatigued; contractions become weak and disorganized, and the heart begins to wriggle or shake rapidly.

The patient now has VF, a condition that can be treated only with defibrillation, which may cause the heart to depolarize and allow the sinoatrial node to resume normal conduction. The best course of action for VF and pulseless VT is immediate defibrillation with 200, then 200 to 300, and then 360 joules in rapid succession (see *Responding to pulseless ventricular tachycardia and ventricular fibrillation*).

If your patient has VT and a pulse along with such signs and symptoms as hypotension, shortness of breath, chest pain, and a decreased level of consciousness, she'll need cardioversion timed to coincide with ventricular systole (her R wave). This timing will help to avoid the possibility of triggering VF by stimulating the ventricle during repolarization (the T wave). In this setting, the defibrillator will discharge the current when it detects the R wave. It may wait a few cycles to learn your patient's rhythm.

If the patient's heart fails to resume a regular rhythm after three defibrillation shocks, you'll

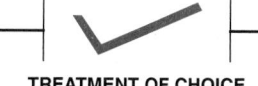

Responding to pulseless ventricular tachycardia and ventricular fibrillation

Cardiac arrest commonly results from ventricular fibrillation (VF), a condition that typically results from pulseless ventricular tachycardia (VT). In most cases, a code team can restore a patient's pulse using these measures:

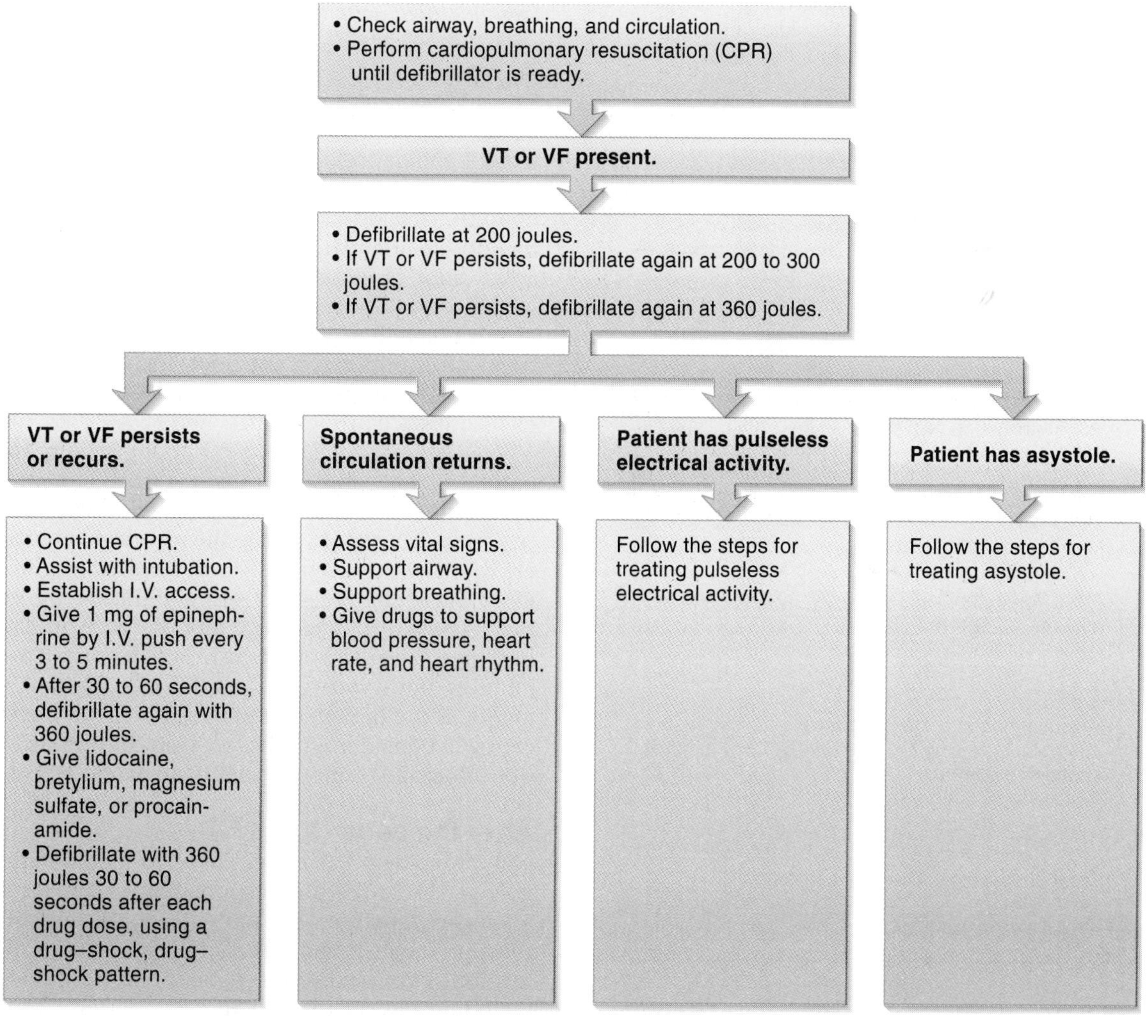

- Check airway, breathing, and circulation.
- Perform cardiopulmonary resuscitation (CPR) until defibrillator is ready.

VT or VF present.

- Defibrillate at 200 joules.
- If VT or VF persists, defibrillate again at 200 to 300 joules.
- If VT or VF persists, defibrillate again at 360 joules.

VT or VF persists or recurs.

- Continue CPR.
- Assist with intubation.
- Establish I.V. access.
- Give 1 mg of epinephrine by I.V. push every 3 to 5 minutes.
- After 30 to 60 seconds, defibrillate again with 360 joules.
- Give lidocaine, bretylium, magnesium sulfate, or procainamide.
- Defibrillate with 360 joules 30 to 60 seconds after each drug dose, using a drug–shock, drug–shock pattern.

Spontaneous circulation returns.

- Assess vital signs.
- Support airway.
- Support breathing.
- Give drugs to support blood pressure, heart rate, and heart rhythm.

Patient has pulseless electrical activity.

Follow the steps for treating pulseless electrical activity.

Patient has asystole.

Follow the steps for treating asystole.

need to follow the AHA's drug protocol in an attempt to chemically convert her heart rhythm back to normal. If the patient has VT and a pulse and is clinically stable, administer lidocaine as ordered.

Pulseless electrical activity
The group of rhythms included in this category generate too weak an impulse and too little blood pressure to sustain life. The category includes idioventricular, ventricular escape, and postdefi-

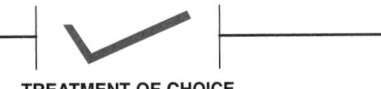

TREATMENT OF CHOICE

Responding to pulseless electrical activity

If your patient has electromechanical dissociation, pseudoelectromechanical dissociation, idioventricular rhythms, ventricular escape rhythms, bradysystolic rhythms, or postdefibrillation idioventricular rhythms, the code team follows these steps:

- Perform cardiopulmonary resuscitation.
- Assist with intubation.
- Establish I.V. access.
- Assess blood flow using Doppler ultrasound, end-tidal carbon dioxide measurements, echocardiography, or arterial line measurements.

- Consider possible causes including acidosis, acute myocardial infarction, cardiac tamponade, hyperkalemia, hypothermia, hypovolemia, hypoxia, pulmonary embolism, tension pneumothorax, and overdose of tricyclic antidepressants, digitalis glycosides, beta-blockers, or calcium channel blockers.

- Give 1 mg of epinephrine by I.V. push every 3 to 5 minutes, as ordered.

- If patient has absolute or relative bradycardia, give 1 mg of atropine by I.V. push every 3 to 5 minutes to a total of 0.03 to 0.04 mg/kg.

- Treat underlying cause, as necessary.

brillation idioventricular rhythms. It also includes electromechanical dissociation, in which the patient has no pulse but shows a heart rhythm on the monitor. In this condition, the conduction system may be working, but the myocardium fails to respond to electrical stimulation. Consequently, never presume that an unconscious patient has a pulse simply because she shows a rhythm on the monitor.

Management of this group of rhythms doesn't involve defibrillation. Instead, the patient should be intubated and receive CPR until the underlying cause of her condition becomes clear. Drugs of choice for pulseless electrical activity include epinephrine, sodium bicarbonate if the patient is acidotic, and atropine (see *Responding to pulseless electrical activity*).

Asystole

At times, an untreated arrhythmia, hypoxia, hypothermia, acidosis, drug overdose, or electrolyte imbalance—such as severe hyperkalemia or hypokalemia—will cause the heart to stop, a condition called asystole. A patient in asystole has no mechanical or electrical cardiac activity and a poor prognosis for recovery. The monitor will show a flat line. (To make sure your patient doesn't have fine VF, turn up the gain, or amplitude, on the monitor and look for small movements. Also, make sure that the lead wires and electrodes are properly attached.)

To treat asystole, perform CPR, make sure the patient is intubated right away, establish I.V. access, and confirm in more than one lead that the patient is in asystole. While the physician considers whether to start transcutaneous pacing, you'll most likely deliver 1 mg of epinephrine by I.V. push every 3 to 5 minutes, as ordered. You also may give 1 mg of atropine by I.V. push every 3 to 5 minutes until you reach a total of 0.03 to 0.04 mg/kg. If the patient doesn't respond, the physician will consider whether to stop the resuscitation effort and pronounce her dead or to continue.

After the code

Fully document the code, the team members involved, their roles and responsibilities, the treatments administered, the patient's responses, and the outcome. Document all follow-up care and teaching provided to the patient and her family, including efforts to help them cope with their fears and emotions.

If the patient didn't survive the cardiac arrest, prepare the body according to your facility's policy. Also, provide support to the patient's family members. As appropriate, allow them to spend time with the patient.

CORONARY ARTERY DISEASE AND ANGINA

Suggested Readings

Braunwald E, et al. *Unstable Angina: Diagnosis and Management.* Clinical practice guideline #10. Rockville, Md: Agency for Health Care Policy and Research and the National Heart, Lung, and Blood Institute, Public Health Service; 1994. US Dept of Health and Human Services AHCPR 94-0602.

Califf R, et al. *Acute Coronary Care.* 2nd ed. St Louis: Mosby, Inc; 1995.

Clinical Practice Guideline, Unstable Angina: Diagnosis and Management. Agency for Health Care Policy and Research, National Heart, Lung, and Blood Institute. US Dept Health and Human Services.

Cummins RO, ed. *Textbook of Advanced Cardiac Life Support.* ACLS/AHA; 1994.

Eckel RH. Obesity and heart disease: a statement for healthcare professionals from the nutrition committee, American Heart Association. *Circulation.* 1997;96(9):3248-3250.

Grundy SM, Balady GJ, Criqui MH, et al. When to start cholesterol-lowering therapy in patients with coronary heart disease: a statement for healthcare professionals from the American Heart Association task force on risk reduction. *Circulation.* 1997;95(6):1683-1685.

Haire-Joshu D. *Management of Diabetes Mellitus: Perspectives of Care across the Life Span.* 2nd ed. St Louis: Mosby, Inc; 1996.

Hartz RS. Minimally invasive heart surgery. Executive committee of the council on cardiothoracic and vascular surgery. *Circulation* 1996; 94(10):2669-2670.

Hennekens CH, Dyken ML, Fuster V, et al. Aspirin as a therapeutic agent in cardiovascular disease: a statement for healthcare professionals from the American Heart Association. *Circulation.* 1997;96(8):2751-2753.

Hjemdahl P, Eriksson SV, Held C, Rehnquist N. Prognosis of patients with stable angina pectoris on antianginal drug therapy. *Am J Cardiol.* 1996;77(16):6D-15D.

Kinney MR, Packa DR. *Andreoli's Comprehensive Cardiac Care.* 8th ed. St Louis: Mosby, Inc; 1995.

Moser DK. Correcting misconceptions about women and heart disease. *Am J Nurs.* 1997; 97(4):26-33.

Ockene IS, Miller NH. Cigarette smoking, cardiovascular disease, and stroke: a statement for healthcare professionals from the American Heart Association. American Heart Association task force on risk reduction. *Circulation.* 1997;96(9):3243-3247.

Olson HG, Aronow WS. Medical management of stable angina and unstable angina in the elderly with coronary artery disease. *Clin Geriatr Med.* 1996;12(1):121-140.

Pearson TA. Alcohol and heart disease. *Circulation.* 1996;94(11):3023-3025.

Rosenfield K, Schainfeld R, Isner JM. Percutaneous revascularization in peripheral arterial disease. *Curr Probl Cardiol.* 1996;21(1):7-93.

Stary HC, Chandler AB, Glagov S, et al. A definition of initial, fatty streak, and intermediate lesions of atherosclerosis. A report from the committee on vasular lesions of the council on arteriosclerosis, American Heart Association. *Circulation.* 1994;89(5):2462-2478.

Valle BK, Lemberg L. Estrogen replacement therapy in women: prevention and treatment of coronary artery disease. *Am J Crit Care.* 1994;3(5):398-401.

Van Horn L. Fiber, lipids, and coronary heart disease: a statement for healthcare professionals from the nutrition committee, American Heart Association. *Circulation.* 1997;95(12):2701-2704.

MYOCARDIAL INFARCTION

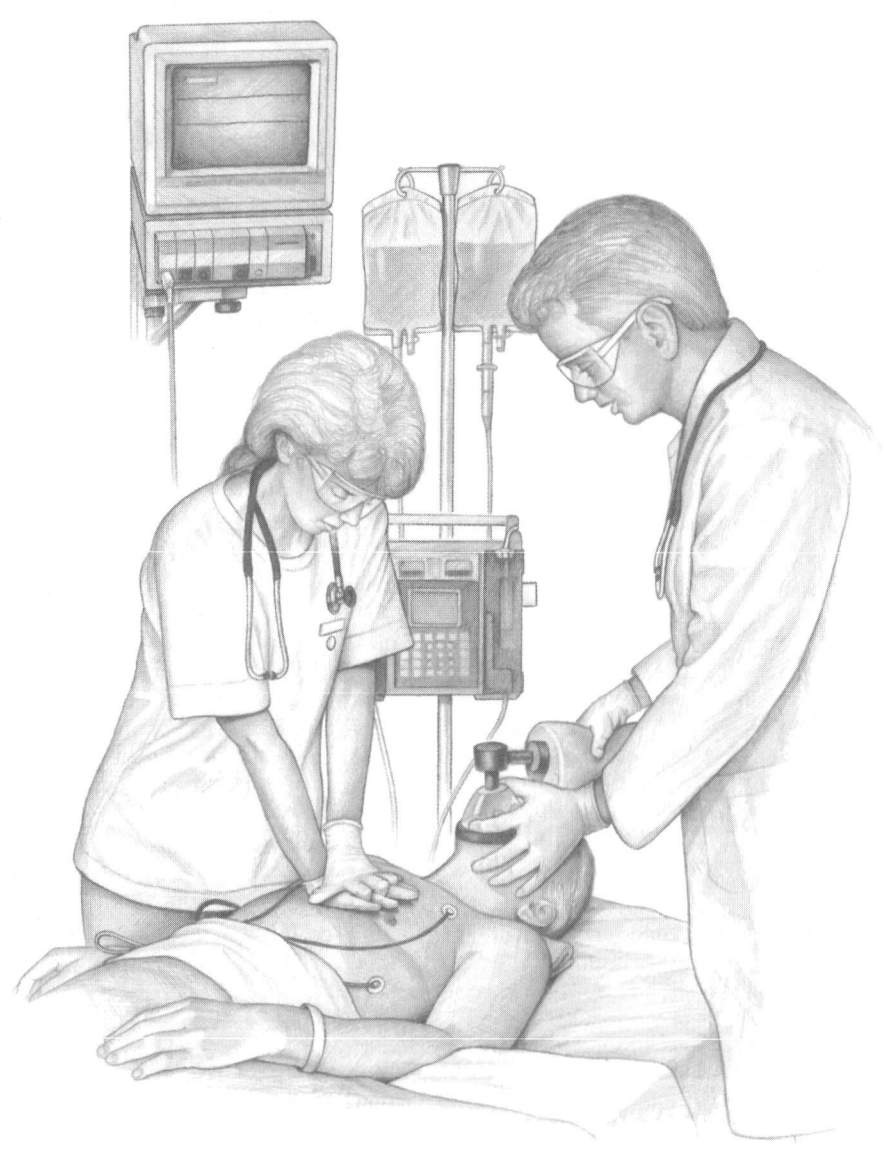

6

MYOCARDIAL INFARCTION

Overview

Each year in the United States, more people die of myocardial infarction (MI) than of any other health problem. About 900,000 Americans have an MI each year, and about 225,000 of them die— more than half before they can reach appropriate medical care.

About 45% of MIs occur in people under age 65, and about 5% occur in people under age 40. Although women have a lower risk of an MI during their younger years, probably because of the protective effect of estrogen, the risk rises to meet and even surpass that of men as they age. Consequently, men and women die of MIs in about equal numbers. Death rates from MIs are higher among African-Americans, both men and women, than among whites.

Clearly, no matter what your patient's age, sex, and race, you must be prepared to differentiate a developing MI from a host of other medical problems. This chapter will help you keep your skills and knowledge fresh by reviewing the pathophysiology of MI, types of MI, and tips for assessing and diagnosing a patient who may be having an MI.

Pathophysiology

In a general sense, the modifiable and nonmodifiable factors that raise the risk of coronary artery disease (CAD) raise the risk of an MI as well. In a more specific sense, however, an MI typically is preceded by a trigger factor that begins the acute infarction process. In fact, up to half the people who have had an MI can identify a specific precipitating factor for it.

Some report engaging in unusually heavy exercise or experiencing extreme mental stress (such as anger) before the signs and symptoms of the MI appeared. What's more, patients hospitalized for the treatment of CAD who also report high levels of stress in their lives face an increased risk of rehospitalization, MI, and death. In all likelihood, these stresses increase the myocardial oxygen demand in a patient at high risk for ruptured atherosclerotic plaque. Other conditions that act as trigger factors by increasing the myocardial oxygen demand include fever and tachycardia.

A decreased circulating blood volume also may trigger an MI. The decrease could result from such problems as acute blood loss caused by surgery or traumatic injury or hypotension caused by hemorrhagic, septic, or anaphylactic shock.

Other factors that may trigger an MI even in a patient who has no history of CAD include the following:
- respiratory infection
- hypoxemia
- pulmonary embolism
- hypoglycemia
- cocaine use
- consumption of ergot preparations, such as ergotamine tartrate for migraine headaches
- consumption of sympathomimetics, such as the nasal decongestant phenylephrine
- traumatic injury to the myocardium or a coronary artery.

The onset of an MI seems to have a strong relationship to circadian rhythms as well. Most MIs begin between 6 A.M. and noon, with 9 A.M. being the most common time. The least common time is 11 P.M. Several physiologic events that take place

What triggers a myocardial infarction?

Any of the following can trigger a myocardial infarction, even in a patient who doesn't have coronary artery disease:
- aortic dissection
- arterial spasm from nitroglycerin withdrawal
- arteritis
- Prinzmetal's angina
- cardiac myxoma
- cardiopulmonary bypass surgery
- coronary arteriography
- emboli from a prosthetic valve
- infective endocarditis
- intracardiac mural thrombus
- anomalous origin of coronary arteries
- coronary arteriovenous fistulas
- coronary artery aneurysm
- coronary artery dissection
- aortic valve insufficiency
- aortic valve stenosis
- carbon monoxide poisoning
- prolonged hypotension
- thyrotoxicosis
- disseminated intravascular coagulation
- hypercoagulability
- polycythemia vera
- thrombocytopenic purpura
- thrombocytosis
- cocaine abuse
- myocardial contusion or other injury
- complication of cardiac catheterization.

in the morning could hold the key to this circadian trigger factor. For example, levels of cortisol and circulating catecholamines increase in the early morning hours. Moreover, assuming an upright position from a recumbent one increases platelet aggregation and blood viscosity, which may promote thrombus formation and precipitate an acute MI (see *What triggers a myocardial infarction?*).

Thrombus formation

Although many factors may trigger an MI, they typically do so via thrombus formation and its consequent obstruction of a coronary artery. A ruptured atherosclerotic plaque can lead to thrombus formation in several ways:
- exposed collagen in the ruptured plaque attracts circulating platelets to form a platelet plug
- thromboplastin released from the ruptured plaque initiates the clotting cascade
- debris from the rupture mechanically obstructs the vessel.

Once formed, the thrombus releases vasoconstrictors, such as thromboxane, serotonin, and thrombin, that further narrow an already narrowed coronary artery.

Coronary artery spasm may play a part in the formation of a coronary thrombus as well by narrowing the arterial lumen, damaging the endothelium, promoting platelet aggregation, and releasing vasoactive substances.

Evolution of a myocardial infarction

As you know, an MI doesn't develop immediately after a thrombus forms. Rather, myocardial cells sustain reversible damage over about the first 20 minutes; then irreversible damage occurs over several hours.

After the obstruction of a coronary artery, the myocardial cells fed by that artery go through a characteristic sequence of events. Between 8 and 10 seconds after the myocardial oxygen supply drops, oxygen reserves are depleted, anaerobic metabolism begins, and myocardial cells become ischemic. Although still alive, the ischemic myocardium doesn't function normally. After about a minute of hypoxia, changes appear on the patient's ECG. After about 20 minutes, ischemic cells begin to die.

If blood flow resumes during that period, the myocardial damage can be reversed, and the myocardium will heal and continue to function. That's why all medical and nursing interventions for a patient with a hypoxic myocardium aim first to restore myocardial blood flow.

Because it has the most tenuous blood supply and the highest oxygen demand, the subendocardial, or innermost area, is where myocardial necrosis begins. Necrotic cells may be interspersed with severely ischemic but living cells in this area, creating small islands of tissue that may either recover or die, depending on how quickly circulation is restored. Over time, the necrotic area may expand, moving like a wave from the subendocardium through to the epicardium, resulting in a full-thickness MI.

Without treatment, the necrotic area will reach its maximum size in about 6 hours—a window of time called the evolving stage. If treatment begins within this 6-hour window, however, and the area is reperfused with blood and oxygen, some of the myocardium can be salvaged. The sooner the reperfusion occurs, the more myocardium can be saved—a realization that led to the adage "time is muscle."

Changes during the evolving stage

Many changes take place at the cellular level during the evolutionary stage of an MI. For one thing, cellular metabolism changes from aerobic to anaerobic, which causes acidosis and electrolyte shifts across the cell membrane. As a result, the cell membranes break and begin to leak enzymes into the bloodstream. They include creatine kinase (CK), lactic dehydrogenase (LD), and aspartate aminotransferase (AST). Although cells across the whole body leak enzymes when damaged, myocardial cells leak particular isoenzymes that can be used as specific markers for diagnosing an MI.

Also, during the evolving phase, the patient experiences an increase in sympathetic nervous system stimulation, especially if he's having an anterior-wall MI. This stimulation creates the fight-or-flight response characterized by an increase in heart rate and myocardial contractility that leads to increased cardiac output (CO). Blood pressure rises as well, from peripheral vasoconstriction.

While this sympathetic response can aid survival in times of danger, it clearly poses its own danger to a person having an MI. Increased catecholamines lead to high myocardial oxygen demands from the resulting tachycardia and increased blood pressure. They also enhance platelet aggregation, raise blood glucose levels, and increase the risk of arrhythmias. High catecholamine levels also may contribute to the anxiety and loss of control that many MI patients feel.

Mechanical changes take place in the heart as well during an acute MI. Myocardial cells suffering from a lack of oxygen, loss of electrolytes, and an acidotic environment lose their contractility, leading to heart failure. The left ventricle loses its ability to pump blood efficiently out of the full heart.

This combination of factors can set the stage for cardiogenic shock, a common complication that involves heart failure and circulatory collapse.

As you assess a patient in the evolving stage of an MI, watch continuously for arrhythmias and for signs of shock that could herald left ventricular pump failure.

Completion of a myocardial infarction

When necrosis has progressed all the way through the area at risk and the outer borders of the infarct become clearly defined, the MI is complete, and the remodeling stage can begin. Remodeling affects both the infarcted area and the ventricular muscle surrounding the infarct. It involves dilation and thinning of the infarcted area and hypertrophy of the remaining myocardium in the left ventricle. The risk of thrombus formation continues in the dilated area where blood flow may be sluggish. Keep in mind that the increased size of the infarcted area doesn't result from continued necrosis.

The infarct can expand, however, probably because damaged muscle cells are no longer bound tightly together. Hypertrophy of the remaining myocardium may result from the extra workload placed on this area by the nonfunctioning infarcted area.

Extension of an infarcted area raises the patient's risk of death considerably. Patients with significant extension also face a higher risk of complications, such as cardiac rupture or a left ventricular aneurysm.

Myocardial repair

Within 24 hours after an MI, the process of repair begins. Leukocytes, especially neutrophils and macrophages, migrate to the necrotic tissue, where they produce proteolytic enzymes that degrade and remove the dead tissue. A collagen matrix forms and eventually turns into scar tissue. By 2 weeks after the MI, the scar has formed but is weak and vulnerable to injury as the patient increases his activity during this time. By 6 weeks after the MI, strong scar tissue has replaced the infarcted area. It's no longer vulnerable, but it also no longer contracts like normal myocardial tissue.

Recognizing a pathologic Q wave

A normal Q wave has less than one-third the amplitude of an R wave and spans less than 0.04 second (one small box on the electrocardiogram paper). After a myocardial infarction, however, Q waves become longer and wider. Be sure to measure amplitude and duration of every Q wave on your patient's electrocardiogram.

Normal Q wave

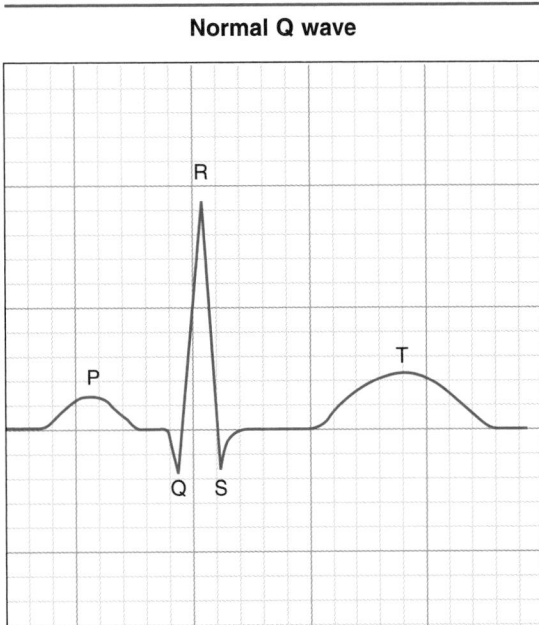

Pathologic Q wave

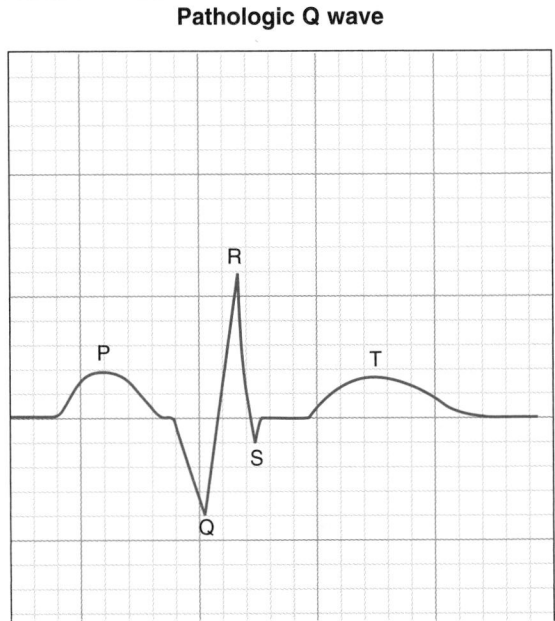

Classifying a myocardial infarction

Many health care professionals classify an MI based on whether it produces Q waves on the patient's electrocardiogram (ECG) and on which area of the heart wall the MI affects. Knowing the classification of your patient's MI gives you a more complete picture of his needs and helps you anticipate treatments and potential complications.

Analyzing Q waves

On a normal ECG tracing, Q waves are small and narrow, and they appear only in certain leads. However, when a person has an MI, Q waves grow larger and appear in any lead that reflects activity in the infarcted area. They're called pathologic Q waves (see *Recognizing a pathologic Q wave*).

In the past, MIs were classified as transmural or subendocardial based on the presence or absence of pathologic Q waves on the patient's ECG. A transmural MI referred to necrosis that extended through all three layers of heart muscle, the presence of pathologic Q waves, and abnormal cardiac enzyme studies. A subendocardial MI referred to necrosis that involved only the innermost layer of the heart, no pathologic Q waves, and abnormal cardiac enzyme studies.

However, Q waves may appear in what used to be called a subendocardial MI and may not appear in what used to be called a transmural MI. Consequently, those terms have been replaced by more accurate terms: *Q-wave MI* and *non-Q-wave*

MI. These ECG-based categories provide useful clinical information because Q-wave MIs usually reflect more damage to the left ventricle and, consequently, a higher risk of death. Interestingly, however, patients with non-Q-wave MIs face a higher risk of extension or reinfarction compared to the risk faced by those with Q-wave MIs. When reinfarction or extension occurs, it usually happens between the 6th and 14th days after the MI.

Locating the infarction

Your patient's MI also can be classified by its location. Knowing the location of your patient's infarct can help you anticipate treatments, common adverse reactions, and complications, which may differ between locations.

To determine the location of your patient's infarction, you'll need to examine his 12-lead ECG for pathologic Q waves and elevated ST segments—the two main electrical clues left by an MI. Remember that ECG changes, which result when damaged myocardial cells disrupt normal depolarization, arise in leads that face the area of infarction (see *Locating a myocardial infarction*). Changes that arise in leads opposite the infarcted areas are referred to as reciprocal changes. Keep in mind that most MIs affect the left ventricle and interventricular septum, although some inferior-wall MIs also involve the right ventricle.

Anterior-wall myocardial infarction
An infarction that affects the front of the heart results from an occlusion of the left anterior descending coronary artery. Because this artery supplies about 40% of the heart's blood, its occlusion can damage much of the myocardial tissue. Indeed, people who have had an anterior-wall MI are more likely to die during the following year than people whose MIs have affected other areas of cardiac tissue.

The ECG changes produced by an anterior-wall MI, such as ST-segment elevation and the development of a Q wave, appear on the leads across the front of the chest: the precordial or V leads, especially V_1 through V_4. Reciprocal changes, such as ST-segment depression, appear in leads II, III, and aV_F.

An anterior-wall MI may cause such arrhythmias as sinus tachycardia, premature ventricular contractions, and atrial flutter or fibrillation. Rapid heart rhythms increase the heart's oxygen demand and reduce the amount of time available for the ventricles to fill during diastole.

Locating a myocardial infarction

When a patient experiences a myocardial infarction (MI), it produces electrocardiogram (ECG) changes. Which leads best show these changes depends on the affected artery and the exact location of the MI. This table gives you a quick reference guide to the relationships among ECG leads, affected arteries, and the locations of MIs.

Leads that show changes	Affected artery	Location of MI
V_1, V_2, V_3, V_4	left anterior descending artery	anterior wall
II, III, aV_F	right coronary artery	inferior wall
V_1, V_2, V_3, V_4	right coronary artery or left circumflex artery	posterior wall
I, aV_L, V_5, V_6	left circumflex artery	lateral wall

This form of an MI also may cause bundle branch blocks because the left anterior descending coronary artery supplies blood to the interventricular septum, where the bundle branches lie. Your nursing interventions will focus on detecting abnormal heart rhythms and treating them promptly.

A patient with an anterior-wall MI may have hypertension, tachycardia, and increased myocardial contractility as a result of increased sympathetic nervous system activity. This sympathetic activity may be a compensatory response to reduced CO by the damaged left ventricle, or it may be a reaction to pain and anxiety. Also, compared with inferior infarctions, anterior-wall MIs cause a higher incidence of pulmonary edema and heart failure.

Inferior-wall myocardial infarction
An inferior-wall MI affects the diaphragmatic surface of the left ventricle and usually results from occlusion of the right coronary artery. The patient's ECG will show ST-segment and T-wave changes

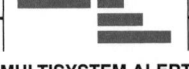

MULTISYSTEM ALERT

Causes of chest pain

Many conditions other than a myocardial infarction can cause chest pain. Use this table to review some of the most important ones.

Condition	Pain characteristics	Other signs and symptoms	Usual treatments
Aortic dissection	• severe stabbing, ripping, or tearing pain in anterior chest • may radiate to shoulders, neck, abdomen, back, or legs as it progresses	• new aortic murmur • reduced or absent peripheral pulses • tachycardia • difference in blood pressure between right and left limbs • altered level of consciousness • paresthesia or paralysis • decreased bowel sounds • oliguria	• blood pressure control • analgesic therapy • surgery
Aortic aneurysm	• substernal chest, abdominal, or back pain, depending on location of aneurysm	• hoarseness and cough • dysphagia • distended neck, chest, or arm veins • dyspnea • pulsating abdominal mass or bruit	• surgery
Pericarditis	• severe, sharp substernal or left-sided chest pain • may radiate to shoulders, arms, neck, and back • worsens with inspiration, coughing, swallowing, moving trunk, and lying down	• fever • friction rub • dyspnea • shallow respirations • ST-segment elevation and T-wave inversion	• position changes • analgesic therapy • anti-inflammatory drugs • antibiotic therapy
Pulmonary embolus	• severe, sharp chest pain	• severe dyspnea • hemoptysis • anxiety • diaphoresis • accentuated pulmonic component of second heart sound • tachycardia • tachypnea • decreased breath sounds	• analgesic therapy • oxygen • anticoagulant therapy • thrombolytic therapy • surgery
Pneumothorax	• mild to severe, sharp or tearing pain on one side of chest	• decreased breath sounds and chest expansion on affected side • dyspnea • cyanosis • tachycardia	• chest-tube insertion
Biliary colic in cholelithiasis	• severe, even excruciating, pain in lower chest around right rib margin • may radiate to back • may occur after eating a heavy meal or while lying down	• tachycardia • diaphoresis • prostration • fever • nausea • vomiting	• analgesic therapy • lithotripsy • cholesterol-lowering drugs • surgery

Causes of chest pain (continued)

Condition	Pain characteristics	Other signs and symptoms	Usual treatments
Costochondritis	• sharp stabbing pain or soreness in rib cage or sternum • worsens with deep inspiration or palpation • doesn't radiate	• shallow respirations • diaphoresis • redness or swelling at site of pain	• position changes • analgesic therapy • corticosteroid therapy
Esophageal spasm	• chest pain similar to Prinzmetal's angina • abrupt pressure, burning, tightness, or squeezing • may radiate to left arm, neck, jaw, or back	• vomiting • dyspnea	• sedative therapy • nitrate therapy • small, frequent feedings of soft foods • surgery
Hiatal hernia	• burning in chest or midepigastric area • may radiate upward • may occur with stress, eating, drinking alcohol, smoking, bending over, or lying down	• heartburn • regurgitation • diaphoresis	• sitting upright • antacid therapy • antisecretory drug • cessation of alcohol use and smoking • surgery

and Q waves in leads II, III, and aV_F. Reciprocal changes appear in the anterior leads V_1 through V_4.

You may see atrioventricular (AV) blocks or sinus bradycardia with an inferior-wall MI because the right coronary artery supplies blood to the AV node in most people and to the sinoatrial node in about half of the people. Inferior-wall MIs also cause parasympathetic nervous system stimulation, which results in hypotension and bradycardia.

Up to 40% of inferior-wall MIs may involve right ventricular infarction as well, a complicating condition that requires different treatment from that used for a typical inferior-wall MI. The patient typically shows signs and symptoms of right ventricular heart failure.

Posterior-wall myocardial infarction
A posterior-wall MI may result from a blockage of either the right coronary artery or the left circumflex artery, depending on which one gives rise to the patient's posterior descending artery, which feeds the posterior wall of the left ventricle. A true posterior-wall MI is uncommon but may accompany an inferior-wall or lateral-wall MI.

Diagnosing a posterior-wall MI by ECG is challenging because no leads face the posterior surface of the heart. Consequently, you have to rely on reciprocal changes that appear in leads V_1 through V_4. They include ST-segment depression, large R waves (which actually are reflected Q waves), and elevated T waves.

Lateral-wall myocardial infarction
An occlusion of the left circumflex artery results in an infarction of the heart's lateral wall on the left side. The ECG changes appear in leads I, aV_L, V_5, and V_6 because they record activity on the heart's far left side. Reciprocal changes appear in leads V_1 through V_3. Occasionally, a patient may have an isolated lateral-wall MI; usually it accompanies an anterior-wall or inferior-wall infarction. A true lateral-wall infarction causes the fewest complications and is least likely to prompt negative hemodynamic responses.

Assessment and diagnosis

When a patient complains of chest pain, your first instinct may be to suspect angina or an MI. But, as you know, not all chest pain is caused by angina or an MI (see *Causes of chest pain*). In-

Facts about women and myocardial infarction

- Women over age 65 are more likely than men to die within a few weeks after a myocardial infarction (MI).
- During the first year after an MI, 44% of women are likely to die compared with 27% of men.
- During the next 6 years after an MI, 31% of women will sustain a second MI compared with 23% of men.
- African-American women ages 35 to 74 have a 38% greater risk of death after an MI than white women do.
- Women are less likely than men to return to work, resume sexual activity, and return to previous social activities after an MI. They may also report more life changes, anxiety, depression, guilt, and marital problems.
- After age 45, women with Type 2 diabetes are twice as likely as men with Type 2 diabetes to have a second MI.
- Women ages 55 and over have higher cholesterol levels than men of similar ages and may need a high-density lipoprotein cholesterol level above 50 mg/dl to receive the same protective benefit men receive at 35 mg/dl.
- Women tend to wait about an hour longer than men before seeking treatment for acute angina.
- Women tend to develop chest pain at rest or under mental stress; men tend to develop it with physical activity.
- Men tend to report severe crushing chest pain; women tend to report nausea, substernal chest or abdominal pain, undue fatigue, and weakness in an arm or a shoulder.
- Women hospitalized for coronary artery disease undergo fewer diagnostic tests and interventions than men.
- Women who undergo coronary artery bypass grafting are more likely than men to die or have unresolved chest pain.
- Women are more likely than men to die in the hospital after percutaneous transluminal coronary angioplasty, possibly because they have smaller arteries and tend to be older and sicker at the time of treatment.

deed, some causes of chest pain have nothing to do with the heart at all. That's why one of your first priorities is to quickly look for clues to other causes of your patient's discomfort. Then you can proceed with a quick but thorough assessment focused on your patient's cardiac status.

Signs and symptoms

Most patients with an acute MI have chest pain—in some cases, an unbearable level of chest pain. More than half of patients with a Q-wave MI (especially an inferior-wall MI) and severe chest pain experience nausea and vomiting as well, probably from vagal stimulation. Remember, too, that opiates commonly given to reduce the pain of an MI can cause nausea and vomiting.

Occasionally, a patient may complain of diarrhea or an urge to defecate during the acute stage of an MI. Other signs and symptoms may include sweating, dizziness, and palpitations, possibly resulting from arrhythmias or cardiogenic shock, a life-threatening complication caused by a decreased CO. Increased catecholamines may produce extreme weakness and a sense of doom.

Remember that the signs and symptoms of an MI may differ somewhat between men and women. For example, about 63% of women don't have previous signs or symptoms, compared with about 48% of men (see *Facts about women and myocardial infarction*).

Chest pain

The typical MI produces precordial or retrosternal chest pain. Your patient may describe it as aching, burning, crushing, tightness, squeezing, or the feeling of a heavy weight on his chest. He may display Levine's sign while describing the pain (a closed fist pressed against his sternum). Keep in mind, however, that a small percentage of patients may have no chest pain at all (see *Signs of a silent myocardial infarction*).

In those who do, the pain typically radiates across the chest and down the medial aspect of the left arm or both arms. It also may extend up to the neck or jaw. Some patients may complain of a tingling, aching, or numbness in the left wrist, hand, and fingers along with severe substernal pain.

Other patients may describe the pain of an MI as indigestion or burning in the upper abdomen. Rarely, a patient may feel pain in his back, particularly between the scapulae. In patients with pre-existing angina, the pain of infarction may affect the same location. Typically, however, it's much more severe, lasts longer, and doesn't respond to rest or nitroglycerin.

Although the pain caused by an MI can vary in intensity, most patients describe it as severe, even unbearable. It may have resolved by the time you see the patient but, usually, it lasts longer than 30 minutes and sometimes up to several hours. Listen for your patient to describe a trigger factor as he explains how, where, and when the MI began.

As with angina, one of the most important assessment steps is to have the patient describe his pain in his own words. Ask him open-ended questions and record the exact words he uses in response. Also, watch his body language for more clues; for example, if he tells you that his pain is "not that bad" but he can't sit still and can't sit up straight, you'll need to investigate further, possibly using different words or comparisons to help him describe the intensity of his pain.

Also, investigate these characteristics of your patient's pain:
• location
• quality
• severity
• onset
• duration
• accompanying signs and symptoms
• factors that cause or contribute to the pain, such as exertion
• factors that reduce or resolve the pain, such as rest.

Keep in mind that both angina and MI pain most likely stem from ischemic or injured tissue rather than infarcted tissue. In fact, restored blood flow should resolve the pain almost immediately. That means that any patient who complains of chest pain is still experiencing ischemia.

General appearance

A patient having an MI usually appears anxious and in considerable distress. His facial expression may look anguished, panicked, or exhausted. He's typically pale, possibly ashen, and beaded with perspiration. You may find him sitting up in bed, gasping for breath, feeling suffocated or at least very short of breath. He may be restless, moving about in bed, trying to find a comfortable

Signs of a silent myocardial infarction

Although most people develop a similar set of signs and symptoms during a myocardial infarction (MI), some have what's called a silent MI. Evidence of a silent MI usually arises well after the fact, during an electrocardiogram ordered for an unrelated reason.

About half of the affected patients can't remember ever having symptoms that could have resulted from an MI. With careful questioning, however, the other half can remember an event that might have been an MI.

Patients most likely to experience a silent MI are those with diabetes or hypertension but no symptoms of angina.

Other patients may have atypical signs and symptoms. For example, elderly patients may have extreme weakness, confusion, and even syncope (signs and symptoms of left ventricular heart failure), rather than chest pain. Patients with cerebral atherosclerosis may have worsening heart failure, pain in an atypical location, apprehension and nervousness, acute indigestion, and signs and symptoms of a cerebrovascular accident.

position. He may massage or clutch his chest while complaining of chest discomfort.

Vital signs

Your patient's heart rate and rhythm offer important indicators of cardiac function in the acute and evolving stages of an MI. Remember that if he has a normal heart rate and rhythm, he isn't experiencing significant hemodynamic compromise. More commonly, however, you'll palpate a pulse that's rapid and regular initially, with the cardiac monitor showing sinus tachycardia. The heart rate will most likely slow down as your patient's anxiety and pain are relieved. Up to 60% of patients with inferior-wall MIs have heart rates between 50 and 70 beats per minute because of the vagal stimulation that accompanies these MIs.

Premature ventricular contractions—QRS complexes that occur earlier than expected—are very common. They appear on the cardiac monitor and you can feel them as an irregular pulse.

Premature ventricular contractions can reduce CO and compromise hemodynamic status.

Most MI patients have a normal blood pressure, although hypertension and hypotension may occur. Anxiety and pain, which increases sympathetic discharge, can elevate the blood pressure. Patients with inferior-wall MIs may have transient hypotension from vagal nerve stimulation. Interestingly, a hypertensive patient's blood pressure may become normal for the first 3 to 6 months after an MI.

Patients who suffer an extensive MI may develop a fever, a nonspecific response to tissue necrosis. It typically begins 4 to 8 hours after the onset of the infarction; the rectal temperature may reach 101° to 102°F (38.3° to 38.9°C). The fever may continue up to a week after the MI, a result of the inflammatory response.

The patient's respiratory rate may be elevated for many reasons, including anxiety and pain. In patients who develop pulmonary edema or left ventricular heart failure, it may exceed 40 breaths/minute.

Physical examination

Despite your patient's alarming symptoms and possibly extensive myocardial damage, his cardiac examination may be quite unremarkable. On palpation, you may find an abnormal pulsation during systole if a portion of the ventricle is dyskinetic; it bulges outward when it should contract inward.

You may notice on auscultation that your patient's heart sounds are soft or muffled immediately after the MI. You also may hear a third heart sound (S_3) just after the second heart sound. It typically reflects severe left ventricular heart failure and indicates a higher risk of death. You'll hear S_3 best with the bell of your stethoscope placed in the area that extends from the lower left sternal border to the apex of the patient's heart. It may be louder on inspiration.

You also may hear a fourth heart sound if you place the bell of your stethoscope on the area of your patient's chest from the lower left sternal border to the apex of his heart. It reflects the atrial contribution to ventricular filling and occurs immediately before the first heart sound. Common among MI patients, it results from decreased left ventricular compliance.

You may hear a systolic murmur when an MI damages the patient's mitral valve. A new, loud holosystolic murmur accompanied by a precordial thrill on palpation may reveal the rupture of a papillary muscle or the development of a new ventricular septal defect.

Extensive myocardial damage may produce a pericardial friction rub that you can hear along the left sternal border to the apex of the heart. You may be able to hear a very loud rub across the whole precordium and over the back. These rubs commonly arise on the second or third day after an MI. A late-onset pericardial rub that arises with chest pain up to 3 months after an MI suggests post-MI (or Dressler's) syndrome.

In a patient with a right ventricular infarction, you may find signs and symptoms of right ventricular heart failure, such as hepatomegaly and a positive hepatojugular reflux. To elicit the hepatojugular reflux, exert gradual, firm pressure over the liver and watch the jugular veins in your patient's neck. If they distend when you apply pressure, you've obtained a positive response. The patient may have peripheral edema as well.

Cardiogenic shock, a life-threatening complication of MI, is caused by left ventricular dysfunction and results in very low CO and circulatory failure.

Diagnostic tests

Several tests—including an ECG, serial cardiac enzymes and proteins, blood tests, chest X-ray, echocardiogram, nuclear scans, and cardiac catheterization—can help confirm a diagnosis of MI and assess the damage.

Electrocardiogram
As myocardial cells become hypoxic and die, they become unable to conduct electricity, a development that produces a series of abnormalities on the ECG tracing (see *Tracking the evolution of a myocardial infarction*). In the hyperacute phase, myocardial cells become ischemic and tall upright T waves appear. In the acute phase, ischemia progresses and ST segments become elevated. If blood flow to the ischemic myocardial cells isn't restored, the cells become injured, which causes ST-segment elevation and T-wave inversion.

In the fully evolved phase a few hours later, necrotic tissue creates Q waves. ST-segment elevation and T-wave inversion continue to indicate ischemia and injury in the area surrounding the infarct. As the myocardium heals, ST segments

Tracking the evolution of a myocardial infarction

You can use your patient's electrocardiogram to track the progression of his myocardial infarction through five phases: the hyperacute phase, early acute phase, later acute phase, fully evolved phase, and healed phase.

Hyperacute phase

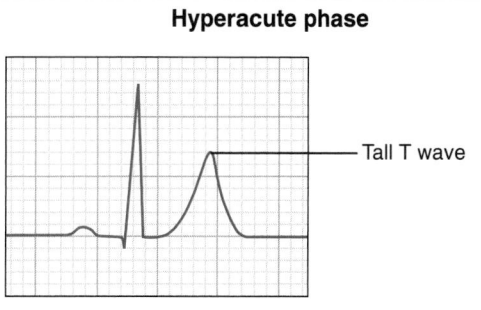

— Tall T wave

Early acute phase

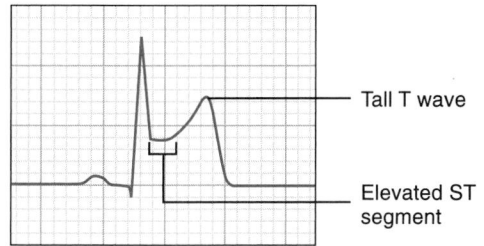

— Tall T wave

— Elevated ST segment

Later acute phase

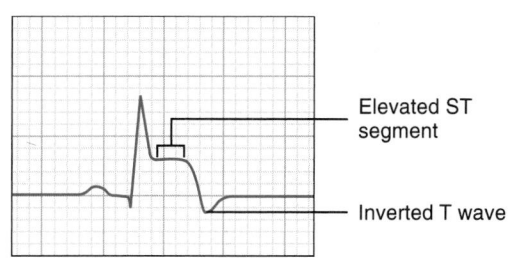

— Elevated ST segment

— Inverted T wave

Fully evolved phase

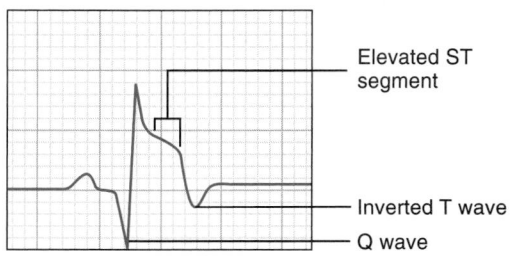

— Elevated ST segment

— Inverted T wave
— Q wave

Healed phase

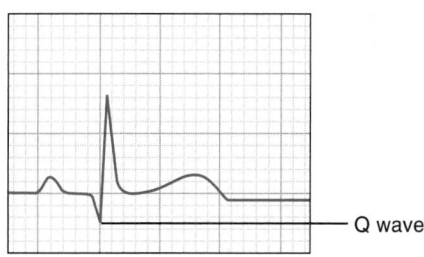

— Q wave

gradually return to baseline, and T waves return to their upright position. Q waves remain as permanent evidence of a previous MI.

Serial enzyme and protein levels

When myocardial cells die, they release enzymes, myoglobin, and contractile proteins. Three enzymes are routinely used to diagnose an acute MI: CK, LD, and AST. Specifically, you'll want to look at myocardial isoenzymes of CK and LD (see *Car-*

diac enzyme trends after a myocardial infarction, page 118).

The most commonly assessed biochemical marker, CK, has three isoenzymes that indicate muscle (MM), brain (BB), and cardiac (MB) origin. Currently, CK-MB is the most specific and sensitive indicator for diagnosing an MI. Serum levels of CK-MB begin to rise 2 to 4 hours after an MI, peak in 12 to 24 hours, and return to normal in 48 hours. Serial serum levels are drawn at ad-

Cardiac enzyme trends after a myocardial infarction

After a myocardial infarction (MI), cardiac enzyme levels show a characteristic pattern, first rising, then peaking, then falling back to baseline. The table below shows the time lines of this pattern for the enzymes and isoenzymes used to diagnose an MI: creatine kinase (CK), CK-MB, lactic dehydrogenase (LD), LD_1, and aspartate aminotransferase (AST).

Cardiac enzyme	Elevation (hr)	Peak (hr)	Return to baseline (days)
CK	4–8	12–24	3–4
CK-MB	2–4	12–24	2
LD	12–48	72–144	8–14
LD_1	12–48	72–144	14
AST	6–10	12–48	3–4

mission and every 4 to 6 hours for 24 hours to monitor their rise and peak.

Five isoenzymes make up LD. When myocardial cells sustain damage, the levels of isoenzymes LD_1 and LD_2 rise, with LD_1 rising higher than LD_2. The normal ratio of LD_1 to LD_2 is less than 1. With an MI, the ratio becomes greater than 1 and is said to be flipped.

Levels of LD rise 12 to 48 hours after an MI and peak in 72 to 144 hours. An LD_1 level that exceeds LD_2 suggests that an MI occurred at least 24 hours earlier. Analysis of LD provides a useful tool when caring for a patient who postponed treatment for 24 hours or more after developing chest pain.

Myoglobin, an oxygen-binding protein found in cardiac muscle, is more sensitive than CK-MB, although not as specific. A rise in myoglobin can be detected as early as 1 hour after an MI, possibly enabling an earlier start for thrombolytic therapy in patients who need it.

Troponin, a contractile protein, may be a more specific indicator of an acute MI than CK-MB because two of its isotypes—troponin T and troponin I—are cardiac specific. Troponin T rises for 3.5 hours to 10 days after an MI. An increasing number of emergency personnel are using measurements of this substance to assist with triage.

Blood tests
After an acute MI, your patient's white blood cell count and erythrocyte sedimentation rate may rise as a result of the inflammatory process. Blood glucose levels may rise from the release of catecholamines, resulting in abnormal glucose tolerance for several weeks.

Chest X-ray
A chest X-ray obtained in the acute stage of an MI may show signs of left ventricular heart failure and cardiomegaly. The degree of congestion and the size of the heart can be useful for identifying patients at highest risk of death. A large heart and signs of severe left ventricular heart failure commonly herald cardiogenic shock, a complication with a high mortality rate.

Echocardiogram
Echocardiography can be useful in assessing a patient with an acute MI by documenting movement in the ventricle wall. It also can detect complications, such as septal or papillary muscle rupture. And it can help assess for other causes of chest pain, such as aortic dissection.

Nuclear scanning
Radionuclide imaging with thallium-201 and technetium Tc 99m pyrophosphate can display dead and damaged areas of myocardial tissue.

Cardiac catheterization
Cardiac catheterization can reveal the exact area and severity of coronary artery obstruction. It also can provide information about heart muscle and ventricular function and about intracardiac pressures and volumes.

7

MYOCARDIAL INFARCTION

Treatment

Once you confirm that a patient has suffered a myocardial infarction (MI), you'll need to quickly take steps to maintain his vital signs, ease his pain, restore myocardial perfusion, and save as much of his heart muscle as possible. Treatment for an MI typically includes administering some or all of the following: oxygen, nitroglycerin, morphine, aspirin, heparin, a thrombolytic drug, a beta-blocker, and an angiotensin-converting enzyme (ACE) inhibitor. The patient also may require percutaneous transluminal coronary angioplasty (PTCA) and cardiac rehabilitation.

Although the goals of treatment have remained virtually unchanged in recent years, the resources available and the procedures recommended for accomplishing those goals continue to evolve (see *Caring for a patient during and after a myocardial infarction,* pages 120 and 121).

Oxygen administration

For some patients after an MI, ventricular function declines, arterial pressures drop, and venous pressures rise. The result is pulmonary edema, which causes a ventilation-perfusion mismatch and hypoxemia. As congestion in the pulmonary vascular bed reduces gas exchange, the patient typically develops tachypnea. Naturally, impaired ventilation, reduced gas exchange, and hypoxemia only aggravate a condition brought on by inadequate delivery of oxygen to myocardial tissues.

That's why your first response to an MI usually involves oxygen administration. For the typical patient, you'll start supplemental oxygen at 2 to 4 L/minute by nasal cannula. Therapy usually lasts 8 to 24 hours. However, it may last longer if the patient's respiratory function, oxygen saturation levels, and arterial blood gas (ABG) levels warrant continued therapy. If his chest pain and shortness of breath continue or recur and he has an oxygen saturation below 92%, you'll probably use a face mask, as ordered, to deliver a higher concentration of oxygen. If the patient's respiratory status declines, he may require endotracheal intubation and mechanical ventilation.

In most cases, you'll give supplemental oxygen even if the patient's ABG measurements remain within normal limits. That's because ABG measurements reflect oxygen levels available to the entire body rather than specifically to the myocardium—a muscle that uses more than an average amount of oxygen. Tachycardia provides a nonspecific but key sign of inadequate oxygen delivery to the tissues.

Throughout oxygen delivery, monitor your patient closely. Check his vital signs, heart rhythm, level of consciousness, pain intensity, and pulse oximetry readings. Remember that both increased and decreased respirations can impair oxygenation.

Also, take steps to ensure the patient's compliance with oxygen therapy. Oxygen tends to dry and irritate the mucosa so much that some patients may try to remove the nasal prongs to reduce the discomfort. You can help avoid this problem by using a saline nasal spray to keep the membranes moist. Tell the patient and his family how profoundly oxygen can influence his condition. And take as much time as you can in this accelerated treatment process to answer questions—

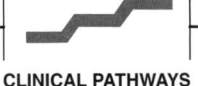

CLINICAL PATHWAYS

Caring for a patient during and after a myocardial infarction

	History and physical examination	Diagnostic tests	Discharge planning
Day 1	• history of angina • history of trigger factor • pain assessment • electrocardiogram (ECG) changes • input and output • vital signs every hour • review of systems every 8 hours	• serial 12-lead ECG • continuous ECG monitoring and rhythm strip every 8 hours • cardiac enzyme levels every 8 hours until they peak • prothrombin time (PT) and activated partial thromboplastin time (APTT) • complete blood count • chest X-ray • electrolyte and glucose levels • blood urea nitrogen level • creatinine level • urinalysis	• Assess support systems available at home. • Consult with social services. • Assess financial status and health insurance.
Day 2	• pain assessment • ECG changes • vital signs every 4 hours • review of systems every 8 hours	• continuous ECG monitoring and rhythm strip every 8 hours • echocardiogram • nuclear scan • cardiac catheterization • electrolyte levels • cardiac enzyme levels every 8 hours until they peak • PT and APTT • complete blood count	• Determine preferred method of teaching for patient and family.
Day 3	• pain assessment • ECG changes • vital signs every 4 hours • review of systems every 8 hours	• continuous ECG monitoring and rhythm strip every 8 hours • electrolyte levels • PT and APTT • complete blood count	• Consult with physical therapist. • Consult with home-care provider. • Consult with cardiac rehabilitation nurse.
Day 4	• pain assessment • ECG changes • vital signs every 4 hours • review of systems every 8 hours	• continuous ECG monitoring and rhythm strip every 8 hours • electrolyte levels • PT and APTT	• Refer patient to local American Heart Association support group.
Day 5	• pain assessment • ECG changes • vital signs every 8 hours • review of systems every 8 hours	• electrolyte levels • telemetry	• Help family manage home modifications.
Day 6	• pain assessment • ECG changes • vital signs every 8 hours • review of systems every 8 hours	• electrolyte levels • complete blood count • thallium stress test to guide cardiac rehabilitation • signal-averaged ECG if appropriate	• Arrange for follow-up visit with physician. • Arrange for home-health visit. • Arrange for cardiac rehabilitation follow-up.

Drugs	Interventions	Patient teaching
• nitrates • 1–3 mg of morphine I.V. over 2–5 minutes, repeated every 5–30 min • 160–325 mg of buffered aspirin crushed or chewed • heparin if patient received alteplase • beta-blocker I.V. followed by oral beta-blocker • angiotensin-converting enzyme (ACE) inhibitor • stool softener • antiemetic as needed • sedative as needed	• oxygen administration as needed • I.V. fluid administration • noninvasive blood pressure monitoring • continuous pulse oximetry • reperfusion therapy with thrombolytic drug or percutaneous transluminal angioplasty • atropine, lidocaine, epinephrine, trans-cutaneous pacing supplies, and defib-rillator kept on hand	• hospital and unit orientation • tests and proce-dures • clinical pathway and plan of care • diagnosis
• enteric-coated aspirin once daily • nitrates • heparin • oral beta-blocker • ACE inhibitor • magnesium as needed • stool softener • sedative as needed	• oxygen administration, as needed • I.V. site maintenance • noninvasive blood pressure monitoring • assistance with activities of daily living and transfers to chair • passive and active range of motion	• pathophysiology of myocardial infarction • diet, drugs, activity
• enteric-coated aspirin • nitrates • heparin • beta-blocker • ACE inhibitor • stool softener • sedative as needed	• oxygen administration, as needed • I.V. site maintenance • assistance with activities of daily living and walking	• steps of cardiac rehabilitation
• enteric-coated aspirin • nitrates • heparin, if necessary • beta-blocker • ACE inhibitor • stool softener	• oxygen administration, as needed • I.V. site maintenance • assistance with activities of daily living and walking	• healthy weight • low-fat diet • cholesterol levels • smoking cessation • exercise • pulse measure-ments
• enteric-coated aspirin • nitrates • beta-blocker • ACE inhibitor • stool softener	• oxygen administration, as needed • I.V. site maintenance • activity increased, as tolerated	• patient and family understanding of previous teaching • discharge planning
• enteric-coated aspirin • nitrates • beta-blocker • ACE inhibitor • stool softener	• oxygen administration, as needed • I.V. access discontinued • telemetry discontinued • activity increased, as tolerated	• patient and family understanding of previous teaching • discharge planning

especially those that could alter the patient's anxiety level and, thus, his oxygen demands.

If you deliver oxygen for 72 hours or more at a rate higher than 4 L/minute, use a humidifier, as ordered, to protect the patient's mucosal lining from becoming dry and irritated.

After the patient's chest pain and shortness of breath subside and his pulse oximetry readings, heart rate, respiratory rate, and blood pressure have returned to normal levels, you can begin weaning him from supplemental oxygen, as ordered. You'll most likely decrease the flow rate in 2-liter increments, assessing the patient frequently to see how well he tolerates each change.

Drug therapy

As soon as possible after starting the patient's supplemental oxygen therapy, you'll begin giving a series of drugs designed to minimize infarct size, reduce complications, and improve his outcome. If your patient hasn't already taken sublingual nitroglycerin, drug therapy probably will start with it.

Sublingual nitroglycerin

The protocol for administering sublingual nitroglycerin to a patient having an MI mirrors that for a patient having an anginal attack. If the patient's chest pain fails to respond to the first dose after 5 minutes, give him another dose and then, if necessary, a third dose, each spaced 5 minutes apart.

Don't give sublingual nitroglycerin to a patient with a systolic blood pressure below 90 mm Hg because it may drive his blood pressure to a dangerously low level. Carefully assess your patient's response to sublingual nitroglycerin.

Angina that doesn't subside or that recurs after rest, oxygen administration, and sublingual nitroglycerin requires more aggressive treatments, possibly including analgesics, thrombolytic therapy, a beta-blocker, I.V. nitroglycerin, heparin, and an ACE inhibitor.

Morphine

The drug of choice for easing the pain of an MI, morphine is an opioid narcotic analgesic that interferes with pain impulses at the cortical level of the brain. It also blocks centrally mediated sym-

pathetic efferent discharge, resulting in peripheral vasodilation. By decreasing systemic vascular resistance (afterload) and ventricular filling pressures (preload), morphine reduces myocardial oxygen consumption. Plus, it helps to reduce circulating catecholamine levels by relieving the patient's pain and anxiety, possibly yielding a reduced risk of catecholamine-induced arrhythmias as well.

For most patients in the acute phase of an MI, you'll give 1 to 3 mg of morphine by I.V. injection over 2 to 5 minutes. Repeat the dose every 5 to 30 minutes as prescribed and needed to control pain. If your patient is over age 65 or debilitated, start with a dose of 2 mg or less to avoid a marked drop in blood pressure. Occasionally, a young, muscular patient may require higher doses to obtain adequate pain relief.

After giving the initial dose, you'll need to titrate a dosage that will help relieve pain and keep the patient's systolic pressure at 90 mm Hg or above. Monitor the patient frequently to maintain these goals. Remember that continued pain indicates continued ischemia; consequently, relieving the patient's pain becomes critically important. A physician may prescribe I.V. nitroglycerin and a beta-blocker to be given along with the morphine. Monitor the patient's reactions carefully and collaborate with the physician to adjust the therapy, as needed.

Most patients require morphine only during the acute phase of an MI; however, a small percentage develop persistent chest pain and may need maintenance doses of 2 to 8 mg every 4 to 6 hours.

Morphine given by slow I.V. injection over 4 to 5 minutes begins to take effect within 10 minutes after administration. It reaches peak effect in 20 to 30 minutes and maintains its analgesic action for about 4 to 5 hours. Its action may be prolonged in elderly patients or shortened in otherwise healthy, young patients. As your patient's pain abates, his vital signs will begin to return to baseline levels.

Adverse effects
Hypotension is one of the chief adverse effects of morphine. Like all of the drug's adverse effects, it varies with the amount given. Other drugs used to treat an MI—including nitrates, beta-blockers, and ACE inhibitors—may also cause or worsen hypotension.

The two keys to avoiding or minimizing hypotension are to titrate morphine in small, incre-

When morphine causes nausea and vomiting

After receiving morphine, many patients become nauseated or vomit. To counteract these adverse effects in a a patient with a myocardial infarction, administer one of these drugs, as ordered.

Drug	Dose	Onset (min)	Duration of action (hr)
diphenhydramine	25–50 mg every 6–8 hr	15	3–6
hydroxyzine	25–100 mg every 6 hr	15–30	4–6
metoclopramide	10–20 mg every 4–6 hr	30–60	1–2
prochlorperazine	5–10 mg every 6–8 hr	30–40	3–4
promethazine	12.5–25 mg every 4 hr	20–30	2–8
thiethylperazine	10 mg every 8–24 hr	30	4
trimethobenzamide	250 mg every 6–8 hr	10–40	3–4

mental doses and to respond quickly if hypotension develops. For example, you may raise the patient's legs or give I.V. fluids to correct his hemodynamic status.

Especially in patients with chronic lung disease, morphine may aggravate hypoxemia by decreasing the rate and depth of respirations. However, only rarely will a patient with severe chest pain or pulmonary edema develop overt respiratory depression when given appropriate amounts of morphine; if he does, prepare to provide oxygen and ventilations with a bag-valve mask device. If his status declines, anticipate endotracheal intubation and mechanical ventilation.

Other common adverse effects of morphine include sedation, nausea, vomiting, dry mouth, constipation, central nervous system (CNS) depression, and euphoria. Elderly patients are particularly susceptible to the constipating effects of morphine and to CNS depression, which usually appears as confusion.

Nursing considerations

To help document your patient's response to morphine and nitroglycerin, teach him how to use a pain rating scale. For example, you might have him rate his pain on a scale of 0 to 10, where 0 represents no pain and 10 represents the worst pain possible. Or you might ask him to mark his pain level on a visual analog scale. No matter which scale you choose, make sure you repeatedly reassess his pain level to track the success of his treatment.

Tell the patient that morphine begins to take effect within about 5 minutes and reaches its peak effectiveness in 20 to 30 minutes. Mention that the drug may make him drowsy.

If the patient becomes nauseated or vomits, give him an antiemetic drug, as prescribed (see *When morphine causes nausea and vomiting*). If your patient has long QT syndrome, use prochlorperazine and promethazine cautiously because they may cause torsades de pointes.

To help prevent straining at stool, give the patient a stool softener, such as docusate sodium 100 mg twice daily, or a laxative.

Avoid giving morphine by rapid I.V. push or by intramuscular (I.M.) injection. The former will cause an immediate drop in blood pressure—a trend poorly tolerated by elderly, hypotensive, or hypovolemic patients—and it could cause respiratory arrest. The latter will falsely raise cardiac enzyme levels.

Rather than giving an increasing amount of morphine to reduce the patient's anxiety, do your best to calm and reassure him. Keep his environment as quiet and controlled as possible to help him stay as calm as possible.

RESEARCH UPDATE

Abciximab to treat a myocardial infarction?

The success of aspirin as a treatment for acute myocardial infarctions (MIs) has prompted researchers to investigate other antiplatelet drugs, including a promising group of drugs called platelet glycoprotein IIb/IIIa receptor antagonists. One drug in this group is already in use: abciximab.

How abciximab works
When an atherosclerotic plaque ruptures, platelets aggregate at the site and become activated. On their exposed surfaces are glycoprotein IIb/IIIa binding receptor sites to which circulating fibrinogen binds, linking the platelets together into a clump and, eventually, into a clot that can obstruct the vessel.

Abciximab halts this process by binding to glycoprotein IIb/IIIa receptor sites on the surface of activated platelets. It blocks the normal binding of fibrinogen, Von Willebrand factor, and other adhesive factors. Consequently, it inhibits platelet aggregation at the site of the ruptured plaque.

Promising results
Typically, physicians prescribe abciximab after a patient undergoes percutaneous transluminal coronary angioplasty or stent placement. However, abciximab also may reduce the risk of death and the extent of damage in a person who's having an MI.

Researchers have found that 0.25 mg/kg of I.V. abciximab followed by a 12-hour infusion at 10 µg/min produces beneficial results. The drug seems to have the greatest benefit when used with aspirin and heparin.

Adverse effects
The most common adverse effect—bleeding—can be minimized with prudent, weight-based heparin dosing. Usually, bleeding develops at the site of the vascular puncture in the patient's groin; it may be difficult to stop. Cerebral hemorrhage may occur as well. Following the guidelines for patients who've had angioplasty can help minimize the risk of bleeding complications.

Give morphine cautiously to any patient with an inferior-wall or right ventricular MI because these problems create the highest risk of hypotension and bradycardia. A physician may prescribe meperidine instead of morphine for a patient with an inferior-wall MI because of the drug's vagolytic properties.

Aspirin

Aspirin blocks the formation of thromboxane A_2, a powerful vasoconstrictor released by platelets clumped at injured arterial walls. By inhibiting thromboxane A_2, aspirin prevents further platelet aggregation and coronary artery vasoconstriction.

Consequently, unless a patient has a documented, life-threatening contraindication to aspirin, you'll want to quickly give it to anyone who may be having an MI. It and perhaps other antiplatelet drugs may provide practical and relatively risk-free improvements in outcome for your MI patients (see *Abciximab to treat a myocardial infarction?*).

Specifically, administer 160 to 325 mg of buffered aspirin as soon as the patient develops signs and symptoms or arrives at the emergency department. It typically takes effect within 20 minutes after ingestion. For faster absorption, have the patient chew a baby aspirin right away as prescribed. Thereafter, give the patient 81 to 325 mg of enteric-coated aspirin daily.

Adverse effects
Aspirin causes gastrointestinal (GI) distress more often than any other adverse effect. However, at a dose of 325 mg or less daily, aspirin creates a minimal risk of adverse effects for your MI patients. Occult GI bleeding and mucosal lesions rarely form at the doses recommended for antiplatelet therapy.

About 1 person in 100 has a sensitivity to aspirin; that number rises to 4 among patients with asthma and to 20 among patients with chronic urticaria. These patients may develop mild to moderate bronchospasm 15 to 30 minutes after ingesting aspirin. Although rarely necessary, an inhaled beta-agonist, such as albuterol, will ease the bronchospasm.

Nursing considerations

To avoid adverse GI effects, urge the patient to take enteric-coated aspirin, and carefully explain why he should do so. Warn him not to crush or chew the coated tablets, but to swallow them whole. Also, urge him to take his aspirin with a full glass of water to prevent the possibility of esophageal erosions.

Tell the patient to take his aspirin with food, milk, or an antacid, as prescribed by his physician, if he develops GI distress.

Elderly patients tend to bruise easily when taking aspirin every day. Most bruises will be superficial and clinically harmless, but the patient should be monitored carefully nonetheless.

Thrombolytic therapy

During the administration of sublingual nitroglycerin, morphine, and aspirin, the patient's physician evaluates whether the patient should receive reperfusion therapy and, if so, whether he should undergo thrombolytic therapy or PTCA.

Most physicians consider a patient a good candidate for thrombolytic therapy if his chest pain started within the previous 12 hours (preferably within 4 hours) and if his ECG shows evidence of hyperacute or acute changes in two or more leads. The physician must then weigh the benefits of saving myocardial tissue against the risk of uncontrolled bleeding.

Most hospitals consider active internal bleeding and acute pericarditis contraindications to thrombolytic therapy. If your patient has one of these conditions, he'll most likely undergo PTCA to open his occluded artery. Most hospitals also maintain a list of relative contraindications; a physician considers the possible effects of these conditions when assessing the patient's overall status. Relative contraindications commonly include the following:
• cardiopulmonary resuscitation that lasted more than 10 minutes
• diabetic hemorrhagic retinopathy
• head injury in the previous month
• cerebrovascular accident in the previous year

• intracranial tumor
• possible aortic dissection
• hypertension above 180/110 mm Hg, especially severe, uncontrolled hypertension
• active peptic ulcer disease
• GI or genitourinary surgery in the previous 6 months
• injury or surgery in the previous 2 weeks
• internal bleeding in the previous 4 weeks
• noncompressable vascular punctures
• pregnancy
• recent transient ischemic attack.

Undoubtedly, the more quickly thrombolytic therapy begins, the better the patient's outcome. In fact, although patients may benefit from thrombolytic therapy even up to 24 hours after the onset of chest pain, the best overall outcomes stem from therapy that begins within 30 minutes after the patient enters the emergency department. Many facilities have developed standing orders, chest-pain algorithms, and assessment criteria sheets to help speed the start of thrombolytic therapy.

Thrombolytic drug options

As you know, a physician may choose among several thrombolytic drugs, including alteplase, anisoylated plasminogen streptokinase activator complex (APSAC), reteplase, streptokinase, and urokinase (see *Doses for thrombolytic drugs,* page 126). Each restores blood flow—and myocardial oxygen supply—by stimulating conversion of plasminogen to plasmin, an enzyme that degrades fibrin, fibrinogen, and other procoagulant proteins, thus causing fresh thrombi to break down. However, these drugs do differ.

For example, because they bind to fibrin in clots rather than to circulating plasminogen, alteplase and reteplase exert a more clot-specific action. Streptokinase may be better able to restore perfusion in patients whose symptoms started 12 to 24 hours earlier. And alteplase may provide better results for patients who have an anterior-wall MI and chest pain that started within the previous 4 hours.

Despite their differences, however, no one thrombolytic drug has proven superior to the others in restoring perfusion among the general population of MI patients. All thrombolytics possess essentially equal patency rates at 24 hours, similar reductions in left ventricular dysfunction, and a nearly identical reduction in death rates.

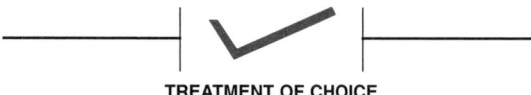

TREATMENT OF CHOICE

Doses for thrombolytic drugs

Drug	Dose
alteplase	• 15-mg bolus followed by 0.75 mg/kg infusion (not to exceed 50 mg) over 30 min, followed by 0.5 mg/kg infusion (not to exceed 35 mg) over 60 min
anisoylated plasminogen streptokinase activator complex	• 30 mg I.V. over 2–5 min
reteplase	• I.V. bolus of 10 units (U) repeated in 30 min
streptokinase	• 1.5 million U over 60 min

Adverse effects

Thrombolytic therapy causes bleeding, usually minor bleeding, in 3% to 10% of patients. Women over age 75 with a history of uncontrolled hypertension, a tendency to bleed easily, a low body weight, diabetic retinopathy, or an international normalized ratio (INR) above 1.0 are most likely to develop it.

A fatal cerebral hemorrhage may develop in up to 2% of patients, a risk that precludes continued or repeated thrombolytic dosing for patients who continue to have chest pain for more than 1 to 2 hours after therapy starts.

In some patients, the newly opened vessel may reocclude. About half of reocclusions take place during the first 24 hours after therapy. Adjunctive therapy with aspirin, heparin, a beta-blocker, and abciximab can help reduce the risk of reocclusion. Patients with continuing chest pain and ECG changes (both indications of reocclusion) will undergo cardiac catheterization in preparation either for PTCA or coronary artery bypass grafting.

All thrombolytic drugs may cause transient hypotension, although it's most common with streptokinase and APSAC. With streptokinase, reducing the infusion rate may reverse the hypotension; volume replacement can resolve it as well. Always assess your patient's fluid volume status before starting thrombolytic therapy. If he's dehydrated, give replacement fluids I.V., as ordered, to prevent hypotension and worsening myocardial ischemia or infarction.

Streptokinase and APSAC may cause mild allergic reactions that include shivering, pyrexia, mild dyspnea or bronchospasm, rash, and flushing. These signs and symptoms can be treated with corticosteroids or diphenhydramine. Although few patients develop true anaphylaxis, exposure to streptokinase or APSAC within the previous 6 months precludes using either drug again. Also, because these drugs are derived from the *Streptococcus* bacterium, they may not be appropriate if your patient has had a *Streptococcus* infection in the previous 6 months.

Nursing considerations

If your patient will be receiving thrombolytic therapy, take time to explain to him the procedure and its goals. Tell him that the drug dissolves blood clots, an action that can help stop his MI but that also can produce some minor bleeding at other locations. Reassure him that you'll monitor him closely for bleeding. Also, encourage him to stay in bed as much as possible to avoid bumps, falls, and other mishaps during the time when he has an increased risk of bleeding.

Before therapy

Before starting thrombolytic therapy, assess the patient's vital signs and neurologic status. Make sure he has two patent I.V. lines with compressible insertion sites. From one of those lines, draw blood samples for baseline tests, including prothrombin time (PT), INR, activated partial thromboplastin time (APTT), complete blood count (CBC), and electrolyte, glucose, blood urea nitrogen (BUN), and creatinine levels. Avoid giving him I.M. injections or performing any nonessential venous or arterial punctures before, during, or within 24 hours after the therapy in vessels that can't be compressed.

When preparing the thrombolytic drug, avoid shaking the vial because doing so will make the drug foam. Instead, roll the vial between your palms to mix the drug. Infuse it over the prescribed length of time, and then flush the tubing to make sure the patient receives the full drug dose.

During therapy

During therapy, assess the patient's vital signs, ECG rhythm and rate, and neurologic status every 15 minutes. Check all puncture sites and the patient's gingivae for bleeding or oozing. Also, watch for blood in his stool, sputum, urine, and vomitus. Don't discontinue I.V. sites, jostle arterial lines, or move the patient unnecessarily. And follow his APTT, hematocrit, and hemoglobin level.

After therapy

Assess the patient's vital signs and neurologic status every 15 minutes for 2 hours after thrombolytic therapy ends, and then every 2 hours for 24 hours. Monitor his APTT, hematocrit, and hemoglobin level for 24 hours. And continue to watch for bleeding for 72 hours. Remember that changes in mental status could signal intracranial bleeding.

If your patient shows signs of bleeding or his hemoglobin level and hematocrit fall, assess him for signs and symptoms (such as hypotension) and report them to the physician. Expect to stop the thrombolytic infusion if it's still running. As prescribed, give fluids and vasopressors I.V., such as dopamine, to raise the patient's blood pressure. Infuse packed red blood cells, as prescribed, to maintain his hemoglobin level and hematocrit—essential for delivering oxygen to the ischemic myocardium. Also, anticipate giving fresh frozen plasma to provide clotting factors.

Occasionally, a patient receiving streptokinase will develop a marked depletion in fibrinogen; if he does, he may need cryoprecipitate along with other blood products. You can raise the patient's fibrinogen level about 0.7 g/L and his factor VIII level about 30% by giving him 10 units of cryoprecipitate. As ordered, maintain his fibrinogen level above 1.0 or 1.5 g/L and his APTT at 1.5 to 2.0 times the control.

If the patient develops minor bleeding or oozing around a catheter or venipuncture site, apply manual pressure to the area for 20 to 30 minutes. If the patient also receives heparin, a physician will order an immediate test of his APTT and, based on the results, may adjust the heparin dosage.

Beta-blockers

Beta-blockers reduce myocardial oxygen demand by decreasing heart rate, electrical impulse conduction, and contractility. They also in- directly increase oxygen supply because the decreased heart rate results in a prolonged filling time, which enhances coronary artery perfusion. Especially in combination with thrombolytic therapy, a beta-blocker can help minimize your patient's infarct size and maximize his outcome.

Using a thrombolytic drug and a beta-blocker together reduces the risk of death by 20% during the first 7 days after an MI. Starting such therapy within the first 6 hours reduces the risk further. However, even when therapy starts 24 hours or more after the initial symptoms, the patient's risks of cardiac arrest and reinfarction decrease.

Used alone, beta-blockers still reduce the risks of nonfatal reinfarction, cardiac arrest, and death. Patients who seem to gain the most benefit from beta-blockers tend to have an anterior-wall MI, hypertension, tachycardia, or some combination of the three.

Drug options

Most patients receive either metoprolol or atenolol I.V. to treat an acute MI. Between 6 and 12 hours later, they switch to oral therapy (see *Administering metoprolol and atenolol,* page 128). If the patient already took a beta-blocker before having an MI, the physician may continue oral therapy with the original drug. In most cases, you'll administer beta-blockers I.V. together with thrombolytics, aspirin, and nitrates.

Patients who respond best to long-term beta-blocker therapy include those with mild to moderate heart failure, abnormal exercise-tolerance test results, and myocardial tissue made dysfunctional by ischemia or infarction. For most patients, oral therapy continues indefinitely.

Avoid giving a beta-blocker I.V. to any patient who has one of the following contraindications:
• pulmonary edema
• hypotension (systolic pressure below 100 mm Hg)
• bradyarrhythmia (heart rate below 50 beats per minute [bpm] without a working pacemaker).
Relative contraindications include asthma or emphysema, conditions in which beta blockade can constrict the airways and lead to bronchospasm.

Adverse effects

Hypotension and bradycardia are the primary adverse effects of beta-blockers. However, only about 1 patient in 10 will be unable to tolerate I.V. therapy when it's administered properly. Pa-

Administering metoprolol and atenolol

To administer one of these beta-blockers safely and effectively to a patient who has had a myocardial infarction, follow these guidelines.

Metoprolol
- Give 5 mg by I.V. bolus over 2 minutes. After 5 minutes, give another 5-mg bolus. After 5 more minutes, give a third 5-mg bolus, for a total dose of 15 mg.
- If your patient has a systolic blood pressure above 100 mm Hg and a heart rate above 55 beats per minute (bpm), administer the first oral dose 15 minutes after the last I.V. dose. Give him 25 or 50 mg every 6 hours.
- If your patient has borderline hypotension or bradycardia, either begin with a low oral dose (12.5 to 25 mg) or withhold the first oral dose until 6 hours after the last I.V. dose. Then start with 25 or 50 mg, and administer the dose every 6 hours.

Atenolol
- Give a 5-mg I.V. bolus over 5 minutes. After 10 minutes, give another 5-mg bolus.
- If the patient has a systolic blood pressure above 100 mm Hg and a heart rate above 55 bpm, administer the first oral dose 15 minutes after the last I.V. dose. Give the patient 25 or 50 mg every 12 hours.
- If the patient has borderline hypotension or bradycardia, either begin with a low oral dose (12.5 mg) or hold the first oral dose until 12 hours after the last I.V. dose. Then start with 25 or 50 mg, and administer the dose every 12 hours.

tients who can't tolerate I.V. therapy should still receive oral therapy within 24 to 72 hours.

Elderly patients tend to be more sensitive to the adverse effects of beta-blockers and may tolerate cardioselective drugs, such as metoprolol and atenolol, slightly better than the others. What's more, elderly patients may vary widely in their response to the chronotropic and hemodynamic effects of these drugs. Adjust the dosage until you reach the lowest effective level possible, a level that achieves the optimal hemodynamic response but causes few or no adverse effects.

Nursing considerations

Tell your patient that he'll be receiving a drug to help reduce his risk of complications. Mention that the drug may cause him to have strange dreams.

Before starting I.V. therapy with a beta-blocker, obtain baseline measurements of the patient's blood pressure and heart rate as well as an ECG strip. If his heart rate exceeds 55 bpm and his systolic blood pressure exceeds 100 mm Hg, you can begin the therapy, as prescribed. If possible, avoid giving morphine injections within 30 minutes of the beta-blocker. Also, avoid giving an ACE inhibitor within 60 minutes before the first dose.

Urge the patient to tell you if he experiences increased shortness of breath or continued chest pain during beta-blocker therapy. If he reports these symptoms, correlate them with his breath sounds, pulse oximetry readings, ABG values, blood pressure, heart sounds, and heart rate and rhythm. If his chest pain continues, obtain a 12-lead ECG and cardiac enzyme tests, as ordered.

To help minimize hypotension and bradycardia, monitor the patient's heart rate, blood pressure, and ECG tracing (for signs of atrioventricular [AV] block) after each I.V. dose. Also, watch for signs and symptoms of worsening heart failure, such as pulmonary congestion or dyspnea. Allow at least 5 minutes to fully assess the hemodynamic effects of each metoprolol dose. Allow 10 minutes to assess the effect of each atenolol dose.

If the patient is receiving nitroglycerin I.V. as well as a beta-blocker I.V., monitor him carefully for changes in blood pressure and heart rate, and respond as outlined below.
- If your patient's systolic blood pressure remains above 100 mm Hg and his heart rate remains above 55 bpm 5 to 10 minutes after the first bolus dose, proceed with the second bolus dose.
- If his pressure drops below 90 mm Hg, stop giving nitroglycerin I.V. during this time, as ordered. Then restart it at half the previous rate.
- If his pressure is between 90 and 100 mm Hg and his heart rate is between 50 and 55 bpm at 15 minutes after the first dose, give half the original bolus amount of beta-blocker as the second dose, as ordered.

If you can't keep the patient's blood pressure at a high enough level, report it immediately because the physician may halt both drugs temporarily or order a different treatment. If the patient's heart rate drops below 50 bpm, or his rhythm suggests a significant delay or block at the AV node, stop the beta-blocker therapy, as ordered. After continued adjustments to his nitroglycerin dosage, you may be able to resume the beta-blocker infusion later.

I.V. nitroglycerin

Even if your patient already received sublingual nitroglycerin, he may receive nitroglycerin I.V. as well. Short-term therapy can help to reduce infarct size, decrease the heart's workload, and increase blood supply by various mechanisms (see *Effects of I.V. nitroglycerin*).

Ideally, nitroglycerin I.V. therapy should begin immediately. A patient with a large anterior-wall MI, left ventricular dysfunction, or persistent ischemia is most likely to receive the greatest benefit from nitrate therapy, both I.V. and oral.

Infuse nitroglycerin cautiously in any patient with a systolic pressure around 90 mm Hg and a normal sinus rhythm. The drug is contraindicated in patients with borderline blood pressure and a fast heart rate because the resulting vasodilation could be life-threatening.

Adverse effects
The higher the dose, the more likely that I.V. nitroglycerin will cause hypotension and tachycardia. Treat them by slowing or stopping the nitroglycerin infusion and giving fluids. When using other drugs that cause hypotension (a thrombolytic, morphine, a beta-blocker, or an ACE inhibitor), titrate the nitroglycerin dosage carefully to keep the patient's blood pressure under control. If hypotension continues despite dosage reductions, you may need to stop the nitroglycerin infusion. Keep in mind that elderly patients may be more sensitive to the hypotensive effects of nitrates because of their decreased baroreceptor response, decreased venous tone, and dehydration.

More than half of patients develop a headache from I.V. nitroglycerin; in about 5%, the pain may be too severe to continue the infusion. For the rest, treat the headache by decreasing the infusion rate and giving acetaminophen, as prescribed.

Less common adverse effects include flushing, dizziness, restlessness, and nausea.

Effects of I.V. nitroglycerin

Nitroglycerin given I.V. can help decrease the heart's workload and increase its blood supply, resulting in a decreased infarct size, fewer complications, and a lower risk of extension and reinfarction. The lists below show you at a glance the effects of nitroglycerin that decrease myocardial workload and increase blood supply.

Decreased myocardial workload
- venous and arterial dilation
- decreased preload and afterload
- increased stroke volume
- improved left ventricular function

Increased blood supply
- coronary artery vasodilation
- decreased coronary artery spasm
- increased collateral blood flow
- increased endothelium-derived relaxation factor activity
- decreased platelet adhesiveness
- increased removal of noxious metabolites

Nursing considerations
Before starting the nitroglycerin infusion, find out whether you'll be mixing the drug yourself or using a premixed formula prepared for I.V. administration. If the former, make sure you dilute the drug in a glass container because nitroglycerin binds with plastic. If you mix it in a plastic container, your patient won't receive his full dose.

Nitroglycerin is compatible with most fluids. Don't add more than 150 mg of nitroglycerin per 250 ml of I.V. fluid. If you notice precipitates or separation after making a solution, discard it and make a weaker solution.

Tell the patient that nitroglycerin tends to cause headaches. Ask him to tell you if he develops one so that you can treat it promptly.

As ordered, start the nitroglycerin infusion at 5 to 10 µg/minute and titrate it upward by 5 to 10 µg/minute every 3 to 5 minutes until the patient reports that his chest pain has subsided, until you reach the desired blood pressure, or until you're giving 200 µg/minute. Because I.V. nitroglycerin has an almost immediate onset of action, you won't need to give a bolus dose. Besides, doing so could cause life-threatening hypotension.

To keep mean blood pressure above 80 mm Hg and systolic pressure above 90 mm Hg, titrate the dosage carefully, especially for elderly patients and those with hypovolemia, a right ventricular MI, or an inferior-wall MI. Titrate up or down by 5 to 10 µg/minute every 5 to 10 minutes.

During the infusion, monitor the patient carefully for changes in blood pressure, then respond as outlined below.

- If his systolic pressure drops below 90 mm Hg, stop the drip and restart at a lower dose when his pressure rises above 90 mm Hg.
- If his mean blood pressure drops below 80 mm Hg, stop and restart at a lower dose as well.
- If his diastolic pressure rises by more than 15 mm Hg, switch to another drug, as ordered.
- If his heart rate increases by 20% above his baseline, check his fluid volume and titrate the nitroglycerin dosage downward.

Continue the infusion for 24 to 48 hours, as ordered. When discontinuing the infusion, titrate downward by 5 to 10 µg/minute every 5 minutes.

Heparin

If your patient received alteplase or reteplase, he also may receive heparin I.V. to reduce the risk of further thrombus formation. Heparin inhibits thrombin and fibrin formation by activating antithrombin III, which in turn inhibits activated coagulation factors of the intrinsic and common pathways, including thrombin, factor Xa, factor IXa, factor XIa, factor XIIa, and kallikrein. It also inhibits the platelet aggregation induced by thrombin.

Anticoagulant dosage levels must vary to keep the patient's clotting time and APTT between 1.5 and 2.0 times the control value. Keep in mind that weight-based dosage protocols may produce fewer adverse effects and a more rapid way to attain a therapeutic APTT. Don't give heparin to a patient with active bleeding or hemorrhage.

Adverse effects

Heparin tends to cause bleeding that may range from minor, acceptable amounts to major, unacceptable amounts (see *Heparin therapy: When is bleeding acceptable?*). Elderly patients, especially women, tend to be more sensitive to heparin; monitor them carefully for bleeding.

Between 5% and 15% of patients receiving heparin develop thrombocytopenia, usually 5 to 9 days after the start of therapy. It occurs more commonly with bovine-derived heparin. Discontinue the heparin, as ordered, if the patient's platelet count falls below 100,000/mm^3.

Nursing considerations

Tell your patient that he'll be receiving a drug that helps prevent blood clots by thinning his blood. Explain that it also raises the risk of bleeding, but that you'll be monitoring him closely to prevent problems. Encourage him to be careful to avoid bumps, falls, and other mishaps that could cause bleeding.

To detect bleeding, assess the patient's puncture sites and gingivae regularly. Also, check his stool, sputum, urine, and vomitus for frank or occult bleeding. Monitor his hemoglobin and platelet levels, hematocrit, and APTT, as ordered. If you detect changes in his mental status, report them immediately; they may signal intracranial bleeding.

Before the continuous infusion begins, give the patient a loading dose of heparin based on his weight—usually 50 to 70 units/kg. If the patient weighs less than 100 kg, you'll probably give an I.V. bolus of 5,000 units. If he weighs more than 100 kg, give a bolus of 7,500 units. Then start the infusion at 1,000 units/hour. Keep in mind that the patient's coagulation status may render a bolus dose unnecessary.

Draw the first APTT sample after 6 hours and continue to do so every 6 hours for 48 hours. Titrate up or down to maintain the appropriate APTT, as outlined below.

- If the patient has an APTT of less than 1.2, give him a 2,500-unit bolus and increase the infusion by 200 units/hour.
- If his APTT is 1.2 to 1.3, increase the infusion by 160 units/hour. If it's 1.3 to 1.5, increase the infusion by 80 units/hour.
- If the patient's APTT is too high, at 2.0 to 2.5, decrease the infusion by 120 units/hour.
- If it's 2.5 to 3.0, decrease the infusion by 200 units/hour.
- If it's above 3.0, stop the drip for 60 minutes and then resume at a rate reduced by 200 units/hour.

After 48 hours, begin testing APTT every 12 hours for 24 hours and once daily thereafter. While the patient is receiving heparin, check his CBC every other day, as ordered.

If the patient develops thrombocytopenia, watch for bleeding and signs and symptoms of emboli. If testing reveals that the patient has heparin antibodies, inform him and tell him to avoid receiving heparin in the future.

Angiotensin-converting enzyme inhibitors

By inhibiting ACEs, drugs in this class block formation of angiotensin II, a potent endogenous vasopressor and modifier of endothelial tone and structure. Angiotensin II also stimulates the sympathetic nervous system and the release of aldosterone, a hormone that retains sodium and eliminates potassium.

By lowering angiotensin production, ACE inhibitors produce acute and sustained reductions in vasoconstriction, thus reducing myocardial oxygen demand. Clinically, they reduce mean arterial pressure, right atrial pressure, and left ventricular end-diastolic volume and pressure, which increases cardiac output and stroke volume. Among other things, these actions serve to limit ventricular hypertrophy and dilation, also known as ventricular remodeling. When given to a patient within 72 hours after the start of an MI, an ACE inhibitor can reduce the risk of death by up to 20%.

Patients who derive the greatest benefit are hemodynamically stable and free from continued ischemic pain, with an ejection fraction below 40%, systolic blood pressure above 100 mm Hg, and no evidence of cardiogenic shock. Giving a nitrate together with an ACE inhibitor may enhance their positive effects as long as the patient's volume and blood pressure don't decline too far. It may take 24 hours or more to make sure your patient is safe from excessive hypotension.

Don't give an ACE inhibitor to a patient with any of the following contraindications:
• bilateral renal artery stenosis
• history of hypersensitivity to the drug, such as a cough or angioedema
• renal failure
• systolic blood pressure below 100 mm Hg.

Therapy almost certainly will begin with a short-acting, low-dose ACE inhibitor (see *Reviewing angiotensin-converting enzyme inhibitors,* page 132). Many physicians prescribe captopril to start because of its short duration of action and flexible dosing. Patients then switch to a longer-acting drug for ongoing therapy. Most patients

Heparin therapy: When is bleeding acceptable?

For a patient receiving heparin, certain types of bleeding are almost unavoidable and therefore acceptable. However, you'll need to monitor your patient for certain other dangerous types of bleeding that require correction.

Acceptable bleeding
• easy bruising
• ecchymosis
• gum bleeding
• hemorrhoidal bleeding
• larger-than-normal bruises
• menstrual bleeding slightly increased for one extra day
• mild hemoptysis
• minor hematoma
• oozing from puncture sites
• petechiae
• pink-streaked nasal discharge
• subconjunctival hemorrhage

Unacceptable bleeding
• adrenal hemorrhage
• black or tarry stools
• bleeding from the nose as if from an open wound, free-flowing and clotless
• cerebral bleeding
• gross hematuria
• gross hemoptysis
• heavy menstrual bleeding that doesn't abate
• hemarthrosis
• hematemesis
• major hematoma
• occult rectal bleeding
• retroperitoneal bleeding

aren't hospitalized long enough to complete the titration process; consequently, they need a series of outpatient visits to adjust the dose needed to maintain systolic pressure above 90 mm Hg. Therapy typically continues for 6 weeks or more; patients with signs and symptoms of left ventricular dysfunction may continue it indefinitely.

Adverse effects
The ACE inhibitors tend to cause hypotension and will do so even with the first dose, especially among patients with hyponatremia, hyperrenine-

Reviewing angiotensin-converting enzyme inhibitors

Drug	Dose	Onset (hr)	Peak (hr)	Duration (hr)
captopril	6.25–50 mg every 8 hr	0.5	1–1.5	8–24
enalapril	2.5–10 mg every 12 hr	3–4	4–8	12–24
lisinopril	2.5–10 mg once daily	3–4	6–8	24
ramipril	1.25–10 mg every 12–24 hr	1–2	2–4	12–24

mia, hypovolemia, or a high ACE-inhibitor dosage. Elderly patients or those with heart failure may be especially sensitive to these drugs and may require smaller doses at longer intervals (6.25 mg of captopril every 12 hours, for example).

Renal insufficiency may develop in a patient taking an ACE inhibitor even if his blood pressure has been normal. If a patient develops signs and symptoms of renal insufficiency, expect to discontinue his ACE inhibitor, as prescribed.

Other adverse effects may include a persistent nonproductive cough, dizziness, angioedema, rash, nausea, a metallic taste, and a headache.

Nursing considerations

Tell your patient that his physician has prescribed a drug to help his heart function more effectively. Mention that it may make him dizzy, especially during the first week of therapy, and urge him to be careful when standing up or getting out of bed. Suggest that he rise slowly to a sitting position and then dangle his feet over the side of the bed before standing up. Also, tell him to call you if he develops any swelling of his face, eyes, or lips after taking the first dose.

Because ACE inhibitors are absorbed at varying rates when taken with food, tell your patient to take his drug in consistent relationship to his meals, either before or after.

If the physician prescribes captopril (the ACE inhibitor usually prescribed for MI patients), start with a test dose of 6.25 mg. Monitor the patient for hypotension and chest pain after giving it, especially during the time of its peak effects 60 to 90 minutes later.

If the patient's systolic pressure remains above 100 mm Hg after the first dose, wait 8 hours and then start giving him 12.5 mg every 8 hours. If his systolic pressure is between 90 and 100 mm Hg after the first dose, wait 8 hours and then start giving him 6.25 mg every 8 hours. And if his systolic pressure drops below 90 mm Hg after the first dose, assess the effects of his other drugs (especially diuretics, which may require a reduced dosage) and adjust their dosages as ordered. After at least 12 hours, preferably 24 to 48 hours, rechallenge the patient with 6.25 mg of captopril.

Once the patient's systolic pressure stays above 90 mm Hg for 48 to 72 hours, double his dose to either 25 mg or 12.5 mg, depending on how his blood pressure responded to the initial dose. Continue this stepped increase on an outpatient basis until the patient takes a maximum of 50 mg every 8 hours with a systolic pressure that remains steadily above 90 mm Hg. If it falls below 90 mm Hg, step back to the previous dosage, assess his other drug dosages, and try again.

Keep in mind that dosage adjustments may take several weeks and that some patients may never be able to take 50 mg of captopril every 8 hours.

Angioplasty

In facilities that have equipment and experienced staff, PTCA offers a proven—possibly a preferable—alternative to thrombolytic therapy for reperfusing the myocardium. In fact, it can reperfuse the affected myocardium within 50 minutes. Plus, the procedure yields patency rates considerably higher than those of thrombolytic drugs, especially in patients with a thrombus in a coronary artery bypass graft.

Nursing considerations

For a patient who's already anxious and fearful, the need for a rapid transition to PTCA can be frightening. As you prepare for the procedure, do your best to comfort and support him. Stay calm and be methodical as you complete your preprocedure tasks.

Before the procedure

Start by finding out which drugs he takes, his current weight, and any other health problems he has. Ask if he's allergic to iodine or contrast dye. Obtain baseline laboratory studies that include a CBC with platelet count, INR, APTT, PT, and myocardial enzyme, electrolyte, BUN, and creatinine levels. Assess whatever hemodynamic data is available.

Start giving fluids and dopamine I.V., as ordered, to ensure adequate blood pressure and perfusion. Also, give a beta-blocker, as ordered, to decrease myocardial workload and oxygen demand. If the patient may be allergic to the dye or to iodine, give corticosteroids as prescribed. Most patients also receive diphenhydramine orally or I.V. Make sure the patient has supplemental oxygen running. And give him a bolus dose of heparin (based on his weight) followed by a continuous infusion, as prescribed. Give him nothing by mouth except drugs and enough water to take them.

Make sure the patient has given written informed consent before he receives his preprocedure sedative. Consent probably will include emergency bypass grafting as well as PTCA.

During the procedure

During the procedure, the patient may receive intracoronary nitroglycerin. He'll also receive an antiplatelet drug, such as aspirin or abciximab. The physician probably will perform angiography on the noninfarcted vessels first so that films will be available in case the patient needs emergency bypass surgery. The physician may place a stent in the occluded vessel to prop it open.

After the procedure

After the procedure, assess the patient continuously for signs and symptoms of reduced perfusion or possible reocclusion. Decreased perfusion to the myocardium may worsen left ventricular function, causing your patient to develop signs and symptoms of worsening heart failure.

Decreased perfusion also may cause renal failure. You'll most likely administer nitroglycerin I.V. to promote coronary perfusion and decrease angina and vasospasm, a common response to PTCA. (Keep in mind that PTCA is contraindicated in a patient whose MI results from vasospasm.)

Also, assess the patient continuously for frank or occult bleeding. Although you must maintain his anticoagulant state to keep the vessel free from thrombi while healing, you must keep his bleeding risk as low as possible at the same time. Take steps to prevent bumps, falls, and mishaps that could cause unwanted bleeding. And carefully monitor the patient's laboratory values every 4 to 6 hours, including his hemoglobin level, hematocrit, PT, APTT, and INR.

Assess the patient's ECG for arrhythmias. Also, use hemodynamic monitoring to guide I.V. fluid replacement and vasopressor therapy.

Until the patient's activated clotting time returns to normal levels, usually about 8 hours, the femoral arterial and venous sheaths used to accomplish PTCA remain in place. While they do, keep the patient on flat bed rest or cautiously elevate his head by no more than 30 degrees, as ordered. Don't allow the patient to raise his head from the pillow to look at the groin site. Take time to explain the importance of immobility to the patient and his family.

Tell the patient to call you if he has any chest pain, needs to change positions, or feels that the groin site may be bleeding. If it begins to bleed, apply direct pressure until it stops. If appropriate, use a mechanical device to apply pressure. Regularly assess the patient's neurovascular status and the pulses distal to the insertion site on his affected limb.

Until the sheaths are pulled, restrict the patient's diet to clear liquids. Insert an indwelling catheter to ease urine retention, as needed. Keep in mind that vomiting can cause a serious groin bleed; give the nauseated patient an antiemetic, as prescribed.

After the sheaths are removed, the patient will remain on bed rest for about 24 hours. Help him with ambulation, as needed. Afterward, assess the groin site for bleeding, hematoma formation, and ecchymosis. Tell him to press on the groin site if he sneezes, coughs, or laughs.

Finally, watch carefully for other complications of bed rest or drugs, including atelectasis, ileus, constipation, and lumbar back pain.

Cardiac rehabilitation

Maximum recovery after an MI depends largely on the patient's willingness and ability to follow through with the lifestyle changes needed to help his heart heal and prevent further ischemia or infarction. If the patient had an uncomplicated MI, he may not need a formal outpatient rehabilitation program. However, he'll almost certainly need inpatient teaching.

Patient teaching

Before the patient leaves the hospital, help him get back on his feet and prepare him for the changes ahead. The first stage involves helping him ambulate on the unit and assessing his heart's response to increasing activity.

Also, provide wide-ranging teaching. For example, he needs to know how to take his drugs properly, what they're for, and what adverse effects he should report. If necessary, construct a drug map to help remind the patient when to take each drug dose. If he requires repeated follow-up checks of his anticoagulation status, explain how, where, and how often to obtain them. Provide him with a phone number he can call to obtain answers to questions after he returns home.

Also, review lifestyle changes that may be helpful in his recovery. Most patients already know about the importance of weight loss, smoking cessation, and stress management. As needed, refer the patient to a dietitian, home health agency, or outpatient clinic to help accomplish needed lifestyle changes and coordinate medical services.

Although exercise forms one important facet of successful recovery after an MI, encourage the patient not to abruptly increase his level of activity once he gets home. Instead, he should maintain his inpatient level of activity for a week or two. After his first follow-up visit with his physician, he may be able to increase his activity level as prescribed. If an outpatient cardiac rehabilitation program is appropriate for the patient and available in his area, urge him to participate once he has his physician's approval.

If possible, provide the patient with written instructions to supplement your verbal teaching. He and his family may better digest the material when they're settled back into their usual environment. Make sure any materials describing exercise include a list of unwanted symptoms, actions to take if they occur, guidelines for a safe walking program, and a log for keeping track of exercise activities, especially walking. A typical log entry includes the patient's heart rate after exercise, the distance covered during the walk, and the time spent walking.

Outpatient activities

For the first few weeks after an MI, the patient's heart remains vulnerable to injury. Indeed, it may continue to heal for 12 weeks or more. That's why some facilities recommend that patients begin outpatient cardiac rehabilitation 2 to 3 weeks after an MI, while others suggest waiting until 6 weeks afterward.

Keep in mind that the exercise program in cardiac rehabilitation poses a greater risk for some patients after an MI than for others. For example, patients with poor left ventricular function have about a 30% chance of dying during the first year after an MI. Those with sustained ventricular tachycardia have an increased risk as well. That's why most patients undergo stress testing, usually with thallium, 7 to 10 days after an MI.

Based on the results of stress testing, physical examination, and history, patients can be classified by their risk of exercise complications, including sudden cardiac death, pulmonary edema, syncope, myocardial ischemia, and another MI. The rehabilitation plan must be adapted accordingly (see *Determining your patient's risk of complications from exercise*). Patients with a moderate or high risk need more frequent or continuous ECG monitoring during exercise. Those with a low risk can safely begin an exercise program with minimal supervision and monitoring. Especially early in rehabilitation, all patients must carefully coordinate all their activities, including exercise.

Activity planning
Encourage your patient to plan his daily activities ahead of time, both to conserve energy and to attempt the most demanding activities at times when he has the most energy. The goal is for the patient to space his activities so that he can rest and avoid becoming too tired.

Explain that he can try to do a little bit more each day. However, if he feels tired the day after increasing his activity level, he should do a little

Determining your patient's risk of complications from exercise

After a myocardial infarction (MI), your patient may face a low, moderate, or high risk of complications from exercise. To determine his risk, review the characteristics listed below.

Low risk
- no ischemia
- no left ventricular dysfunction
- ejection fraction above 50%
- no significant arrhythmias
- activities that exceed 7.5 metabolic equivalents 3 weeks after the MI

Moderate risk
- angina or ST-segment depression of 1–2 mm caused by exercise
- mild left ventricular dysfunction
- history of heart failure
- ejection fraction of 35%–49%
- nonsustained ventricular arrhythmias
- activities between 4.5 and 7.5 metabolic equivalents 3 weeks after the MI

High risk
- hypotension or ST-segment depression of more than 2 mm caused by exercise
- ischemia caused by light exercise
- severe left ventricular dysfunction
- ejection fraction below 35%
- sustained ventricular arrhythmias
- activities of less than 4.5 metabolic equivalents 3 weeks after the MI

less that day. Urge the patient to think about taking slow, steady breaths during his activities. Also, suggest that some of his activities involve enjoyable diversions or hobbies.

Tell the patient to avoid lifting, pushing, pulling, and any other activity in which he might find himself holding his breath and straining—a combination he should avoid. Urge him to use healthy body mechanics. For example, if he must lift something, tell him to bend his knees before doing so rather than lifting with his back. Urge him to divide a load and make several trips whenever possible. If he must move something heavy, tell him to push rather than pull it. And warn him to avoid working for long periods in a stooped position.

Self-monitoring

In any exercise program, the patient must learn and practice self-monitoring skills. For example, he must take his own pulse and accurately assess and respond to any signs or symptoms that arise during exercise. Warning signs and symptoms that the patient's heart isn't tolerating the exercise include the following:
- angina
- an inappropriately fast heart rate
- dizziness
- loss of coordination
- nausea and cool, moist skin

- shortness of breath
- sudden sweatiness.

If these signs or symptoms arise, the patient must stop exercising, rest, and take nitroglycerin if prescribed. He also should call his physician. If you don't feel that the patient can or will recognize and respond properly to these signs and symptoms, you should consider him a moderate or high risk even if, physically, he fits the low-risk category.

Heart rate

When teaching the patient how to check his pulse, show him how to find his radial pulse first, although the pulses in his neck or temple offer acceptable alternatives. Tell him to use his first two fingers (not his thumb), to apply gentle pressure, and to count the heartbeats for 10 seconds. Then he should multiply the resulting figure by 6 to obtain his pulse rate. Make sure the patient knows his resting heart rate and the target rate for which he should strive during exercise. The target rate varies with the patient's age, heart condition, prescribed drugs, and diagnosis, but typically it should rise by 20 to 30 bpm over the resting rate during exercise.

Perceived exertion

If your patient has trouble counting his heart rate, consider having him use a perceived exertion scale instead. On this scale, the patient chooses words, numbers, or colors to describe his perception of exercise difficulty. Reassure the patient that mild to moderate exercise is effective; he'll gain virtually no added benefit from strenuous exercise.

Describe some other subjective measures of exercise intensity as well. For example, tell the patient to avoid becoming so breathless that he can no longer converse while exercising. Counting, humming, and singing also can help keep his breathing easy and relaxed. Advise him to walk slowly for 2 to 3 minutes to warm up before he begins exercising at a somewhat higher level. He should feel warm at this higher level, but not hot. He shouldn't sweat or feel flushed.

Precautions

Especially early in rehabilitation, the patient is better off taking two to four short walks rather than one long walk. He should avoid walking in very cold or very hot weather. And he should avoid steep inclines. Tell him to drink plenty of water and to follow sensible safety practices. For example, he should walk with a buddy, tell someone when he expects to return home, wear comfortable but sturdy shoes, and avoid dangerous areas or those with inadequate paving or lighting. Tell him to consider wearing or carrying medical identification, especially if he's taking an anticoagulant.

Over time, the patient can extend the length and distance of his walk as his heart tolerates it. He should continue to walk at a comfortable pace, however, and he should stop right away if he develops unwanted signs or symptoms. The next day, he should resume walking at a lower intensity level. In general, the patient should engage in an activity safely and successfully for 2 weeks before increasing its level of intensity.

Lifestyle changes

The need for lifestyle changes varies widely among patients who have had an MI. For each patient, you can help determine which aspects of his lifestyle need to change, how they need to change, and in what priority they need to change. Then help the patient devise a plan for change that includes realistic, prioritized goals.

In devising such a plan, take the patient's resources and support structure into account. Does he have supportive family members who will help him change his diet habits? Do other people in his home smoke? Will his family and friends give him the positive feedback and encouragement he needs to successfully navigate the changes ahead?

Whether or not the patient has supportive family members at home, he probably will benefit from charting his lifestyle changes. Suggest that he keep a diet diary and an exercise log to help motivate himself and track his progress. Help him learn to quickly detect and change negative thinking patterns that can reduce his chance of success in all areas of lifestyle change. And help him identify ways to use humor, prayer, or diversionary leisure activities to cope with change and reduce stress.

Also, mention that many patients experience a period of depression after having an MI. He may feel overly fatigued, dejected, and irritable, and he may feel a decrease in energy and libido. This condition is called vital exhaustion; if it lasts too long or becomes too intense, the patient's risk of death increases. Urge him and his family members to obtain counseling or medical intervention if the patient becomes depressed.

Over time, as the patient's heart muscle heals and he makes healthy changes in his lifestyle, he may find himself feeling better than ever.

8

MYOCARDIAL INFARCTION

Complications

After a patient suffers a myocardial infarction (MI), his survival may well depend on your quick, effective response to complications. That's why you need to watch for dangerous complications and be ready to promptly administer the treatments required throughout an MI patient's hospitalization.

This chapter reviews some of the most common—and most deadly—complications you'll encounter when caring for MI patients: arrhythmias, cardiogenic shock, myocardial rupture, pericarditis, ventricular aneurysm, cerebral embolism, and right ventricular infarction.

Arrhythmias

Arrhythmias affect more than 75% of patients who've had an MI. Some develop relatively harmless arrhythmias; others develop life-threatening ones. In general, you'll need to respond any time an arrhythmia impairs your patient's hemodynamic status, threatens the myocardium by raising oxygen demand, or increases the probability of advancement to a life-threatening rhythm.

Commonly, a patient with an arrhythmia displays signs and symptoms, such as syncope, hypotension, angina, confusion, and evidence of heart failure.

Obviously, your patient's electrocardiogram (ECG) also provides crucial information in your effort to detect arrhythmias. It can reveal rhythm disturbances, conduction problems, hypertrophy of the left ventricle, and ectopy of the atria and ventricles. A physician may also order a signal-averaged ECG to detect late potentials that can warn of impending ventricular tachycardia.

Some patients may wear a Holter monitor in the hospital. Over a 24-hour to 48-hour recording period, the patient logs his activities and any symptoms that arise. Then, an examiner analyzes the ECG recording along with the patient's log.

Your patient's electrolyte levels provide diagnostic data as well. Abnormal levels can influence or cause several arrhythmias, including life-threatening ventricular tachycardia and ventricular fibrillation. For example, hypokalemia, which develops in up to 25% of patients after an MI, raises the risk of both arrhythmias. Likewise, hypomagnesemia may lead to ventricular arrhythmias, torsades de pointes, and sudden death.

Electrophysiology studies also may yield valuable diagnostic data. During this invasive test, a physician inserts electrophysiology catheters into the patient's right atrium and ventricle by way of a peripheral vein. The catheters record electrical activity in the heart. Then, using programmed electrical stimulation, the physician triggers the arrhythmia, measures the hemodynamic effects, and assesses the patient's response to interventions, such as drugs and pacing.

These diagnostic tests may reveal acute tachyarrhythmias or bradyarrhythmias that arise after an MI. They also can help point the way to an effective treatment.

Tachyarrhythmias

During and after an MI, especially an anterior-wall MI, sympathetic stimulation attempts to compensate for decreased cardiac output (CO). How-

Recognizing sinus tachycardia

In sinus tachycardia, the sinoatrial node paces the patient's heart at 100 or more beats per minute (bpm). You'll see a regular rhythm with a P wave for every QRS complex.

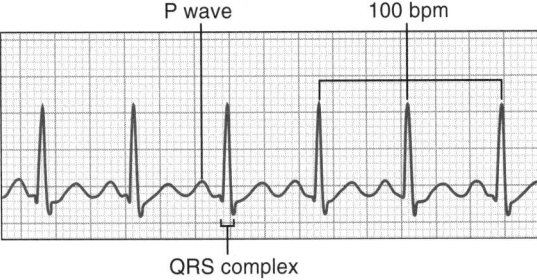

ever, that stimulation also raises the patient's risk of acute tachyarrhythmias, such as sinus tachycardia, atrial fibrillation, atrial flutter, ventricular tachycardia, and ventricular fibrillation. These arrhythmias may create hemodynamic instability that requires a swift and accurate response. Sometimes the response involves drug administration. Sometimes it involves cardioversion or defibrillation.

Sinus tachycardia

Characterized by its regular rhythm and increased rate, sinus tachycardia develops in nearly a third of patients who experience an MI—even more in patients who have an anterior-wall MI. In an attempt to maintain an adequate CO, the sinoatrial (SA) node paces the patient's heart at 100 or more beats per minute (bpm). The ECG strip shows a regular rhythm with a P wave for every QRS complex (see *Recognizing sinus tachycardia*).

The danger of sinus tachycardia results from the shortened diastolic filling time it creates. If filling time becomes too short, the coronary arteries may receive too little blood to perfuse the myocardium, causing or worsening myocardial ischemia. Plus, the ventricle has too little time to fill and ejects too little blood, which decreases CO and blood pressure even more. To make matters worse, the increased heart rate also increas-

es the heart's oxygen consumption at a time when less oxygen may be available.

To reduce the increased rhythm, treat the underlying cause, as prescribed. For example, if your patient feels pain or anxiety, you may give morphine to calm him, relax vascular smooth muscle, and decrease circulating catecholamines. Also, expect to administer a beta-blocker to decrease his heart rate, slow the conduction of atrioventricular (AV) impulses, and decrease the force of myocardial contractility.

Atrial fibrillation and atrial flutter

Roughly 15% of MI patients develop atrial fibrillation or, occasionally, atrial flutter (see *Recognizing atrial fibrillation and atrial flutter*). In these arrhythmias, the atria produce chaotic electrical signals either from multiple reentry points inside the atria or from multiple ectopic foci. Either way, the atrial beat is so rapid and so uncoordinated that it's more like a quiver.

In an MI patient, atrial fibrillation or atrial flutter may stem from atrial enlargement caused by heart failure or pericarditis related to the MI. Just after an MI, atrial fibrillation may result from occlusion of the right coronary artery or the proximal left circumflex artery.

In atrial fibrillation, numerous sites in the atria fire spontaneously, producing rates as high as 400 uncoordinated impulses per minute. As a result, the atria quiver and fail to contract effectively. Not all of the atrial impulses proceed through the AV node, which results in an irregular ventricular rate of 100 to 200 bpm. Several factors cause the patient to have increasing hemodynamic instability:
- the quivering atria no longer contribute to ventricular filling
- the increased rate decreases ventricular filling time
- irregular conduction causes irregular and insufficient filling of the ventricle from beat to beat.

In atrial flutter, which affects less than 1 in 100 MI patients, the atria typically produce 250 to 350 bpm. The ventricular rate usually remains regular and produces F waves, which have a sawtooth appearance, on the patient's ECG rather than P waves. The PR interval may be regular or it may vary.

For a patient with atrial fibrillation or atrial flutter and hemodynamic instability, the physician may order electrical cardioversion. However, if the patient has minimal hemodynamic insta-

Recognizing atrial fibrillation and atrial flutter

If your patient has atrial fibrillation, you'll see an irregular rhythm, an atrial rate that's too fast to count, and a ventricular rate as high as 180 beats per minute (bpm). You won't see P waves; instead, the baseline will show fine or coarse fibrillatory waves. Also, you won't see T waves, and the QT interval will be unmeasurable.

Atrial fibrillation

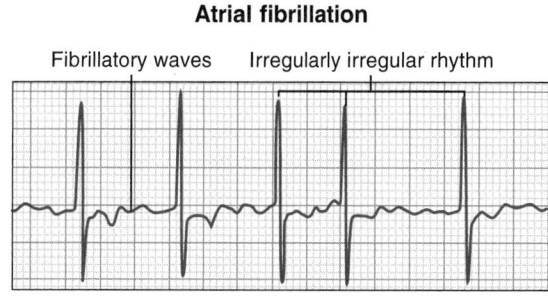

If your patient has atrial flutter, his rhythm may be regular or irregular. The atrial rate typically reaches 250 to 300 bpm, while the ventricular rate remains at 50 to 75 bpm. You'll notice that P waves have been replaced by F waves, giving the tracing a sawtooth appearance. The PR interval may be regular, or it may vary.

Atrial flutter

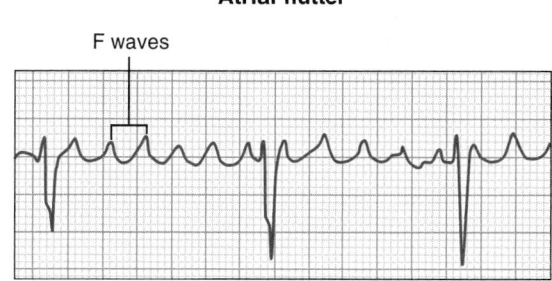

---

bility, your first priority is to slow the ventricular rate rather than to convert it to a sinus rhythm. That's because the heart may convert to a sinus rhythm spontaneously once the rate approaches normal. To slow the ventricular rate, give a calcium channel blocker (usually diltiazem or verapamil), a beta-blocker (usually metoprolol, esmolol, or atenolol), or a short-acting digitalis glycoside preparation (digoxin), as prescribed.

Remember that patients with atrial fibrillation or atrial flutter face a higher risk of embolic complications because blood tends to pool in the atria. As ordered, start anticoagulation therapy as soon as possible after the onset of the arrhythmia.

Ventricular tachycardia and ventricular fibrillation

Most common during the acute phase of an MI, ventricular tachycardia and ventricular fibrillation also may arise up to 14 days after the infarction and may have serious, possibly deadly, consequences for your patient.

You'll know the patient has ventricular tachycardia when you see a run of three or more ventricular beats at a rate of 100 bpm or more on his ECG tracing (see *Recognizing ventricular tachyarrhythmias,* page 140). Because ventricular beats originate in the ventricle and move from cell to ventricular cell rather than following the normal conduction pattern through the bundle branches and Purkinje fibers, the ECG shows bizarre ventricular complexes that measure more than 0.12 second in width. The rhythm may be regular or slightly irregular. Not every QRS complex has a P wave, and T waves typically deflect in the opposite direction from the QRS complex.

For the MI patient, ventricular tachycardia may degrade rapidly into ventricular fibrillation, a deadly chaotic rhythm that halts CO. Indeed, ventricular fibrillation is the most common arrhythmia caused by an MI and the most common cause of death for patients who die before obtaining emergency care. You'll know it by the highly irregular rhythm and variable size and

Recognizing ventricular tachyarrhythmias

If your patient has ventricular tachycardia, you'll see a run of three or more ventricular beats at a rate of more than 100 beats per minute (bpm). The QRS complexes will be bizarre and measure 0.12 second or more. T waves will deflect in the opposite direction of the QRS complex. The rhythm usually is regular, but it may be slightly irregular.

Ventricular tachycardia

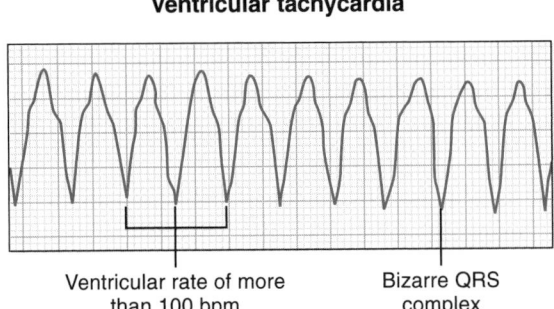

Ventricular rate of more than 100 bpm

Bizarre QRS complex

If your patient has ventricular fibrillation, you'll see a grossly irregular rhythm but no QRS complexes or P waves. The rate typically becomes too high and disorganized to count. You may see coarse fibrillation, as shown here, or fine fibrillation.

Ventricular fibrillation

Coarse fibrillatory waves

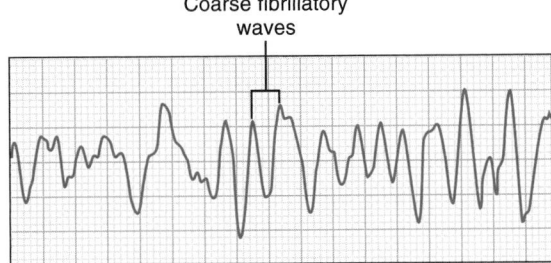

If your patient has torsades de pointes, you'll see a gradual alteration in the amplitude and direction of electrical activity. Consequently, the QRS complexes appear to be twisting around the isoelectric line. You'll see an irregular rhythm and either a fast or slow rate but no P waves.

Torsades de pointes

Irregularly irregular rhythm

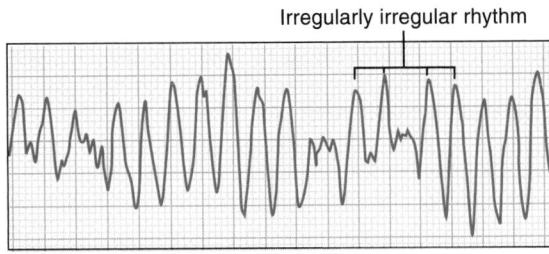

shape of the QRS complexes; none are normal. Typical QRS complexes aren't even discernable. You'll see no P waves, and the rate may be too rapid and disorganized to count.

Ventricular tachycardia and fibrillation may result from a number of MI-related problems. For example, the increase in circulating catecholamines may change the automaticity of myocardial cells by altering the influx of sodium ions, thus allowing groups of affected cells to depolarize at different rates.

These arrhythmias may also result when ischemic tissue conducts impulses at a slower rate than that of the surrounding normal tissue. Thus, the normal tissue may repolarize while the ischemic tissue is still depolarizing. The initial depolarizing current may then reenter the normal tissue during its repolarization phase, yielding a chaotic, ineffective rhythm. In effect, the ventricles quiver rather than contract.

Treatment
Both ventricular tachycardia and ventricular fibrillation require a rapid, effective response. Start by checking the patient's airway, breathing, and circulation. If you can't find a femoral or carotid pulse, treat the patient as though he has ventricular fibrillation.

If you can find a pulse, the patient has ventricular tachycardia and probably will undergo synchronized cardioversion. In this procedure, the patient's heart receives a direct current timed to coincide with depolarization—the R wave. Delivering the current at precisely this time avoids the possibility of delivering it during repolarization, which could cause ventricular fibrillation.

You also may give lidocaine, bretylium, or another antiarrhythmic drug to a patient with ventricular tachycardia and a pulse. Anticipate giving a beta-blocker and managing the patient's electrolyte levels as well.

Ventricular fibrillation typically requires immediate defibrillation. If the arrhythmia arose more than 72 hours after the MI took place, assess carefully for recurrent ischemia and abnormal electrolyte levels. The patient may require cardiac catheterization and serial measurement of his cardiac enzyme levels to reveal the cause of this late-onset fibrillation. If the problem doesn't stem from ischemia or abnormal electrolyte levels, the patient may need electrophysiologic testing and an implantable cardioverter-defibrillator.

A surgeon implants a transvenous cardioverter-defibrillator under the skin, typically below the left subclavian vein. He then threads wires from the device into the subclavian vein, through the superior vena cava, and into the right side of the heart. Or a surgeon may implant an epicardial cardioverter-defibrillator in the abdomen, and then perform a median sternotomy or left-sided thoracotomy, attach patches to the patient's ventricles, and tunnel the connecting wires to the patient's abdomen. The device activates when it senses ventricular tachycardia or defibrillation. Naturally, the patient needs your teaching and support before receiving the device (see *Teaching your patient about his implantable cardioverter-defibrillator,* page 142).

Torsades de pointes
Torsades de pointes literally means twisting of the points. As its name implies, this arrhythmia causes an ECG in which cycles of QRS complexes seem to be twisting around the isoelectric line. No P waves appear on the tracing. You'll see an irregular rhythm and a rate that may be fast or slow.

Torsades de pointes typically results from drug toxicity; reaction to antiarrhythmic drugs, such as quinidine or procainamide; or abnormal electrolyte levels. Because it prolongs the QT interval, its treatment differs from that used for ventricular tachycardia or fibrillation.

Anticipate giving the patient magnesium sulfate I.V. You may also give isoproterenol, a beta agonist that increases CO and contractions. Don't give isoproterenol to a patient with ischemia, however, because it increases myocardial oxygen demand.

Most patients with torsades de pointes undergo overdrive pacing, usually at 170 to 180 bpm, to suppress the arrhythmia, shorten the QT interval, and allow the heart's intrinsic rhythm to return. For a prolonged arrhythmia, a patient may need cardioversion. However, even if these interventions correct the arrhythmia, it probably will return unless the underlying cause is corrected.

Bradyarrhythmias

After having an MI, your patient also faces a risk of acute bradyarrhythmias, in which his heart rate drops below 60 bpm. They include sinus bradycardia, AV blocks, and asystole.

Sinus bradycardia
About a third of all MI patients and more than half of those who sustain a posterior-wall or an inferior-wall MI develop sinus bradycardia. By definition, *sinus bradycardia* refers to a decrease in the rate of atrial depolarization caused by slowing of the SA node (see *Recognizing sinus bradycardia,* page 143). On the patient's ECG, you'll notice little more than a rate slowed to

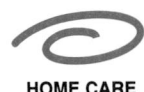

HOME CARE

Teaching your patient about his implantable cardioverter-defibrillator

If your patient is going home with an implantable cardioverter-defibrillator, be sure to teach him about the device. Start by showing him a picture of it and reviewing its parts and its function.

Next, assure him and his family that household appliances—such as toasters, microwaves, vacuums, and televisions—won't affect his defibrillator. However, he should avoid touching a running motor that contains spark plugs. Also, tell him to avoid strong magnetic fields, such as those used in magnetic resonance imaging machines and airport security wands. Reassure him that sexual activity and routine contact with another person won't activate the defibrillator or shock the other person.

Tell him to avoid clothing that puts pressure on the defibrillator. And tell him to report signs and symptoms of infection: redness, swelling, drainage, and pain at the incision site and a fever above 100.5°F (38.1°C).

Explain that if the device fires, he'll feel a thump in his chest or back. Encourage him to call his physician anytime this happens.

Also, tell his family to call his physician right away if the patient loses consciousness or if he thinks the device may be malfunctioning. Suggest to family members that they attend a class in cardiopulmonary resuscitation. Encourage the patient to carry or wear medical identification at all times.

If your patient seems overly anxious about the device, help him learn to use relaxation techniques and coping strategies to reduce his stress. And refer him and his family to a support group for people with implantable cardioverter-defibrillators.

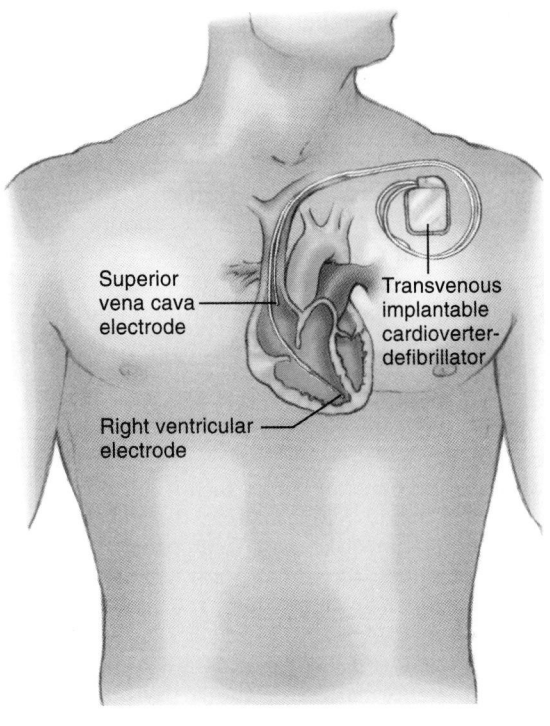

Superior vena cava electrode

Transvenous implantable cardioverter-defibrillator

Right ventricular electrode

---

60 bpm or less. The rhythm, QRS complexes, and P waves all will be normal.

Administer treatments for sinus bradycardia only when it produces signs and symptoms—a development that signals a rate too slow to provide adequate tissue perfusion. Such signs and symptoms include chest pain, escape ectopy, hypotension, an altered level of consciousness, and pulmonary edema.

Although atropine is usually the treatment of choice for patients with sinus bradycardia, you'll need to administer it with care. The reflex tachycardia it creates could worsen the patient's ischemia and extend his infarction. If atropine is too dangerous or the patient needs longer-term control, he'll probably undergo transvenous pacing.

Keep in mind that the patient may need other treatments as well. For example, if increased vagal tone causes nausea, give an antiemetic, as prescribed. For chest pain, give fluids and low-dose dopamine therapy I.V., as ordered; a patient with sinus bradycardia may not tolerate nitroglycerin or morphine until after receiving treatments to support his blood pressure.

Atrioventricular blocks

Common during an MI, an AV block results from a delay or interruption in impulse conduction between the atria and ventricles. It may occur at the level of the AV node, bundle of His, bundle branches, or Purkinje pathways.

Atrioventricular blocks may range from mild to severe and include first-degree, second-degree types I and II, and third-degree (or complete) blocks. They commonly improve over a few hours or days; occasionally, however, patients with a second-degree type II or third-degree AV block may need permanent pacing even for transient arrhythmias.

First-degree block

You'll know first-degree AV block by its prolonged PR interval (greater than 0.20 second). The QRS complexes will be normal, the rhythm will be regular, and every P wave will be followed by a QRS complex (see *Types of atrioventricular block,* page 144). This arrhythmia usually causes no symptoms and therefore requires no treatment.

Second-degree block type I

When some impulses are conducted and some are blocked, the patient has second-degree AV block, Mobitz type I, also known as Wenckebach block. It occurs at the level of the AV node and may result from increased parasympathetic tone or drug effects. Usually transient, it causes progressive prolongation of the PR interval until an impulse is completely blocked. Then the pattern repeats. Usually only a single impulse is blocked and the pattern repeats itself.

Second-degree block type II

This block, called Mobitz type II block, arises just distal to the AV node and results from ischemic damage to the right bundle branch and the left anterior fascicle of the left branch. You may see a normal or a wide QRS complex. Each P wave is followed by a QRS complex except the blocked one. The PR interval may be normal or prolonged. Unpredictable, this block can deteriorate to a complete heart block.

Third-degree block

Also known as complete heart block, a third-degree AV block allows no electrical conduction

Recognizing sinus bradycardia

If your patient has sinus bradycardia, you'll see a rate that's less than 60 beats per minute (bpm) and a regular rhythm. The P waves and QRS complexes will be normal.

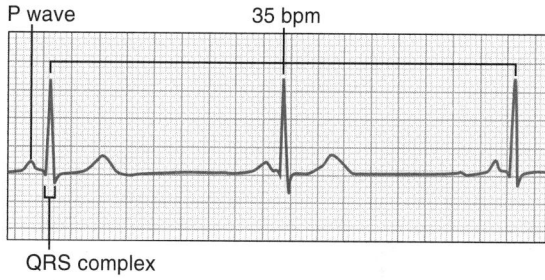

between the atria and ventricles, which creates independent beats in the atria and ventricles. This block occurs at the level of the AV node, bundle of His, or bundle branches. The atrial rate may remain at 60 to 100 bpm, but the ventricular rate may drop below 40 bpm.

Third-degree AV block commonly produces chest pain, loss of consciousness, and profound hypotension. Some patients may maintain marginal perfusion as long as they remain still and in bed. Treatment includes atropine, dopamine or epinephrine, and transcutaneous or transvenous pacing.

Treatment

For patients with bradyarrhythmias, cardiac pacing may be the treatment of choice. A pacemaker uses a battery-operated generator to deliver shocks to the patient's heart via one or more electrodes placed in the heart or on the patient's body. A pacemaker may be used permanently or temporarily, and it may pace continually or only as needed.

Many physicians prescribe temporary cardiac pacing for patients with a bradyarrhythmia while deciding whether or not to implant a permanent pacemaker. Patients who receive permanent pacemakers typically have a chronic, severe brady-

Types of atrioventricular block

First-degree atrioventricular block

In first-degree atrioventricular (AV) block, you'll see a PR interval that's prolonged beyond 0.20 second. The rhythm will be regular. P waves and QRS complexes will be normal.

PR interval of more
than 0.20 second

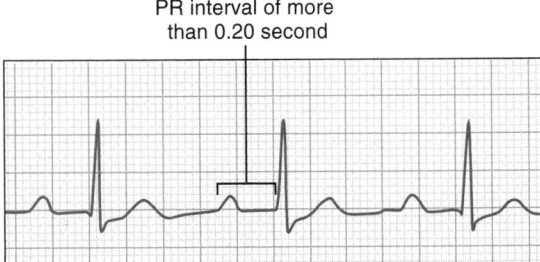

Second-degree atrioventricular block type I

In second-degree AV block type I, you'll see a pattern of progressively prolonged PR intervals, followed by a dropped QRS complex. The atrial rhythm will be nearly regular.

Pattern of progressively   Dropped
prolonged PR intervals   QRS complex

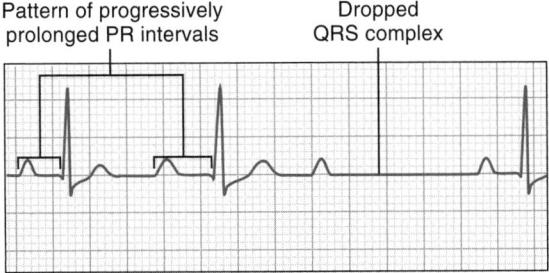

Second-degree atrioventricular block type II

In second-degree AV block type II, the PR interval doesn't lengthen before one or more QRS complexes are dropped. The atrial rhythm will be regular, but the ventricular rhythm will be irregular. The QRS complex may be normal or wide.

Constant PR   Dropped
intervals   QRS complex

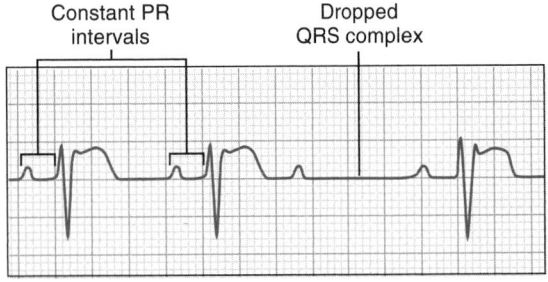

Third-degree atrioventricular block

In third-degree AV block, atrial and ventricular rates are regular, but the atrial rate will be 60 to 100 beats per minute (bpm), and the ventricular rate will be 20 to 40 bpm. The PR interval will vary. The QRS complex may be normal or wide.

Ventricular rate of   Atrial rate of
30 beats/minute   80 beats/minute

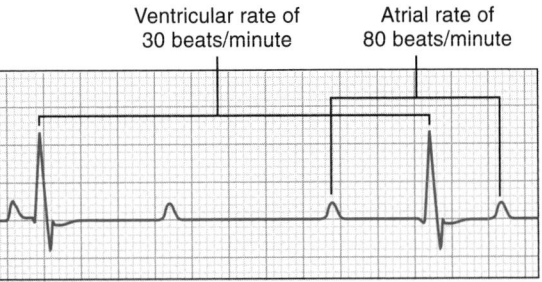

arrhythmia from an AV block or SA node malfunction.

When teaching your patient, make sure you include appropriate family members, and take time to explain why the pacemaker is necessary and how to live with it. For example, explain the rhythm problem that resulted in the patient's need for a pacemaker. Outline how and when the pacemaker works. Talk about any diet restric-

tions and other lifestyle changes the patient needs to make, including smoking cessation.

Review the drugs your patient will be taking, including their names and how and when to take them. Explain their possible adverse effects and tell the patient which effects should prompt a call to his physician. Encourage the patient to keep all follow-up appointments.

Teach the patient how to check his own pulse

rate and rhythm and explain when and why he should do so. Also, talk about methods the patient can use to conserve energy. Tell him to stop any activity that causes chest discomfort, fatigue, shortness of breath, pain, palpitations, or light-headedness.

If the patient will be wearing a Holter monitor, tell him not to take a bath or shower during the 24 to 48 hours he'll be wearing it. Also, teach him how to keep a log of his activities and symptoms during that time.

Encourage the patient's family members to learn basic life support. And help the patient and his family find the resources they need to obtain information and emotional support.

Asystole

Also called ventricular standstill, *asystole* refers to the absence of a heartbeat and a flat line in at least two leads on the patient's ECG tracing. You'll see no QRS complexes and detect no electrical activity.

Asystole requires immediate cardiopulmonary resuscitation (CPR) and immediate transcutaneous pacing or surgical repair. Don't defibrillate the patient because doing so could prevent the return of spontaneous cardiac activity. Instead, give atropine and epinephrine, as ordered, to stimulate contraction of the myocardium. Keep in mind, however, that because asystole represents extensive myocardial ischemia and injury and because it tends to take place after ventricular rupture, the patient has a poor prognosis.

Cardiogenic shock

This life-threatening complication arises in 5% to 15% of MI patients and reflects the heart's inability to maintain enough tissue perfusion to meet the body's metabolic needs. Despite significant advances in treatment, cardiogenic shock continues to carry a high death rate.

When more than about 40% of the left ventricle is infarcted, its ability to pump declines dramatically, along with CO, oxygen delivery, and tissue perfusion. The decline in tissue perfusion affects all the body's organs and prompts a series of compensatory mechanisms that attempt to restore perfusion, especially to vital organs.

For example, increased catecholamine levels shift fluid into the vascular compartment, thus ex-

panding the blood volume. Hypoperfusion stimulates the sympathetic nervous system, which prompts the adrenal medulla to secrete epinephrine and norepinephrine, increasing blood flow to the heart, brain, and other vital organs and decreasing it elsewhere. Epinephrine and norepinephrine also directly increase CO and myocardial contractility.

Decreased kidney perfusion activates the renin-angiotensin-aldosterone system, which causes the kidneys to reabsorb sodium and water and to secrete potassium, an action that helps to maintain intravascular volume but may lead to hypokalemia.

Finally, hypotension caused by shock causes the posterior lobe of the pituitary gland to release antidiuretic hormone, which leads to reabsorption of sodium and water in the renal tubules.

Working together, these mechanisms may compensate for the heart's inadequate pumping ability, but only temporarily. Eventually, their effects will become detrimental because they create an imbalance between oxygen supply and demand, leading to even more ischemia. Increased ischemia hampers myocardial contractility, further decreasing coronary artery perfusion, stroke volume, and output. Without an adequate supply of oxygen, the body's cells switch from aerobic to anaerobic metabolism. Lactic acid builds up in the blood and eventually causes metabolic acidosis.

Signs and symptoms

A patient with cardiogenic shock has a systolic blood pressure below 90 mm Hg (more than a 30% decline in a hypertensive patient) and tachycardia. He'll have a weak and thready pulse and marked pallor and cyanosis of the lips and nail beds. His skin will feel cool and clammy; it may appear mottled. The patient probably will seem anxious.

Your physical examination will most likely reveal jugular vein distention. You may auscultate third and fourth heart sounds (S_3 and S_4), the former from vibration of ventricle walls caused by overfilling and the latter from vibration of atrial walls as they contract forcefully at the end of diastole to move blood into the stiff ventricles. You may not be able to hear the first heart sound, which marks the closure of mitral and tricuspid valves, because of the decrease in contractility. You may hear a holosystolic murmur of mitral regurgitation and possibly an ejection murmur of septal rupture.

Auscultation of the patient's lung fields will reveal inspiratory crackles. You may hear expiratory grunting and see pink, frothy sputum. You may even hear diffuse wheezing if your patient has severe left ventricular heart failure.

A prolonged capillary refill time, decreased urine output, and altered level of consciousness all reflect the patient's impaired organ perfusion. You'll also find a cardiac index (CI) of less than 2.2 L/minute/m^2 and a pulmonary artery wedge pressure (PAWP) above 15 mm Hg.

Diagnostic tests

Tests used to confirm and monitor cardiogenic shock include the ECG, chest X-ray, arterial blood gas measurements, other laboratory tests, and pulmonary artery catheterization.

Electrocardiogram

Early in cardiogenic shock, the patient's ECG may look normal, or it may reveal sinus tachycardia. Over time, however, you'll see indications of ischemia, such as ST-segment and T-wave changes. Usually in cardiogenic shock, the patient has a transmural infarction and develops large Q waves.

Chest X-ray

The patient's chest X-ray will reveal early interstitial pulmonary edema and enlargement of the heart, both indications of heart failure.

Arterial blood gas studies

Arterial blood gas measurements help to determine the patient's oxygenation, ventilation, and metabolic state. Arterial blood gases drawn during cardiogenic shock typically indicate respiratory alkalosis (pH above 7.45 and bicarbonate level above 28 mEq/L) progressing to metabolic acidosis (pH below 7.35 and bicarbonate level below 24 mEq/L). This occurs initially as a compensatory mechanism to blow off carbon dioxide because of increasing lactic acid levels. As shock progresses, however, metabolic acidosis develops as respiratory compensation fails.

Laboratory tests

Serum electrolyte levels may be increased or decreased depending on the stage of shock and its compensatory mechanisms. Cardiac enzyme levels will be increased from the MI. Blood urea nitrogen and creatinine levels may be increased as well, indicating renal impairment caused by shock.

Pulmonary artery catheterization

Monitoring your patient's pulmonary artery pressure, CO, and other hemodynamic values allows for rapid identification of complications after an MI, provides a direct means for assessing the patient's progress and response to fluids and drugs, and permits careful dosage adjustments. An invasive technique, pulmonary artery catheterization requires percutaneous insertion of a catheter into the right side of the heart. Typically, monitoring for such a patient takes place in the critical care unit.

Treatment

The goals of treatment for a patient in cardiogenic shock include the following:
- to preserve as much myocardium as possible through early reperfusion
- to stabilize cardiac function with drugs and mechanical assist devices
- to stimulate myocardial contractility in an effort to maximize systolic function and reduce pulmonary venous congestion and afterload.

For most patients, the mainstays of treatment are vasoactive drugs and intra-aortic balloon counterpulsation.

Vasoactive drugs

Drugs used to treat cardiogenic shock include nitroglycerin, sodium nitroprusside, dopamine, dobutamine, epinephrine, norepinephrine, phenylephrine, and amrinone (see *Reviewing vasoactive drugs*).

Nitroglycerin dilates veins, which reduces preload. It also improves myocardial perfusion by dilating coronary vessels. Usually, you'll give it with other drugs.

Sodium nitroprusside, commonly the drug of choice in cardiogenic shock, dilates both venous and arterial beds, therefore reducing preload and afterload. Because the drug can worsen hypotension, give it with dopamine, as prescribed.

Dopamine stimulates dilation of renal, splenic, and mesenteric arteries when given in low doses (2 to 5 µg/kg/minute), improving perfusion to the kidneys and intestine. As the drug takes effect, the patient's heart rate and blood pressure rise slightly and his urine output increases.

A powerful vasoconstrictor when administered in high doses, dopamine has a highly toxic effect on healthy tissue. That's why you give it through a central venous line, not a peripheral

Reviewing vasoactive drugs

Drugs	Actions	Adverse effects	Nursing interventions
nitroglycerin	• coronary artery dilation • venous dilation	• hypotension • reflex tachycardia	• Use cautiously in patients with hypotension. • Monitor patient for reflex tachycardia. • Monitor heart rate and blood pressure. • Assess chest pain.
sodium nitroprusside	• arterial dilation • venous dilation	• hypotension • ventilation-perfusion mismatch • increased ischemia • thiocyanate toxicity	• Use cautiously in patients with hypotension. • Protect drug from light. • Monitor heart rate and blood pressure with direct intracardiac monitoring. • Assess chest pain.
dopamine	• increased blood pressure, urine output, and cardiac output (CO) • alpha, beta, and dopaminergic receptor stimulation	• hypertension • tachycardia • increased ischemia	• Correct hypovolemia and tachycardia. • Monitor cardiac status. • Document heart rate, blood pressure, urine output, and peripheral circulation. • Administer phentolamine mesylate for extravasation.
dobutamine	• increased CO and mean arterial pressure without increased heart rate • increased urine output	• reflex tachycardia • enhanced arrhythmias • increased ischemia	• Monitor cardiac status. • Monitor heart rate, blood pressure, CO, pulmonary artery wedge pressure, and urine output. • Monitor patient for arrhythmias. • Check for signs and symptoms of ischemia.
epinephrine	• vasoconstriction • increased contractility • increased heart rate, blood pressure, and CO • increased myocardial oxygen demand	• increased ischemia • arrhythmias • gluconeogenesis	• Monitor cardiac status. • Check blood pressure every 2 minutes until stable, then every 15 minutes. • Correct acidosis. • Monitor patient for arrhythmias. • Monitor blood glucose level.
norepinephrine	• increased systemic vascular resistance and myocardial contraction	• reflex tachycardia • arrhythmias • decreased blood flow to peripheral and renal vasculature	• Protect drug from light. • Monitor cardiac status. • Check blood pressure every 2 minutes until stable, then every 15 minutes. • Correct acidosis. • Monitor patient for arrhythmias. • Monitor blood glucose level.
phenylephrine	• vasoconstriction	• reflex tachycardia • arrhythmias • decreased blood flow to peripheral and renal vasculature	• Monitor cardiac status. • Check blood pressure every 2 minutes until stable, then every 15 minutes. • Correct acidosis. • Monitor patient for arrhythmias. • Monitor blood glucose level.
amrinone	• increased CO • decreased preload • decreased peripheral vascular resistance	• reflex tachycardia • increased ischemia • thrombocytopenia	• Monitor cardiac status. • Initiate bleeding precautions if platelet count decreases.

I.V. line. At 5 to 10 µg/kg/minute, dopamine stimulates beta-adrenergic receptors, which slightly increases blood pressure, heart rate, and CO but decreases blood flow to the kidneys and skin.

In doses of 10 to 20 µg/kg/minute or more, dopamine becomes a pure alpha agonist, which causes blood pressure and heart rate to remain elevated, urine output to decrease, and arrhythmias to develop from increased myocardial oxygen consumption.

Dobutamine is a synthetic catecholamine that increases CO and mean arterial pressure and reduces ventricular filling pressures—without significantly increasing the heart rate. It also increases urine output, thereby boosting excretion of excess body fluids. Typically, you'll give a low dose of 7.5 µg/kg/minute together with dopamine.

Epinephrine, norepinephrine, and phenylephrine are potent vasoconstrictors typically used when dopamine and dobutamine achieve little or no effect. These three drugs cause pronounced vasoconstriction of peripheral arteries and veins, thus shunting more blood to the heart, lungs, and brain.

Amrinone, a phosphodiesterase inhibitor, allows calcium to improve myocardial contraction, easing the heart's workload. It also causes vasodilation and doesn't change the heart rate significantly. Remember, however, that amrinone may cause thrombocytopenia.

Intra-aortic balloon counterpulsation

To counteract a failing left ventricle, the patient may undergo intra-aortic balloon counterpulsation. The device consists of a polyurethane balloon mounted on the distal end of a vascular catheter and connected at its proximal end to a console.

A physician positions the balloon-tipped catheter in the patient's descending aorta and sets the console to inflate the balloon during diastole and deflate it during systole. Inflation moves blood forward into the coronary circulation and brain and backward to the renal and mesenteric arteries (see *Intra-aortic balloon pump in action*). As a result, diastolic blood pressure and coronary artery perfusion increase. Oxygen demand and afterload decrease.

Nursing considerations

If your patient develops cardiogenic shock, assess his oxygenation, ventilation, and perfusion. Provide supplemental oxygen and prepare him for intubation. Monitor his pulse oximetry readings often. Also, monitor his electrolyte levels and take aggressive steps to correct any imbalances, as ordered. Insert a peripheral I.V. line and administer fluids as prescribed, such as crystalloids, colloids, or blood products. Then prepare the patient for transport to the critical care unit.

Naturally, patients with cardiogenic shock and their families tend to be overwhelmed, anxious, and upset. Also, the patient's level of consciousness may be affected by poor CO. Explain all procedures and interventions to your patient and his family, but remember to relate your teaching to your patient's individual situation.

If the patient recovers from cardiogenic shock, focus your discharge teaching on the drug he'll be taking and the adverse effects it can cause. Discuss the lifestyle alterations the patient will need to make and risk factors for further trouble. Review the signs and symptoms of myocardial ischemia. Tell the patient to notify his physician if he develops chest pain, shortness of breath, light-headedness, excessive sweating, or the feeling that he's going to faint.

Provide family members with referrals to classes in CPR. Also, provide a list of community resources that offer information and emotional support.

Myocardial rupture

Although rare, myocardial rupture is a serious complication of an MI that can quickly result in the patient's death. It may affect the interventricular septum, the left papillary muscle, or the ventricular wall. In most cases, only immediate surgical correction can save the patient's life.

Septal rupture

A rupture of the interventricular septum typically creates a single perforation that's one to several centimeters in diameter. Blood shunts from the higher-pressure left ventricle to the lower-pressure right ventricle through the hole, increasing the right ventricle's workload. Naturally, the size of the perforation determines the extent to which blood moves from the left ventricle to the right.

Your assessment of a patient with ventricular septal rupture will reveal a new pansystolic mur-

Intra-aortic balloon pump in action

After the balloon has been positioned in the aorta, the pump inflates the balloon during diastole and deflates it during systole. As a result, the balloon forces more blood to the coronary arteries, brain, and renal arteries. And it decreases preload and afterload. In these illustrations, the descending aorta is shown in front of the heart to clearly depict this relationship between balloon inflation and blood flow.

Diastole	Systole
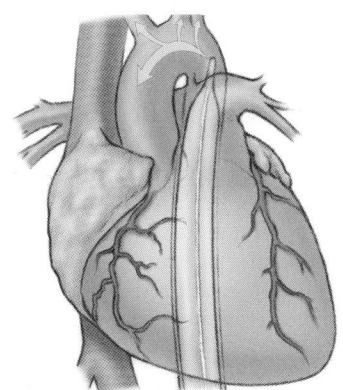	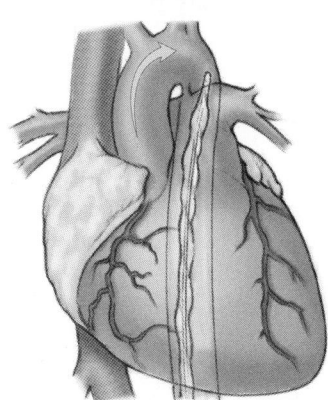

mur that's loud and harsh; heart failure, possibly with pulmonary edema; shock; shortness of breath; and a cough.

Noninvasive tests used to help confirm the diagnosis include echocardiography with Doppler ultrasound. If the images from these tests aren't adequate, the patient probably will undergo transesophageal echocardiography to obtain better ones.

Treatment aims to maintain hemodynamic support until the patient can undergo surgical correction of the rupture. Take time to explain to the patient and his family what has happened and to describe the surgery he needs. Tell the patient what to expect afterward and describe the intubation, ventilator, and hemodynamic monitoring he'll need.

Papillary muscle rupture

Acute injury or necrosis may, on rare occasions, cause the left ventricular papillary muscle to partially or totally rupture. Partial rupture causes severe mitral regurgitation. Complete rupture is rapidly fatal. Unlike ventricular septal rupture, which occurs in large infarctions, papillary muscle rupture occurs in relatively small infarctions.

Suspect a papillary muscle rupture if your patient develops a loud, systolic murmur of mitral regurgitation followed by the sudden onset of signs and symptoms of severe heart failure, such as tachycardia, adventitious breath sounds, extra heart sounds, dyspnea, or edema. You'll auscultate crackles in the patient's lung fields, extra heart sounds, and a midsystolic ejection click. Diagnostic tests for papillary muscle rupture include transthoracic and transesophageal echocardiography.

Treatment for a papillary muscle rupture involves immediate surgical correction and a possible valve replacement. Until surgery can take place, the patient may benefit from medical treatments that support oxygenation, afterload reduction, and blood pressure—such as intra-aortic balloon counterpulsation.

Teach the patent and his family members about what has happened and about the tests and treatments he'll need. Prepare the patient for his postoperative course, including his recovery, rehabilitation, and drug regimen.

In your discharge teaching, stress the importance of frequent and regular appointments with his physician. Outline signs and symptoms that could indicate surgical complications, and tell the patient when and how to seek medical assistance. Review all the drugs the patient will be taking, including their dosing schedules, actions, and adverse effects. Describe any limitations the patient should place on his activities. And provide a list of community resources that provide information and emotional support.

Ventricular rupture

If a necrotic area of the free ventricular wall ruptures, blood will flow into the pericardium, rapidly causing cardiac tamponade and death. Only immediate detection and treatment can save the patient's life.

Signs and symptoms of ventricular rupture include persistent, vague chest pain; unexplained hypotension; sudden hemodynamic deterioration, especially with a new systolic murmur; and asystole and cardiac arrest. The patient may undergo immediate bedside echocardiography to confirm the diagnosis and assess the extent of hemodynamic compromise. Cardiac catheterization can also confirm the diagnosis, but usually there isn't time for this procedure.

Once rupture of the ventricular free wall is confirmed, the patient must undergo immediate surgical correction. Supportive medical treatments can help to maintain his hemodynamic and physiologic status in the meantime.

Patients who experience myocardial rupture won't be able to respond to preoperative teaching, so your teaching must address the family. Explain what has happened and which treatment the patient needs. The emergent nature of this condition only increases the importance of allowing family members to express their feelings and ask questions. Answer them as best you can.

For a patient who survives ventricular rupture and the ensuing surgery, provide teaching similar to that required by any patient who undergoes open-heart surgery. Review the procedure itself. Explain diet and fluid restrictions. Outline each drug the patient will be taking, including its purpose, dosage, adverse effects, and the need for

any special follow-up laboratory tests or physician visits.

Talk with the patient about any activity limitations he must undertake. Instruct him to increase his activity level gradually and to rest between activities. Emphasize the importance of avoiding fatigue. Tell him to avoid lifting more than 10 pounds for 4 to 6 weeks after surgery. Also, tell him to avoid driving for 4 to 6 weeks or until cleared by his physician.

Teach him how to care for his incision. Tell him to wash it with soap and warm water, allow the shower to run over it, pat the incision gently to remove most of the moisture, and then allow it to air dry. Urge him to avoid taking baths because of the increased risk of infection caused by stagnant water.

Tell the patient to call his physician if he develops a fever that's higher than 101°F (38.3°C), a cough that produces sputum, pain and swelling at the incision site, or drainage from the incision. Urge him to seek emergency care if he develops chest pain and shortness of breath.

Pericarditis

Pericarditis may develop within a few days after having an MI (early pericarditis) or 2 to 10 weeks afterward (late pericarditis). The former results from a direct inflammatory response to transmural myocardial damage. The latter probably results from an autoimmune response to necrotic tissue at the infarct site. In both cases, chest pain typically differs from that caused by an MI. For most patients, it's worse on inhalation, and it varies with position changes.

Signs and symptoms

Signs and symptoms of early pericarditis include some or all of the following: dyspnea, cough, pallor, tachycardia, fever, friction rub over the anterior chest wall, and pain that's aggravated by turning, lying down, and taking deep breaths and somewhat relieved by sitting up and leaning forward.

Signs and symptoms of late pericarditis include fever, a white blood cell (WBC) count above 20,000/mm^3 (leukocytosis), malaise, and dull chest pain that varies with position changes and worsens with deep inhalation.

In both early and late pericarditis, an ECG may

reveal diffuse ST-segment elevation in many leads during the acute phase. When the ST segment returns to normal, the T wave will invert in most leads. Within days or weeks, the T wave will then return to baseline.

Treatment

The treatment goal for both early and late pericarditis is to decrease the inflammatory response, thereby reducing the level of pain. As prescribed, give the patient 650 mg of aspirin every 4 hours, 25 to 50 mg of indomethacin three times daily, 400 to 800 mg of a nonsteroidal anti-inflammatory drug (usually ibuprofen) every 6 hours, or corticosteroids.

Late pericarditis typically resolves on its own and requires no further intervention. Early pericarditis, on the other hand, may progress to the point where it compresses the heart. Consequently, you'll want to watch carefully for signs and symptoms of infection, including a persistent fever, a WBC count above 20,000/mm^3, and chills. These signs suggest the development of purulent pericarditis and effusion.

If a pericardial effusion develops, the patient may need pericardial drainage to reduce the pressure on his heart. It may take place via pericardiocentesis, in which a surgeon inserts a large-bore needle into the pericardium and extracts fluid. Or it may take place via a pericardial window procedure, in which a surgeon makes an incision over the anterior left fifth rib or xiphoid process, exposing the pericardium and anterior surface of the heart. After cutting away a portion of the pericardium to make a window, the surgeon then removes fluid through the window and closes the incision without closing the pericardium.

Nursing considerations

If your patient develops chest pain days or weeks after having an MI, your first priority is to help distinguish the pain of pericarditis from the pain of ischemia or continued infarction. To start, find out whether the pain varies with the patient's position. Also, ask him whether the pain worsens when he takes a deep breath.

If the patient's pain stems from pericarditis, help him into a position that minimizes his pain and administer an anti-inflammatory drug as prescribed. Use continuous cardiac monitoring to detect arrhythmias. Carefully explain the differ-

ence between the patient's current chest pain and the pain he experienced during his MI.

Explain to the patient and his family all the treatments and procedures the patient will need and any preoperative requirements the patient must follow. Provide emotional support to the patient and his family.

Before discharge, talk with the patient and his family about the underlying cause of his pericarditis and about what caused his pain. Tell them that the signs and symptoms of inflammation may recur for up to about 2 weeks. Urge him to avoid heavy lifting and overexertion during that time. And tell him to contact his physician if his symptoms continue or get worse.

Review the patient's drugs, including their names and intended effects. Explain how and when to take them and which adverse effects to watch for and report. If he had surgery, teach him and his family how to care for the wound and which signs of infection to watch for and report. Emphasize the importance of continued follow-up appointments with a physician. And tell the patient about community resources available to provide information or emotional support.

Ventricular aneurysm

In the area of the ventricle scarred by an MI, pressure from inside the heart may cause the thin tissue to form an aneurysm. In fact, it does so in 12% to 15% of MI patients. Without treatment, the patient may develop angina, heart failure, arrhythmias, embolism, or possible hemopericardium and cardiac tamponade from a ruptured ventricular wall.

Signs and symptoms

A ventricular aneurysm causes anginal chest pain, arrhythmias, and signs and symptoms of heart failure. They include tachycardia, adventitious breath sounds, extra heart sounds, dyspnea, and edema. Plus, because the bulging aneurysm retains blood that otherwise would contribute to CO, the patient may develop hypotension, decreased CO, and possible thrombus formation on the inner wall of the aneurysm.

To confirm the presence of a ventricular aneurysm, the physician most likely will order transthoracic or transesophageal echocardiography and cardiac catheterization.

Treatment

Until the patient can undergo surgery to correct the aneurysm, he'll receive treatment for his heart failure and anginal symptoms. He'll receive prophylactic anticoagulation to prevent systemic emboli. And he'll receive antiarrhythmic therapy. Surgery aims to remove the dysfunctional ventricular tissue while maintaining the ventricle's natural configuration.

Nursing considerations

Before the patient undergoes surgery, review the procedure with him and his family. Explain the need for the procedure and its risks and possible complications. Tell the patient to inform you of increased chest pain, increased shortness of breath, palpitations, or any other unusual symptom.

After surgery, the patient will undergo hemodynamic monitoring, mechanical ventilation, and vasoactive drug therapy in the critical care unit. As you would for any patient who has undergone open-heart surgery, encourage the patient to cough frequently and perform deep-breathing exercises. Provide routine wound care and encourage ambulation as soon as the patient can tolerate it.

Before discharge, review the patient's drugs, including their names, intended effects, how and when to take them, and which adverse effects to watch for and report. Emphasize the importance of continued follow-up visits with a physician. And make sure the patient and his family know which signs and symptoms warrant seeking medical care.

Cerebral embolism

After an MI, the risk of systemic embolism rises, either from thrombi formation in the heart's chambers or valves or from unstable plaques in the coronary arteries. If an embolus occludes a blood vessel in the patient's brain, he'll have a cerebrovascular accident (CVA). The signs, symptoms, and long-term effects of the CVA depend largely on the area of the brain affected and the amount of brain tissue deprived of oxygen. In general, patients with atrial fibrillation and heart failure face the highest risk of cerebral embolism.

Signs and symptoms

If your patient has a CVA, he'll complain of a headache, his neurologic status will decline, and he may have seizures. These signs and symptoms will arise abruptly. The specific neurologic deficits created will correspond to the portion of his brain affected (see *Effects of cerebral embolism*). Depending on the size and location of the infarction, the CVA may be mildly to severely debilitating.

To confirm a cerebral embolism, a physician most likely will order computed tomography scanning, which reveals areas of cerebral ischemia, infarction, and bleeding. The patient also may undergo magnetic resonance imaging, which reveals areas of edema and gross changes in cerebral blood flow. And he may undergo cerebral angiography, which reveals vasospasms and hemorrhage.

Treatment

Treatment aims to prevent further deficits by limiting the size of the brain infarction. It involves hemodynamic, physiologic, and ventilatory support. Thrombolytic drugs can dissolve the embolus and restore blood flow to the affected area. Remember, however, that you must monitor the patient frequently during thrombolytic therapy because these drugs can disrupt clots throughout the body, including those at invasive sites and necrotic areas, thus raising the risk of continued embolization.

Nursing considerations

If your patient develops a cerebral embolism, give corticosteroids and anti-inflammatory drugs to decrease cerebral edema and inflammation, as prescribed. Give vasoactive drugs, such as dopamine and epinephrine, for hemodynamic support. Monitor the patient's hemodynamic and ventilatory status closely.

If the brain infarction is large enough to impair his ability to breathe, anticipate the need for endotracheal intubation and mechanical ventilation. Monitor the patient closely for cardiac arrhythmias and assess his neurologic status frequently.

Prepare for cerebral angiography and thrombolytic therapy, if indicated. During or after thrombolytic therapy, administer anticoagulation therapy to prevent more emboli from forming.

If the CVA leaves chronic neurologic deficits, take steps to minimize the effects of confusion and disorientation. Ensure the patient's continued safety. And coordinate the launch of multidisciplinary care to provide for the patient's neurologic, physiologic, and emotional needs.

Physical or occupational therapists usually take part in this aspect of care and can assist with patient and family teaching. Patients who suffer disabling CVAs usually receive several weeks of intensive physical and occupational therapy. Families should be encouraged to attend these sessions and interact with the patient.

Before discharge, family members may need to make a difficult decision about whether to bring the patient home or transfer him to an extended care facility, a nursing home, or a rehabilitation center. Do your best to support the family's decision. If they request it, involve a cleric or social worker. If the patient goes home, help the family arrange for home care, possibly including visiting nurses, home health aides, and physical therapists. Provide information about services available in the community.

Right ventricular infarction

Especially among patients with acute inferior-wall and posterior-wall MI caused by occlusion of the right coronary artery, a right ventricular infarction may complicate the healing process by raising the risk of several other complications, including these:
- rupture of the interventricular septum
- rupture of the free wall of the heart
- high-grade AV block, including complete heart block
- atrial septal defect resulting from the infarction or hypoxemia resulting from right-to-left shunting across a patent foramen ovale.

A right ventricular infarction causes hypotension, reduces CO, and renders the infarcted right ventricle unable to fill the left ventricle adequately.

Signs and symptoms
The signs and symptoms caused by a right ventricular infarction mirror those of right ventricular heart failure and include an increased jugular venous pulse during inhalation, an S_3 and an S_4, a systolic murmur of tricuspid insufficiency, a widely split second heart sound (from increased right ventricular volume and delayed closure of the pulmonary valve), hypotension, oliguria, dizziness, nausea, diaphoresis, a positive hepatojugular reflux from liver engorgement, a paradoxical pulse, and cardiogenic shock. The patient will have little or no pulmonary congestion.

Effects of cerebral embolism

The neurologic deficits created by a patient's cerebral embolism correspond to the brain hemisphere deprived of oxygenated blood. Here's a quick review.

Right hemisphere
An infarction in the right hemisphere may leave the patient unaware that he has a neurologic deficit. Indeed, he may be unaware of the entire left side of his body. He may turn his eyes to the right, ignoring the left side of the room. And he may have left homonymous hemianopia—blindness in the left halves of both visual fields. If you ask him to copy a picture, he may fail to draw the left side.

Left hemisphere
An infarction in the left hemisphere creates right-to-left disorientation. Thus, when you touch one of the patient's fingers, he won't be able to tell you whether it was on his right or left hand. He may have right homonymous hemianopia. And he may have expressive, receptive, or global aphasia.
- With expressive aphasia, a patient is unable to speak, write, or identify familiar objects. He does understand what you say to him, though.
- With receptive aphasia, a patient is unable to understand spoken or written words and may speak in garbled sentences.
- With global aphasia, a patient displays qualities of both expressive and receptive aphasia.

Diagnostic tests
Because the standard 12-lead ECG offers no specific indicators for right ventricular infarction, you'll need to obtain a right-sided 12-lead ECG. If the patient has had a right ventricular MI, you'll see ST-segment elevation of at least 1 mm in leads V_3R through V_6R.

Echocardiogram findings typical of right ventricular infarction include right ventricular enlargement, abnormalities of right ventricular wall motion, and paradoxical septal wall motion. Tricuspid regurgitation may appear in some patients.

Technetium Tc 99m pyrophosphate imaging produces abnormal results 48 to 72 hours after the infarction; these results remain abnormal until about the seventh day after the infarction. Multiple gated acquisition scans, also using technetium 99m, can help to evaluate regional ventricular wall motion. The patient most likely has a right ventricular infarction if his scan shows a lack of movement or abnormal movement in the right ventricular wall, if he has an elevated right atrial pressure, and if his right ventricular ejection fraction is less than 40%.

Hemodynamic measurements can help diagnose a patient's right ventricular infarction by showing an increased right atrial pressure, an increased right ventricular end-diastolic pressure, a decreased or normal PAWP, and a normal pulmonary artery pressure.

Treatment

With right ventricular infarction, the damaged right ventricle prevents the left ventricle from filling properly. So therapy aims to improve left ventricular filling, increase CO, and improve peripheral perfusion.

If the patient has both left ventricular dysfunction and right ventricular dysfunction, anticipate administering diuretics and vasodilators to reduce preload and afterload. The patient also may undergo intra-aortic balloon counterpulsation to increase his CO.

Patients who survive the acute phase of right ventricular infarction typically have a good prognosis if they sustained no significant left ventricular dysfunction.

Nursing considerations

Because the patient will need continuous hemodynamic monitoring, prepare him for transfer to the critical care unit. Administer fluids to increase his right ventricular output, as ordered. If volume alone can't improve his CI, give dopamine or dobutamine as prescribed.

Monitor the patient's electrolyte levels and correct any imbalances. Also, monitor the patient for arrhythmias—especially complete heart block and bradyarrhythmias. Anticipate the use of a transvenous pacemaker because many patients with right ventricular infarction who develop heart block don't respond to atropine. As indicated, prepare the patient and his family for cardiac catheterization, percutaneous transluminal angioplasty, or thrombolytic therapy.

Before discharge, explain to the patient and his family what has happened to his heart. Discuss the signs and symptoms of heart failure, including the ones he should report to his physician: chest pain, dyspnea, and edema. Urge the patient to weigh himself daily to check for fluid retention. And emphasize the importance of any necessary lifestyle changes, such as quitting smoking, following a low-sodium diet, avoiding alcohol, exercising regularly, and reducing stress.

MYOCARDIAL INFARCTION

Suggested Readings

Abrams J. The role of nitrates in coronary heart disease. *Arch Intern Med*. 1995;155(4):357-364.

Amsterdam EA. Controlled trials comparing reteplase with alteplase and streptokinase in patients with acute myocardial infarction. *Pharmacotherapy*. 1996;16(5 Pt 2):137S-140S.

Antman E, Braunwald E. Acute myocardial infarction. In: Braunwald E, ed. *Heart Disease: A Textbook of Cardiovascular Medicine*. 5th ed. Philadelphia: WB Saunders Co; 1996.

Ball SG, Hall AS. Who should be treated with angiotensin-converting enzyme inhibitors after myocardial infarction? *Am Heart J*. 1996;132(1 Pt 2 Su):244-250.

Bassand JP. Left ventricular remodelling after acute myocardial infarction: solved and unsolved issues. *Eur Heart J*. 1995;16(Suppl I):58-63.

Califf R, et al. *Acute Coronary Care*. 2nd ed. St Louis: Mosby, Inc; 1995.

Comparison of coronary bypass surgery with angioplasty in patients with multivessel disease. *N Engl J Med*. 1996;335(4):217-225.

Eisenberg MJ, Topol EJ. Prehospital administration of aspirin in patients with unstable angina and acute myocardial infarction. *Arch Intern Med*. 1996;156(14):1506-1510.

Every NR, Parsons LS, Hlatky M, Martin JS, Weaver WD. A comparison of thrombolytic therapy with primary coronary angioplasty for acute myocardial infarction. Myocardial infarction triage and intervention investigators. *N Engl J Med*. 1996;335(17):1253-1260.

Frishman WH, Burns B, Atac B, Alturk N, Altajar B, Lerrick K. Novel antiplatelet therapies for treatment of patients with ischemic heart disease: inhibitors of the platelet glycoprotein IIb/IIIa integrin receptor. *Am Heart J*. 1995; 130(4):877-892.

Grines CL. Should thrombolysis or primary angioplasty be the treatment of choice for acute myocardial infarction? Primary angioplasty: the strategy of choice. *N Engl J Med*. 1996; 335(17):1313-1316.

Krumholz HM, Radford MJ, Ellerbeck EF. Aspirin for secondary prevention after acute myocardial infarction in the elderly: prescribed use and outcomes. *Ann Intern Med*. 1996; 124(3):292-298.

Phalen T. *The 12-Lead ECG in Acute Myocardial Infarction*. St Louis: Mosby, Inc; 1995.

Ryan TJ, Anderson JL, Antman EM, et al. ACC/AHA guidelines for the management of patients with acute myocardial infarction: a report of the American College of Cardiology/American Heart Association task force on practice guidelines (committee on management of acute myocardial infarction). *J Am Coll Cardiol*. 1996;28(5):1328-1428.

Talbert RL. Strategies in the management of acute myocardial infarction. *Pharmacotherapy*. 1996;16(5 Pt 2):127S-136S.

Tootill DM. Thrombolytic therapy: nursing strategies for successful patient outcomes. *Prog Cardiovasc Nurs*. 1995;10(1):3-12.

Turner DM, Turner LA. Right ventricular myocardial infarction: detection, treatment, and nursing implications. *Crit Care Nurse*. 1995; 15(1):22-27.

Wenger N, et al. *Cardiac Rehabilitation as Secondary Prevention*. Clinical practice guideline. Quick reference guide for clinicians, No. 17. Rockville, Md: Agency for Health Care Policy and Research and the National Heart, Lung, and Blood Institute, Public Health Service; 1995. US Dept of Health and Human Services publication AHCPR 96-0673.

HEART FAILURE

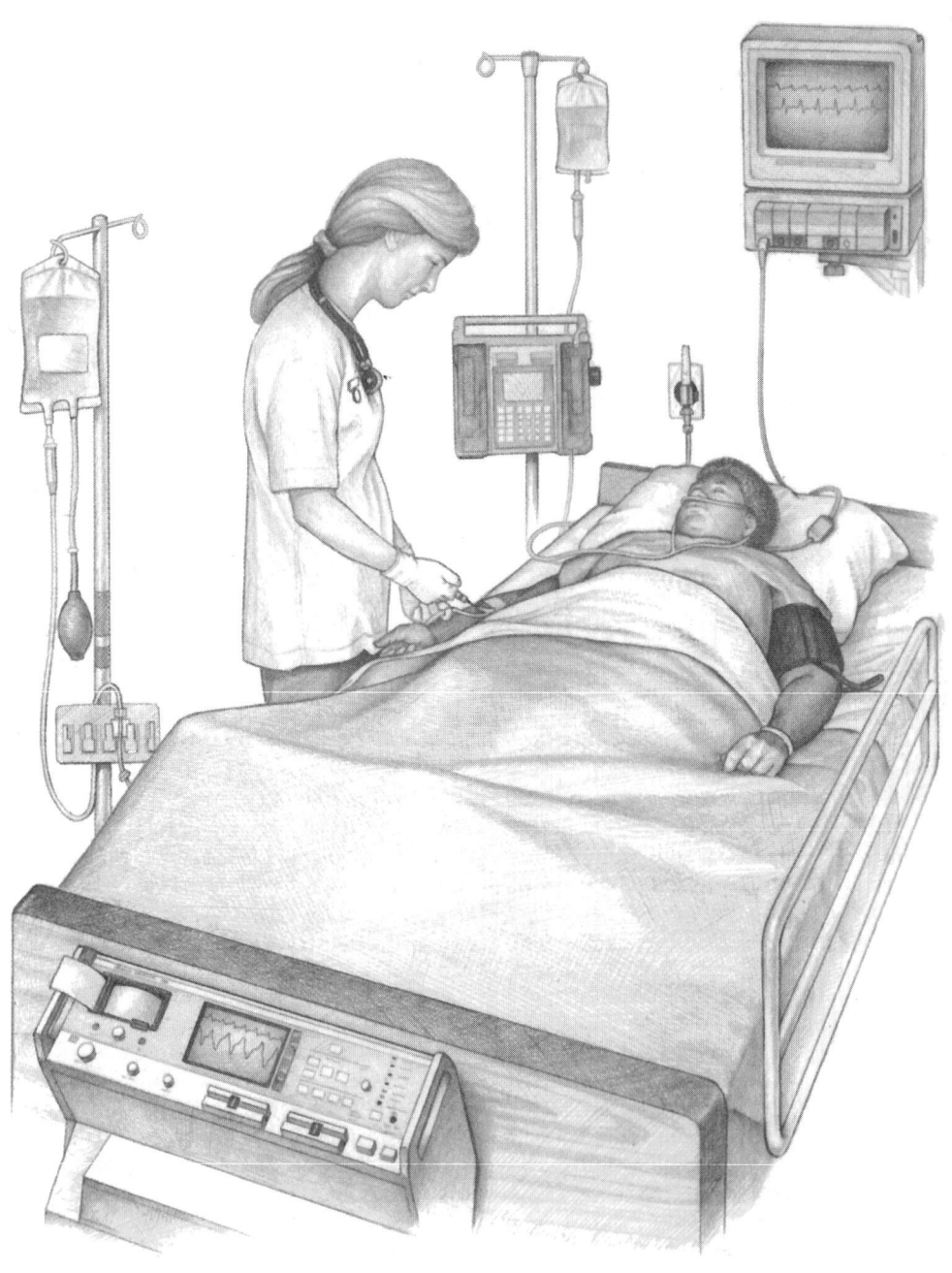

9

HEART FAILURE

Overview

As more and more people survive what once were fatal cardiac disorders, the number left with heart failure continues to grow. In the United States alone, 5 million people have heart failure, and 875,000 people, most over age 65, are admitted to hospitals for heart failure every year.

Clearly, your understanding of heart failure and your ability to care for the patients it affects are more important than ever. In this chapter, you'll find a brief overview of the causes of heart failure and the body's intricate response to them. Plus, you'll review the steps needed to assess your patient efficiently and accurately.

Classifying heart failure

The term *heart failure* refers to a complex set of causes and effects that surround the heart's inability to pump sufficient blood to the body's tissues. Partly because of the complexity that underlies this process of heart failure, several classification systems have been used to describe the disorder.

Systolic and diastolic failure

The preferred classification system describes heart failure according to the part of the cardiac cycle in which the primary dysfunction occurs: systole or diastole.

In systolic heart failure, the heart doesn't eject enough blood from the left ventricle into the systemic circulation with each contraction. As a result, blood backs up into the pulmonary vasculature. As pressure rises in the pulmonary vessels, fluid leaks into the alveoli, and your patient develops signs and symptoms of heart failure, such as shortness of breath and fatigue.

Systolic heart failure may stem from a number of causes. For example, after a myocardial infarction (MI), the scarred left ventricle may lose its ability to contract forcefully. In dilated cardiomyopathy, the expanding ventricle receives progressively larger volumes of blood—too large to pump effectively. In both cases, blood eventually backs up into the pulmonary vasculature.

In diastolic heart failure, the ventricle can't relax fully, which impairs ventricular filling. Consequently, less blood can be pumped out to the systemic circulation. Chronic hypertension may be the most common cause of diastolic heart failure because it leads to ventricular hypertrophy, a condition that limits the ventricle's ability to relax during diastole.

Although systolic and diastolic heart failure may develop as singular disorders, they also commonly develop together. For example, besides reducing contractility in the left ventricle, an MI leaves a necrotic area that doesn't stretch or relax properly.

Left ventricular and right ventricular heart failure

This system classifies heart failure by the side of the heart initially affected.

In left ventricular heart failure, the left ventricle has difficulty pumping blood into the systemic circulation. Consequently, your patient may develop pulmonary congestion and activity intolerance. Eventually, the right ventricle may fail as well because it must work harder to offset the left ventricular failure.

Right ventricular failure causes blood to back up into the venous circulation and produces such signs as edema, hepatomegaly, and jugular vein distention. Right ventricular heart failure may occur without left ventricular heart failure in such conditions as pulmonary hypertension, pulmonary embolism, or right ventricular infarction.

Functional ability

A system originated by the New York Heart Association classifies heart failure according to the level of activity restrictions it imposes. Useful for obtaining a general idea of your patient's condition, this system describes the amount of activity she can perform before symptoms arise. Basing your results on a specific energy measure, such as metabolic equivalents of a task (METs), can increase the objectivity of this system and allow you to place a patient in one of four functional classes:

- Class I. No activity limitation. The patient can perform activities of seven METs or more, such as walking briskly uphill or bicycling at 10 miles per hour (mph) or faster.
- Class II. Slight symptoms with ordinary activities. The patient can perform activities that require five to seven METs, such as doing yard work or housecleaning.
- Class III. Activities limited by symptoms. The patient can perform activities that require two to five METs, such as walking at 2 to 3 mph, cooking, or doing light housecleaning.
- Class IV. Symptoms with all activities and possibly at rest. The patient can't perform activities that require one to three METs, such as bathing or dressing.

What causes heart failure

No matter which system you use to describe heart failure, remember that the disorder you're describing is a multifaceted syndrome, not a single disease. In fact, any condition that impairs heart rate, myocardial contractility, preload, or afterload will reduce cardiac output (CO)—thus causing heart failure or raising the patient's risk of developing it.

In general, the problems that lead to reduced CO and heart failure can be grouped into four categories. They include abnormal cardiac muscle, abnormal left ventricular volume, abnormal left ventricular pressure, and abnormal left ventricular filling.

Abnormal muscle

If the heart muscle can't contract forcefully enough to eject blood from the ventricle, CO falls. Commonly, reduced pumping ability results either from the scars left by an MI or from cardiomyopathy. Cardiomyopathy can take several forms, each of which can profoundly impair CO. The three most common are dilated cardiomyopathy, hypertrophic cardiomyopathy, and restrictive cardiomyopathy (see *Reviewing cardiomyopathies*).

In dilated cardiomyopathy, the most common form, the left ventricle becomes grossly overstretched and holds a large volume of blood. The ventricle can't pump this large volume forward, so blood backs up, resulting in pulmonary congestion.

In hypertrophic cardiomyopathy, the left ventricular muscle enlarges, becoming stiff and noncompliant. Too little room remains in the ventricle to receive an adequate volume of blood during diastole, thus reducing CO.

Restrictive cardiomyopathy develops after myocardial infiltrates stiffen the walls of the heart, rendering it unable to fill and contract normally.

You may hear the term *ischemic cardiomyopathy* as well. It refers to a condition that resembles dilated cardiomyopathy. Ischemic cardiomyopathy can result from prolonged periods of myocardial ischemia, usually from coronary artery disease. In response to chronic ischemia, the heart muscle gradually reduces its contractility in an effort to conserve energy—a process called myocardial hibernation.

The heart muscle may respond in a similar manner to the restoration of blood flow to functioning myocardial tissue after an acute injury, such as an MI. This tissue may respond by reducing contractility—a condition called myocardial stunning. The hibernating or stunned myocardium may gradually improve its contractility if adequate myocardial blood flow can be restored through angioplasty, bypass surgery, or another intervention.

Reviewing cardiomyopathies

Cardiomyopathies can lead to heart failure by altering the structure and function of heart muscle. Use this table to review the three most common types: dilated, hypertrophic, and restrictive cardiomyopathy.

	Normal heart	Dilated cardiomyopathy	Hypertrophic cardiomyopathy	Restrictive cardiomyopathy

Characteristics			
Ventricles	• greatly increased chamber size • thinning of left ventricular muscle	• normal or decreased chamber size • left ventricular hypertrophy • thickened interventricular septum	• decreased ventricular chamber size • left ventricular hypertrophy
Atrial chamber size	• increased	• increased	• increased
Myocardial mass	• increased	• increased	• normal
Preload	• increased	• normal	• increased
Ventricular inflow resistance	• normal	• increased	• increased
Contractility	• decreased	• increased or decreased	• normal or decreased
Possible causes	• viral infection • bacterial infection • chemotherapy • hypersensitivity to penicillin, tetracycline, or sulfonamides • peripartum syndrome related to toxemia	• genetic susceptibility • poorly controlled hypertension • obstructive valvular disease • thyroid disease	• amyloidosis (hyaline deposition) • sarcoidosis (interstitial infiltrates) • hemochromatosis (iron accumulation) • infiltrative neoplastic disease

Abnormal volume

Heart failure also may result from conditions that prevent the smooth forward flow of adequate volumes of blood through the heart. For exam- ple, mitral valve insufficiency may allow blood to flow backward into the left atrium with each ventricular contraction. This problem decreases the volume of blood moving forward through the heart, reduces CO, causes blood to back up into the pulmonary vasculature, and results in interstitial edema. Insufficiency of any heart valves may lead to this reduction of forward flow and backup of blood.

Also in the category of abnormal volume conditions are those that raise the body's metabolic demand beyond what the heart can accommodate, placing the patient in a high-output state. These conditions include chronic anemia, arteriovenous (AV) fistula, thyrotoxicosis, pregnancy, septicemia, beriberi, and a recent infusion of large volumes of I.V. fluids over a short period of time.

Abnormal pressure

The most common reason for abnormal pressure in the heart is systemic hypertension. That's because the muscle becomes hypertrophied as the left ventricle continually ejects blood against high arterial pressures. In turn, myocardial oxygen demand rises as the heart works harder under increased stress. Ultimately, the heart loses its ability to meet these high demands and heart failure sets in.

Pulmonary hypertension causes a similar problem for the heart's right ventricle. Patients with chronic obstructive pulmonary disease may have increased pulmonary resistance that leads to cor pulmonale, a form of right ventricular heart failure.

Stenosis or narrowing of the aortic and pulmonary valves also can create increased pressure on the ventricles by making it more difficult to eject blood across the altered valve openings. Eventually, this increase in pressure causes changes similar to those of hypertension.

Abnormal filling

When the ventricle doesn't fill with sufficient blood, stroke volume declines and CO drops. Abnormal ventricular filling can result from obstruction or impaired relaxation.

For example, a stenotic mitral valve can reduce the passive flow of blood into the left ventricle. Atrial contraction won't completely fill the ventricle either, which leads to atrial volume overload, a reduced ventricular volume, and lowered CO. Over time, the left atrium may become enlarged and

prone to atrial fibrillation. Loss of the atrial kick reduces ventricular volume—and CO—even more.

Tricuspid stenosis produces the same results on the heart's right side. And eventually, of course, a reduced right ventricular volume will reduce the left ventricular volume as well.

Although rare, an atrial myxoma, a large benign tumor, may affect the filling of the heart chambers. Ultimately, the tumor limits ventricular filling and, therefore, decreases stroke volume and CO. In some cases, an elongated tumor can move across the mitral or tricuspid valve and impair blood flow through the valve. The tumor may even move into the ventricle and obstruct filling directly.

Finally, the ventricle will be unable to fill normally if the muscle doesn't relax fully during diastole. This problem can occur in hypertension as well as in myocardial hibernation or myocardial stunning.

What happens in heart failure

Regardless of the underlying cause, the body reacts to heart failure with a similar set of compensatory and counterregulatory actions in an attempt to offset a declining CO.

Compensatory mechanisms provide a temporary boost to CO. They include stimulation of the sympathetic nervous system, activation of the renin-angiotensin-aldosterone system, and hypertrophy and dilation of the ventricles. To counteract the negative effects of these compensatory mechanisms, the body also produces prostaglandins and atrial natriuretic factor. Because of these intertwined pathophysiologic responses, heart failure is now considered to be a neurohormonal disorder.

Sympathetic stimulation

When CO falls, the sympathetic nervous system engages several mechanisms to increase the heart's chronotropic (rate) and inotropic (contractile) responses.

Baroreceptors in the aortic arch sense the decrease in aortic pressure and prompt the pituitary gland to release arginine vasopressor. Also called antidiuretic hormone, arginine vasopressor promotes vasoconstriction and sodium and water reabsorption in the kidneys.

Sympathetic nervous system stimulation causes the adrenal medulla to release the catecholamines epinephrine and norepinephrine, which increase contractility, heart rate, and vasoconstriction.

Also, the release of norepinephrine from synaptic nerve endings stimulates alpha-adrenergic and beta$_1$-adrenergic receptors. Stimulation of alpha receptors in the arterioles produces vasoconstriction, increasing circulating volume and preload and shunting blood from nonessential tissues to the heart and other vital organs.

Stimulation of beta$_1$ receptors, which are mainly in the heart, increases contractility and heart rate and, therefore, increases CO. Over time, in patients with heart failure, these beta$_1$ receptors lose their responsiveness to this stimulation. This phenomenon is called down regulation. Treatment with a beta-blocker, such as propranolol, may help increase the number and function of beta$_1$ receptors.

Although sympathetic nervous system stimulation succeeds for a time in supporting CO, it eventually taxes the heart more than the original mechanical problems that reduced CO. For example, vasoconstriction increases afterload and myocardial oxygen consumption. An increased heart rate increases oxygen demand as well and also reduces ventricular filling time.

Plus, because the patient develops an increased heart rate even at rest, she may have little reserve left to respond to increases in activity or emotional stress. Specifically, heart failure restricts heart rate variability by limiting parasympathetic stimulation (which reduces heart rate) and promoting sympathetic stimulation. This reduced variability offers a clue to the severity of your patient's heart failure. It also may raise the patient's risk of sudden death from ventricular tachycardia and ventricular fibrillation.

Renal response

Another type of neurohormonal compensatory mechanism prompted by heart failure is the renin-angiotensin-aldosterone system (see *Steps in the renin-angiotensin-aldosterone system,* page 162). When the kidneys sense a decrease in in-coming blood flow, they begin to secrete renin, an enzyme that converts angiotensinogen to angiotensin I, which then rapidly forms angiotensin II. A potent vasoconstrictor, angiotensin II promotes the release of aldosterone by the adrenal cortex. In turn, aldosterone promotes sodium and water retention. The resulting increase in intravascular volume leads to an increase in preload and eventually an increase in CO.

Although effective for a time, this mechanism eventually causes heart failure to worsen as the heart becomes unable to pump effectively against the increased volume. That's because contractility declines and CO falls when preload increases beyond a certain point. This eventual failure of the renal response is why patients with heart failure receive angiotensin-converting enzyme inhibitors to block the conversion of angiotensin I to angiotensin II.

Ventricular enlargement

In time, the volume and pressure changes that result from sympathetic nervous system stimulation and renin secretion will cause hypertrophy and dilation of the myocardium. In hypertrophy, the myocardial muscle thickens in response to increased pressure and stress on the chamber walls. It does so in heart failure because of the increased afterload, but the larger muscle mass requires more oxygen and eventually may worsen the patient's heart failure rather than improving it.

In dilation, increased pressure stretches the myocardial muscle fibers, elongating the chamber to accommodate the increased intravascular volume. Over time, however, the muscle fibers become overstretched and their contractility declines.

Counterregulatory substances

Heart failure also prompts the body to produce counterregulatory substances, including renal prostaglandins and atrial natriuretic factor. Both work to reduce volume overload and ease vasoconstriction.

Prostaglandins
Later in the sequence of physiologic changes that mark heart failure, the kidneys release the prostaglandins prostacyclin and prostaglandin E$_2$. These

Steps in the renin-angiotensin-aldosterone system

When cardiac output (CO) decreases, the kidneys respond by secreting the enzyme renin, which is converted to angiotensin II, a powerful vasoconstrictor that prompts the release of aldosterone. By promoting sodium and water retention, aldosterone increases intravascular volume, preload, and CO.

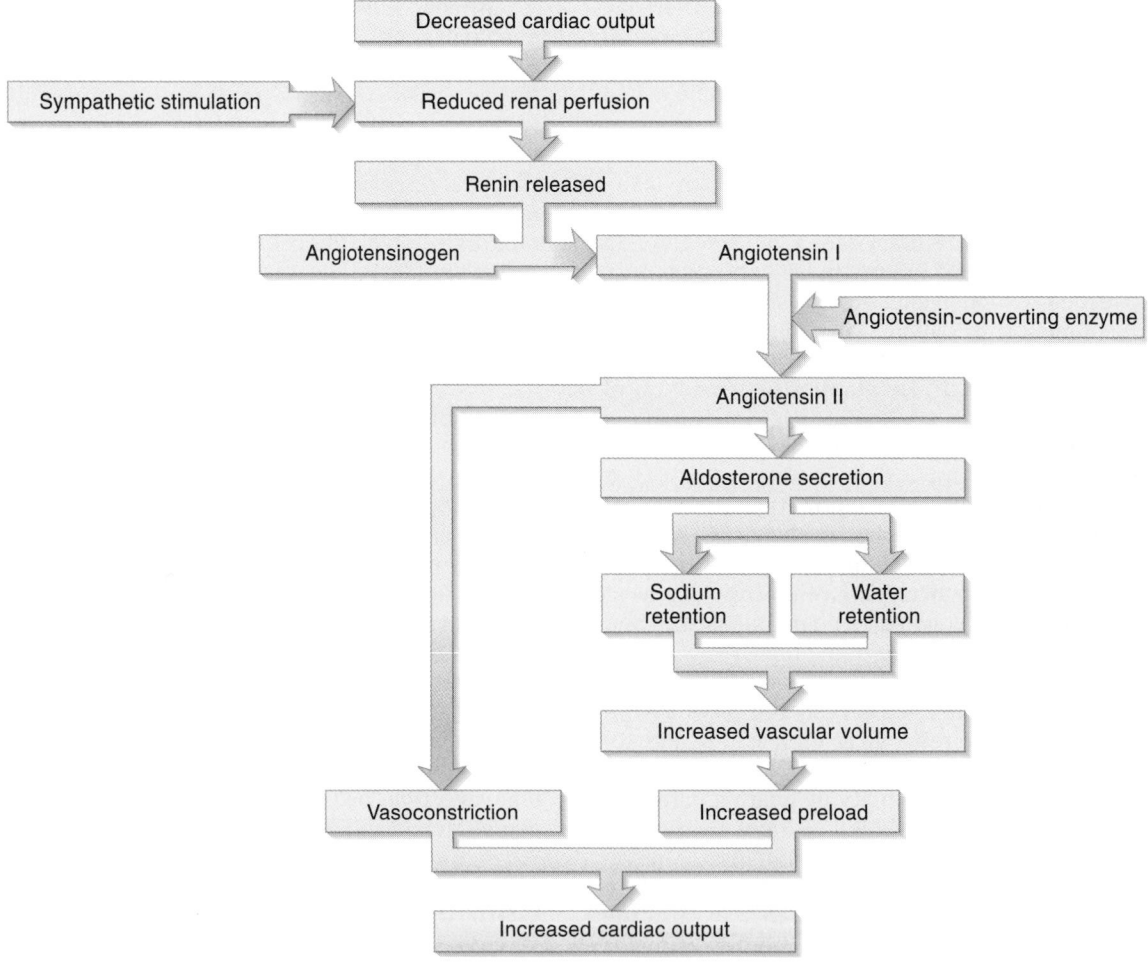

substances maximize the positive effects of the renin-angiotensin-aldosterone system and minimize the negative effects.

In healthy people, prostaglandins exert a mild vasodilatory effect. In people with vasoconstriction, however, they exert a potent vasodilatory effect. Prostaglandins also inhibit sodium and water reabsorption in the kidneys, thus reducing the volume overload caused by the renin-angiotensin-aldosterone system.

Prostaglandins work with angiotensin II in the kidneys to promote glomerular filtration. Normally, the afferent arteriole going into the glomerulus is larger than the efferent arteriole exiting it. This discrepancy increases pressure in the glomerulus, promoting filtration of fluid from the blood. Prostaglandins promote glomerular filtration by dilating the afferent arteriole while angiotensin II constricts the efferent arteriole.

Atrial natriuretic factor

Atrial natriuretic factor, a hormone secreted by atrial and sometimes ventricular tissue, probably helps to counteract the body's response to sympathetic nervous system stimulation and the renin-angiotensin-aldosterone system. Its secretion is prompted when stretch receptors in the chamber walls sense stress caused by excess intravascular volume. The hormone promotes vasodilation and diuresis, reducing the heart's workload.

What triggers heart failure

Many factors can trigger or worsen heart failure, especially those that increase the heart's workload. Keep in mind that any increase in the body's metabolic demands increases the heart's workload. Conditions that can trigger or worsen heart failure include arrhythmias, hypertension, cardiac inflammation and infection, high-output conditions, multisystem complications, adverse drug effects, and noncompliance.

Arrhythmias

Arrhythmias can trigger or worsen heart failure by decreasing CO or upsetting oxygen supply and demand.

Tachyarrhythmias reduce the length of diastole, thus reducing ventricular filling time. In fact, rapid heart rates reduce stroke volume so much that the increased number of beats per minute doesn't make up for the overall loss of CO. Atrial fibrillation may be the most ominous; loss of synchronous atrial and ventricular contractions can reduce CO up to 30%.

Bradyarrhythmias also can reduce CO. Although a slowed heart rate usually increases the volume of blood ejected into the systemic circulation by increasing ventricular filling time, a severe bradyarrhythmia won't produce enough beats to maintain CO.

Hypertension

Hypertension increases the heart's workload by increasing afterload. Hypertensive crisis, a severe and sudden rise in blood pressure, may cause acute, overwhelming failure in a heart with an underlying problem.

Cardiac inflammation and infection

Myocarditis (inflammation of the myocardium) and infective endocarditis (infection of the endocardium and valves) impair CO because inflammation decreases contractility and valve dysfunction leads to ventricular dysfunction. Plus, inflammation and infection increase myocardial oxygen demand.

High-output conditions

High-output heart failure occurs when the heart can't supply the body with enough blood and oxygen even with a sufficient circulating blood volume, normal myocardial contractility, and the ability to increase the heart rate. Many conditions—such as fever, anemia, AV fistula, thyrotoxicosis, sodium-water imbalance, and nutritional changes—can result in high-output heart failure. Each condition causes an increase in myocardial workload and, in chronic conditions, can eventually lead to heart failure.

Fever

As you know, fever increases the body's metabolic rate. Specifically, an increase of 1.8°F (1°C) can increase metabolism by 5%. The body attempts to dissipate heat by increasing blood flow through dilated cutaneous vessels and raising the heart rate along with the body temperature.

Anemia

In tissues chronically deprived of oxygen from low hemoglobin levels, the body initially responds by increasing the heart rate and stroke volume. Metabolic acidosis develops as the body switches to anaerobic metabolism, producing lactate and other metabolites that have a vasodilatory effect.

When hemoglobin levels fall below 7 g/dL, blood viscosity also declines, reducing the resistance against which the heart must eject blood into the circulation. This means that afterload declines even more than what you'd expect from the vasodilation caused by the buildup of cellular metabolites. However, the volume returning to the heart is increased.

In severe, chronic anemia, structural changes may occur in the heart muscle itself. When hemoglobin levels drop to about 5 g/dL, the left ventricle may enlarge from fluid overload, the contracting wall may thicken from stress, and the heart's weight may increase by as much as 50%.

Anemic patients without heart disease may adapt to these changes without any overt signs or symptoms of heart failure. However, those patients who develop signs and symptoms have a high likelihood of undetected cardiac disease.

Arteriovenous fistula
An AV fistula may be congenital or acquired and may vary in size. In all cases, blood flows from the high-pressure artery to the low-pressure vein, creating an area of hyperdynamic circulation. Examples of large fistulas with significant hemodynamic effects include hepatic hemangioendotheliomas, vascular lesions on the skin surface, and Wilms' tumor, a cancer that occurs in young children.

High-output failure may arise in infancy or early childhood during periods of rapid growth. That's because the child's metabolic needs increase during growth spurts, even as more blood flows through the fistula, thus rendering the heart unable to meet the child's high metabolic demand. High-output failure also commonly arises in patients with renal failure after construction of an AV shunt for hemodialysis.

Thyrotoxicosis
Also known as hyperthyroidism, thyrotoxicosis increases the body's metabolic demand, causing tachycardia and increasing the heart's workload. Most people with normal hearts can tolerate these increases. However, two groups may have an increased risk of heart failure: neonates and elderly patients.

Neonates with hyperthyroidism may develop heart failure because they have such high resting heart rates that their hearts can't increase the rate further to meet the demands of hyperthyroidism.

Elderly patients may develop apathetic hyperthyroidism. Such a patient may have atrial fibrillation, chest pain, and signs and symptoms of heart failure, but she won't have signs and symptoms of

thyrotoxicosis, such as palpitations or diaphoresis. These effects may be diminished because of an age-related blunting of the sympathetic nervous system's response.

Sodium-water imbalance
A large intake of sodium (such as a bolus of high-sodium I.V. fluid) over a short period of time can cause sudden and severe fluid retention. If the patient can't eliminate the fluid at a rapid enough rate, the dramatic increase in preload may be more than her heart can tolerate. Her ventricle may simply be distended too much by this large fluid load. The fibers become overstretched, contractility declines, and CO falls.

Nutritional changes
Patients with vitamin B_1 (thiamine) deficiency, a condition called beriberi, are prone to develop high-output heart failure because thiamine deficiency causes massive peripheral vasodilation that leads to reflex tachycardia and decreased systemic vascular resistance. In turn, this reduced systemic vascular resistance increases CO. Sodium and water retention by the kidneys also creates an excessive circulating volume. Severe heart failure may arise suddenly, primarily from the increased volume.

In the United States, thiamine deficiency is more commonly associated with chronic alcohol use, but you may see it in people who follow a diet high in carbohydrates and low in thiamine. Suspect thiamine deficiency in those who follow fad diets high in unenriched rice or those who eat mainly junk food. Keep in mind that a patient who develops heart failure for another reason may become sicker if she also has a thiamine deficiency.

Multisystem complications

The increased demands imposed by the development of another disease, cardiac or not, can prompt an episode of heart failure. The increased workload may result from heart rate, preload, afterload, or contractility demands that can no longer be met.

In particular, renal problems, hepatic disease, pulmonary disorders, traumatic injury, or burns can lead to heart failure, especially if the patient receives large volumes of replacement fluid. Even normal physiologic events, such as pregnancy, can raise the metabolic demand high

Signs and symptoms of heart failure

Signs and symptoms of heart failure vary depending on the affected ventricle. If the right ventricle is impaired, you'll find evidence of venous congestion and peripheral edema. If the left ventricle is impaired, you'll find evidence of decreased cardiac output and pulmonary congestion.

Right ventricular heart failure
- anasarca
- anorexia
- ascites
- dependent edema
- elevated central venous pressure
- enlarged liver
- enlarged right atrium and ventricle
- hepatojugular reflux
- indigestion
- jaundice
- jugular vein distention
- nausea
- nocturia
- parasternal heave
- right upper quadrant pain

Left ventricular heart failure
- alternating pulse
- angina
- crackles
- dizziness
- dyspnea
- enlarged left atrium and ventricle
- fatigue
- hemoptysis
- nocturnal cough
- oliguria
- pallor
- point of maximal impulse enlarged and shifted to left
- restlessness
- tachycardia
- tachypnea
- third or fourth heart sound
- weakness

enough to cause heart failure in a person with only minor valve or muscle dysfunction.

Adverse drug effects

Several drugs can depress myocardial contractility and eventually produce heart failure in a person whose heart can't compensate. Antiarrhythmics and calcium channel blockers, primarily verapamil, can cause myocardial depression. Doxorubicin, an antineoplastic drug, weakens the heart muscle, which can lead to heart failure. Anabolic steroids, estrogen, and androgens can worsen heart failure in some patients by causing excessive fluid retention. Finally, alcohol has a negative inotropic effect and directly depresses myocardial contractility.

Noncompliance

As you know, patients with heart failure require individualized treatment to maintain the highest

possible functional level for their specific cardiac dysfunction. If the patient purposely or inadvertently reduces her therapy, you should naturally expect to see her heart failure worsen.

Recognizing heart failure

Because heart failure stems from many problems and may arise through a number of mechanisms, you may see patients with a wide range of signs and symptoms (see *Signs and symptoms of heart failure*). Some people have no signs or symptoms, even though they've been diagnosed with heart failure. To confirm your suspicion of heart failure based on the patient's signs and symptoms, perform a physical assessment and note the results of the patient's diagnostic tests.

Signs and symptoms

When assessing a patient who may have heart failure, note such signs and symptoms as dyspnea, orthopnea, paroxysmal nocturnal dyspnea, cough, fatigue, and nocturia.

Dyspnea

Shortness of breath or labored breathing may be the first symptom your patient notices. She may feel it at rest or only during exertion. Almost certainly, however, it will slowly worsen. That's because dyspnea typically results from pulmonary congestion caused by excess blood volume backed up from the left ventricle into the pulmonary vasculature. Eventually, increased volume and pressure in the pulmonary vessels causes fluid to shift into the alveoli.

You can measure the severity of your patient's dyspnea using a scale of perceived exertion, which allows your patient to describe her level of dyspnea in relation to her usual activities. Also, consider using a 100-ml visual analog scale to rate her dyspnea. Simply show the patient a horizontal line with "not breathless" written at one end and "extremely breathless" at the other end. Then ask her to place a mark at the place along the line that best represents her level of dyspnea. Both scales allow you to follow and document changes in your patient's condition over time.

Orthopnea

Ask the patient if she gets breathless when she lies down. If so, her impaired heart probably can't tolerate the increased preload that results from this position. Many patients with heart failure sleep propped up on several pillows, raise the head of the bed, or sleep sitting in a chair.

Paroxysmal nocturnal dyspnea

Ask if the patient awakens breathless, anxious, and feeling suffocated in the night. If she does, it may stem from several mechanisms:
- slow reabsorption of interstitial fluid from her limbs
- sudden elevation of intrathoracic pressure when lying down
- reduced sympathetic nervous system activity during sleep
- nocturnal depression of the respiratory center.

Most patients report that symptoms ease after they sit up for 30 minutes or so.

Cough

Ask if your patient has a persistent dry cough. If she does, it may result from fluid accumula-

tion and elevated pressures in the pulmonary system.

Fatigue

Most people who have heart failure report considerable fatigue. Your patient may say that her arms and legs feel heavy, a sensation that may stem from increased fluid volume and edema. Also, over time, impaired oxygenation may decrease the ability of skeletal muscles to continue taking up and metabolizing oxygen, a trend that only worsens activity intolerance. Plus, reduced activity compounds the problem by causing reduced muscle tone, strength, and mass.

Nocturia

Your patient may report that she voids infrequently during the day but wakes up six or more times at night to urinate. If so, it means that fluid is shifting from the interstitial to the vascular space when she lies down, increasing blood flow to her kidneys.

Assessment

The findings of your physical examination will vary based on the specific disorder that reduced the patient's CO. As always, conduct your examination in an orderly manner, including inspection, palpation, percussion, and auscultation. And remember that systolic blood pressure usually declines in a patient with heart failure, but diastolic pressure tends to rise, reducing the normal pulse pressure.

Inspection

On inspection, a patient with heart failure may appear quite normal if her condition is mild. Over time, however, the fluid excess may cause her to look puffy despite an overall loss of muscle mass from cardiac cachexia.

During your examination, watch the patient for shortness of breath with even limited activity. If necessary, slow the pace of your examination or allow for frequent rest periods.

Also, observe your patient's skin color carefully. If she has liver congestion, her skin or sclera may look jaundiced. Peripheral vasoconstriction caused by sympathetic nervous system stimulation and renin-angiotensin-aldosterone system activation may cause cyanosis.

Rating pitting edema

Your patient has pitting edema if you leave an indentation when you press your fingertip into her edematous skin. Use this scale to rate the severity of such edema.

Grade +1	Grade +2	Grade +3	Grade +4
• indentation up to ¼ inch • quickly returns to baseline	• indentation ¼ to ½ inch • returns to baseline in 10 to 15 seconds	• indentation ½ to 1 inch • returns to baseline in 1 to 2 minutes	• indentation more than 1 inch • takes more than 2 minutes to return to baseline

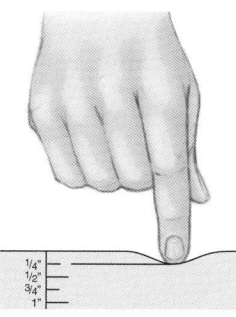 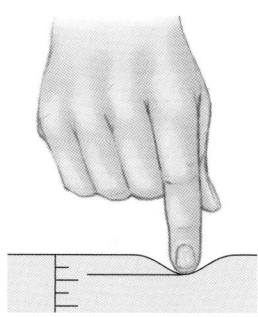 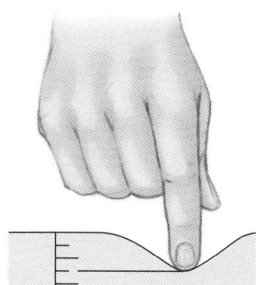 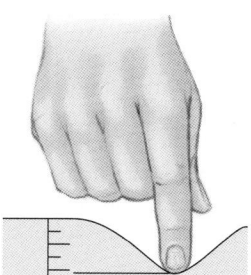

If the patient has fluid overload, you'll observe distended neck veins and possibly protruding eyeballs. Extra or exaggerated waves in the venous pulsations may suggest arrhythmias, valve dysfunction, or right ventricular filling defects.

Palpation

Edema develops as pressure in the blood vessels increases and forces fluid into the interstitial space. Keep in mind, however, that the degree of the fluid shift doesn't necessarily reflect the degree of your patient's heart failure.

Assess the patient's edema by pressing one or two fingertips into an edematous area. If you leave an indentation, the patient has pitting edema, a condition that you'll want to rate carefully (see *Rating pitting edema*). Remember that edema appears only after the patient has gained at least 5 pounds of fluid.

Reduced CO may weaken your patient's peripheral pulses; high-output failure, on the other hand, may strengthen the patient's peripheral pulses. As you palpate, you may detect a paradoxical pulse, a regular pattern of alternating stronger and weaker pulsations. This pulse reflects the heart's inability to maintain contractions of consistent strength.

In a normal patient, you'll palpate the point of maximal impulse (PMI) in the fifth intercostal space near the midclavicular line. You can feel a tapping sensation less than 2 centimeters in diameter against the palmar surface at the base of your fingers. In a patient whose heart is enlarged because of heart failure, the PMI may be displaced toward the left anterior axillary line. Also, you may palpate a PMI that's more than 2.5 centimeters in diameter.

Your patient with heart failure also may have hepatomegaly and a positive hepatojugular reflux from increased venous congestion. Assess her for hepatojugular reflux by placing her in the semi-Fowler position and pressing over her liver for 30 seconds. If you see the distention of her neck veins move up her neck during palpation, she has a positive hepatojugular reflux. This reflux occurs because the right atrium can't accept the extra volume of blood from the liver. During palpation, your patient may complain of tenderness in her right upper quadrant; it results from liver engorgement. With deep palpation, you may be able to feel the edge of her engorged liver against your fingertips.

Percussion

When you percuss over the heart of a patient with heart failure, you'll find the width of her heart to be more than a third the width of the chest wall.

When you percuss over her abdomen, you may hear dullness several centimeters below the right costal margin, an indication of an enlarged liver.

Auscultation

Crackles in your patient's lung bases suggest fluid overload in her pulmonary vasculature. As her heart failure worsens, the crackles will move higher in her lung fields. Gurgling sounds suggest pulmonary edema.

Listen for extra heart sounds as well. A third heart sound results from rapid ventricular filling and a fourth heart sound results from the contraction of an atrium forcing blood into a noncompliant ventricle.

Diagnostic tests

The patient will undergo several diagnostic tests to help confirm her heart failure. A chest X-ray may show that she has pulmonary venous congestion and interstitial edema. If she has systolic ventricular failure, the film will show an enlarged heart as well.

An echocardiogram can provide data on heart chamber size, valvular disease, left ventricular hypertrophy, and left ventricular contractile function.

Radionuclide angiocardiography, an invasive test involving injection of radioactive material, can help assess right ventricular function.

Both echocardiography and radionuclide ventriculography can be used to measure the patient's ejection fraction—the left ventricle's performance as a pump. If the patient has heart failure from systolic dysfunction, you may see an ejection fraction below 40% rather than one between 60% and 75%, which you'd see in a normal patient. Keep in mind, however, that a patient with diastolic dysfunction may have a normal ejection fraction.

A number of laboratory tests may return abnormal results for a patient with heart failure. For instance, renal and hepatic dysfunction from decreased organ perfusion will cause these abnormal findings:
- proteinuria
- elevated urine specific gravity
- elevated blood urea nitrogen levels
- elevated creatinine levels
- elevated bilirubin levels
- elevated serum enzyme levels, such as aspartate aminotransferase and alanine aminotransferase levels
- elevated prothrombin time and partial thromboplastin time.

Heart failure is a syndrome with many possible causes and assessment findings. Despite the diversity, however, you can find pathophysiologic changes common to virtually all heart failure patients as their bodies attempt to compensate for inadequate CO. Detecting these common changes early in the process of heart failure will help you maximize each patient's outcome through prompt, effective treatment.

10

HEART FAILURE

Treatment

No matter what the cause of your patient's heart failure, the main goal of her therapy remains the same: to improve cardiac output (CO) by reducing myocardial workload and optimizing pump performance. Achieving this goal usually requires a combination of drug therapy and diet adjustments. Some patients also need invasive support or surgical intervention.

Naturally, if your patient has acute heart failure, you'll need to act quickly to stabilize her condition with I.V. vasoactive drugs, hemodynamic monitoring, oxygen, respiratory monitoring, and if necessary, mechanical ventilation (see *Caring for a patient with heart failure,* pages 170 and 171). If the patient requires invasive monitoring, her treatment most likely will take place in a critical care unit.

After the patient's condition stabilizes, you can focus on long-term goals, such as managing symptoms, promoting optimal cardiac function, and enhancing your patient's quality of life.

Drug therapy

Drug therapy forms the cornerstone of treatment for acute and chronic heart failure. A physician may prescribe one or more drugs from the following classes: nitrates, diuretics, inotropic drugs, angiotensin-converting enzyme (ACE) inhibitors, and beta-blockers.

Nitrates

Nitrates dilate blood vessels by relaxing the smooth muscle that lines them. As a result, pe-

ripheral resistance drops, cardiac workload declines, and CO improves. As a group, nitrates are most effective for treating acute left ventricular heart failure and pulmonary edema.

Some nitrates, such as nitroglycerin and isosorbide, reduce preload by dilating veins, thus increasing venous pooling and decreasing blood return to the heart. Others, such as hydralazine, reduce afterload by dilating arteries; myocardial workload declines because the heart pumps against reduced resistance.

Sodium nitroprusside dilates both arteries and veins. Usually, however, you'll give it to reduce afterload. It's particularly effective for patients with both acute heart failure and hypertension.

Adverse effects and interactions

The most common adverse effects caused by nitrates include headaches, skin flushing, dizziness, and hypotension. These effects usually diminish after several days, although they may limit the usefulness of nitrates in some patients. The most severe complications of nitrates include decreased consciousness and cardiovascular collapse. Keep in mind that patients who take a nitrate for a long time commonly develop a tolerance to the drug's effects.

Also, remember that several substances alter the effects of nitrates. Alcohol, haloperidol, antihypertensive drugs, beta-blockers, calcium channel blockers, and phenothiazines increase the effects of nitrates. Antidepressants and antihistamines decrease the absorption rates of transdermal and transmucosal nitrates. Also, absorption of oral nitrates declines if the patient has food in her stomach when she takes the drug.

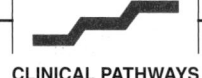

CLINICAL PATHWAYS

Caring for a patient with heart failure

	History and physical examination	Diagnostic tests	Discharge planning
Day 1	• blood pressure, heart rate, and respiratory rate on admission, after 1 hour, then every 2 hours until condition is stable • weight on admission • code status • advance directive • chest pain assessment with vital signs every hour, as appropriate • breath sounds every 4 to 8 hours. • level of consciousness assessment every shift	• 12-lead electrocardiogram (ECG) • complete blood count and electrolyte, blood urea nitrogen (BUN), creatinine, and cardiac enzyme levels • international normalized ratio (INR), prothrombin time (PT), or partial thromboplastin time (PTT), if receiving anticoagulant • urinalysis • pulse oximetry or arterial blood gas measurements • chest X-ray, echocardiography, and cardiac catheterization with angiography, if needed	• Assess home care needs; focus on physical environment, such as location of bathroom and number of stairs. • Assess family support system and other available resources.
Day 2	• chest pain assessment with vital signs every hour, as appropriate • blood pressure, heart rate, and respiratory rate every 4 hours • breath sounds every 4 to 8 hours • level of consciousness every shift • daily weight • activity tolerance, emotional status, social function, and cognitive abilities	• 12-lead ECG • BUN, creatinine, and electrolyte levels • cardiac enzyme levels, if elevated • INR, PT, or PTT, if receiving anticoagulant • echocardiography, if not done on day 1 • multiple gated acquisition scan	• Arrange for social services consultation, if indicated. • Arrange for cardiac rehabilitation consultation. • Arrange for occupational therapy consultation, if needed.
Day 3	• chest pain assessment with vital signs every hour, as appropriate • blood pressure, heart rate, and respiratory rate every 4 hours • breath sounds every 4 to 8 hours • daily weight • activity tolerance, emotional status, social function, and cognitive abilities	• 12-lead ECG • BUN, creatinine, electrolyte, and digoxin levels • cardiac enzyme levels, if elevated • INR, PT, or PTT, if receiving anticoagulant	• Collaborate with social services to plan appropriate home care services, including homemaker, nursing assistant, occupational therapist, and physical therapist.
Day 4	• chest pain assessment with vital signs every hour, as appropriate • blood pressure, heart rate, respiratory rate, and breath sounds every 8 hours • daily weight • activity tolerance, emotional status, social function, and cognitive abilities	• 12-lead ECG, if indicated • BUN, creatinine, and electrolyte levels • cardiac enzyme levels, if elevated • INR, PT, or PTT, if receiving anticoagulant	• Follow up with social services.
Day 5	• chest pain assessment with vital signs every hour, as appropriate • blood pressure, heart rate, respiratory rate, and breath sounds every 8 hours • daily weight • activity tolerance, emotional status, social function, and cognitive abilities	• digoxin level, if indicated	• Arrange for follow-up appointment with physician. • Arrange for follow-up to laboratory tests.

Drugs	Interventions	Patient teaching
• diuretic (thiazide, loop, or potassium sparing) • inotropic drug (digoxin, dopamine, dobutamine, amrinone, or milrinone) • preload reducer (nitrate or morphine) • afterload reducer (angiotensin-converting enzyme inhibitor, hydralazine, sodium nitroprusside, or prazosin) • anticoagulant (heparin or warfarin) • potassium supplement, if indicated • stool softener	• oxygen via nasal cannula, as needed • continuous ECG monitoring • intake and output monitoring • fluid restriction and 2-gram sodium diet • intermittent I.V. access device or I.V. fluid administration at keep-vein-open rate • indwelling urinary catheter, if indicated • endotracheal intubation and mechanical ventilation, as indicated • intra-aortic balloon counterpulsation, if needed • thrombolytic therapy, if needed	• Review plan of care with patient and family. • Orient patient to hospital and room. • Explain procedures and treatments. • Explain importance of reporting chest pain and other symptoms.
• diuretic • inotropic drug • preload reducer • afterload reducer • anticoagulant • potassium supplement • stool softener	• oxygen via nasal cannula, as needed • continuous ECG monitoring or telemetry • intake and output monitoring • fluid restriction and 2-gram sodium diet • intermittent I.V. access device • bed rest with bathroom privileges • indwelling catheter removal • range-of-motion exercises • skin care	• Review pathophysiology of heart failure. • Explain causes of signs and symptoms and effects of weight gain and sodium retention. • Review drugs. • Explain low-sodium diet and fluid retention.
• diuretic • inotropic drug • preload reducer • afterload reducer • anticoagulant • potassium supplement • stool softener	• no supplemental oxygen if saturation > 94% • telemetry as needed • intake and output monitoring • fluid restriction and 2-gram sodium diet • intermittent I.V. access device • skin care • ambulation 3-4 times daily for short distances • pulmonary hygiene	• Teach ways to conserve energy. • Explain weight monitoring and activity restrictions. • List signs and symptoms that require medical attention.
• diuretic • inotropic drug • preload reducer • afterload reducer • anticoagulant • potassium supplement • stool softener	• telemetry discontinued, if indicated • intake and output monitoring • fluid restriction and 2-gram sodium, low-cholesterol diet • intermittent I.V. access device discontinued, if indicated • ambulation in room with frequent rest periods	• Reinforce all teaching with patient and family.
• diuretic • inotropic drug • preload reducer • afterload reducer • anticoagulant • potassium supplement • stool softener	• intake and output monitoring • fluid restriction and 2-gram sodium, low-cholesterol diet • ambulation in room with frequent rest periods • change to oral drug administration, as prescribed	• Review discharge instructions. • Provide written instructions.

Don't give nitrates to patients who are hypersensitive to them or to patients who have severe anemia, increased intracranial pressure, or cerebral hemorrhage.

Nursing considerations

Depending on your patient's condition, you may administer one of several different nitrates. Each has its own characteristics of onset and action—and its own nursing considerations.

Intravenous nitroglycerin

Because I.V. nitroglycerin can change a patient's cardiac status swiftly, treatment typically takes place in a critical care unit or an emergency department with continuous monitoring in place.

If you're responsible for administering your patient's nitroglycerin I.V., make sure the order specifies the starting dose and the amount by which her mean arterial pressure (MAP) should drop. For example, the order may say, "Administer nitroglycerin I.V. at 10 µg/minute until MAP declines by 10%."

Tell your patient why she needs nitroglycerin, which adverse effects to expect, and which signs and symptoms to report to you. Assure her that you'll monitor her closely throughout therapy.

Before giving the drug, check your facility's policy for preparing and administering it. Because plastic absorbs some of the drug, dilute it in a glass bottle with either 5% dextrose in water (D_5W) or normal saline solution. Use an infusion pump to deliver the drug and vented tubing to draw it from the vacuum-sealed glass bottle, according to policy.

Before discharge, you may need to switch the patient from her I.V. nitrate to the oral or topical form that she'll be taking at home. As ordered, start the oral or topical drug while the I.V. form is still running. Then discontinue the I.V. after a specified period of time has passed, usually several hours.

Intravenous sodium nitroprusside

If the physician orders sodium nitroprusside I.V., dilute the drug in D_5W and don't combine or infuse it with any other drugs. Deliver it with an infusion pump. Because of its instability, you'll need to mix a new solution every 3 to 4 hours. Make sure you keep the resulting solution bag covered with aluminum foil because the drug degrades rapidly in light. The newly prepared solution may have a slightly brown tint. However, if it becomes dark brown, blue, or green, discard it and prepare a new solution.

Remember that a patient receiving I.V. nitroprusside will be in a critical care unit on continuous hemodynamic monitoring. You'll need to titrate the dosage according to the patient's blood pressure and pulmonary artery wedge pressure. As ordered, give dopamine I.V. in conjunction with sodium nitroprusside I.V. to optimize the patient's hemodynamic status.

Sublingual nitroglycerin

If your patient complains of chest discomfort or other symptoms of angina, place a nitroglycerin tablet under her tongue. Ask if she feels a burning or stinging sensation as the tablet dissolves. If not, replace it; the tablet may have lost its effectiveness. If she still feels chest pain after 5 minutes, place another tablet under her tongue. Continue this pattern until you've given 3 or 4 tablets over 15 to 20 minutes, as prescribed.

Monitor the patient's blood pressure closely before and after giving each dose. Also, give the patient nothing by mouth while she has a sublingual tablet in place.

Store sublingual nitroglycerin in its original container, tightly closed to maintain its potency. Protect the container from light and avoid carrying it in a pocket against your body because sunlight and heat can inactivate the drug.

Topical and transdermal nitroglycerin

A physician may prescribe topical or transdermal nitroglycerin to treat the symptoms of acute (not chronic) heart failure. If so, remember to apply each new dose to a new skin area to minimize irritation and redness. Choose hairless sites on the upper arms, chest, or back for optimal absorption.

For the paste form, measure the prescribed length onto a premeasured paper or plastic wrap, and then tape it to the patient's skin. To remove the paste, gently dab it from the skin with a tissue. Wear gloves to avoid absorbing the drug through your own skin. Then carefully wash the area with soap and water. Look for any other paste or patches left on the skin, clothing, or bed before applying the next dose.

Monitoring tips

To assess the effectiveness of nitrate therapy, look for changes in the patient's signs and symptoms. For example, look for an improved respiratory quality and rate, decreased blood pressure, and increased activity level and exercise tolerance. The patient's urine output may increase from improved renal perfusion. And her peripheral edema may subside.

Hemodynamic signs of a nitrate's effectiveness include improved CO and decreased systemic vascular resistance and intracardiac pressures.

Patient teaching

When starting nitrate therapy, tell your patient about the adverse effects she might experience. Explain that a headache is the most common adverse effect because the drug dilates blood vessels, which can create pressure and pain in her head. Reassure her that the headaches usually subside as her body becomes accustomed to the drug. Tell her to report any adverse effects to you. Also, tell her to ask for an analgesic if she needs one for her headache. Make sure you have an order to provide an analgesic, such as acetaminophen or propoxyphene.

If a physician prescribes sublingual nitroglycerin for the patient to use at home, tell her to store it in its original container. Tell her to keep the container tightly closed and protected from light. Also, tell her not to carry the container in a pocket next to her body. Urge her to replace the drug every 3 to 6 months to ensure its potency if and when she needs it.

If a physician prescribes oral nitrate tablets for chronic heart failure, tell the patient to take the tablet at least 1 hour before a meal or 2 hours afterward with a glass of water. If she'll be taking a sustained-release version of the drug, tell her not to break, crush, or chew the pills. Remember that chewable tablets are available; tell her to chew them thoroughly before swallowing.

Encourage your patient not to smoke because nicotine raises blood pressure. Smoking also raises the risks of heart disease and speeds up its progression. Plus, smoking alters the effectiveness of vasodilators.

Tell the patient to avoid activities that could prompt episodes of hypotension, such as rising quickly from a seated or lying position, drinking alcoholic beverages, or exercising in hot weather.

To help her avoid dizziness, instruct your patient to sit or lie down before taking her nitrate and to stay that way for 15 minutes afterward.

Also, tell her to stop or avoid any hazardous activities if she feels dizzy.

Diuretics

As a group, diuretics increase the volume of urine eliminated from the body, thus reducing overall fluid and electrolyte levels. Although different types of diuretics affect different portions of the renal tubule, most work by inhibiting tubular reabsorption of sodium in the kidneys, which increases sodium excretion (see *How diuretics work,* page 174). Because water tends to move with sodium, increased sodium excretion causes increased water excretion.

By increasing the amount of fluid that the kidneys remove from the bloodstream, diuretics reduce fluid congestion in the lungs and peripheral tissues. A decreased circulating fluid volume also reduces preload. Consequently, diuretics help to relieve signs and symptoms for patients who have moderate to severe heart failure.

Several categories of diuretics are available to treat heart failure, including thiazide, loop, and potassium sparing diuretics.

Thiazide and loop diuretics reduce pulmonary edema, peripheral edema, and symptoms of fluid retention. They're especially effective when used together with ACE inhibitors. Their rapid action makes them useful in emergency situations, such as acute respiratory failure from pulmonary edema. Hydrochlorothiazide is the most commonly prescribed thiazide diuretic; furosemide is the most commonly prescribed loop diuretic.

Potassium sparing diuretics—such as spironolactone, triamterene, or amiloride—are most effective in treating heart failure when used in combination with an ACE inhibitor, a loop diuretic, and digoxin.

Adverse effects and interactions

Thiazide diuretics can cause hypokalemia, nausea, vomiting, and anorexia. They also may cause urinary frequency, hyperglycemia, hyperuricemia, dizziness, fatigue, or weakness. The most serious adverse effects include hepatitis, uremia, and blood dyscrasia, including anemia (aplastic or hemolytic), agranulocytosis, thrombocytopenia, and neutropenia.

Loop diuretics tend to cause nausea and electrolyte imbalances, including hypokalemia, hy-

How diuretics work

Diuretics work by altering the reabsorption and excretion of water and electrolytes at specific sites along the nephron.

Loop diuretics
Loop diuretics work in the ascending loop of Henle. They inhibit the reabsorption of sodium and chloride, enhancing their excretion and that of magnesium and potassium. When given I.V., these drugs have a rapid onset and a short duration of action. They're effective in emergency situations and for patients with a glomerular filtration rate (GFR) below 20 ml/minute.

Thiazide diuretics
Thiazide diuretics block reabsorption and cause the excretion of roughly equal amounts of sodium and chloride in the thick portion of the distal convoluted tubule on the ascending loop of Henle. They also prompt the excretion of potassium, bicarbonate, and magnesium. Thiazide diuretics can't be used for patients with a GFR below 30 ml/minute.

Potassium sparing diuretics
Potassium sparing diuretics work in and near the collecting duct, competing with aldosterone to interfere with sodium-potassium exchange. They prompt the excretion of sodium, chloride, bicarbonate, calcium, and water and the retention of potassium, phosphate, and hydrogen. These relatively weak diuretics can be used to enhance the action of a potassium-wasting diuretic.

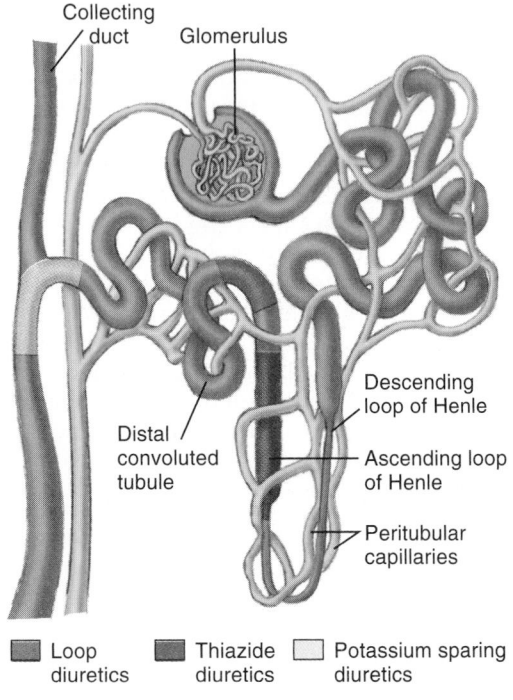

pochlorhydria, hypomagnesemia, hyponatremia, hypocalcemia, and hyperuricemia. Patients with impaired glucose tolerance may develop glycosuria and, consequently, increased urine output. More serious adverse effects include circulatory collapse, hearing loss (transient or permanent), renal failure, Stevens-Johnson syndrome, and several hematologic reactions similar to those caused by thiazide diuretics.

Potassium sparing diuretics can cause adverse effects similar to those listed so far, but the most common and most serious is hyperkalemia.

All patients taking diuretics, especially elderly ones, face an increased risk of orthostatic hypotension caused by rapid fluid loss. The concurrent use of a diuretic and an ACE inhibitor compounds the problem.

Don't give a thiazide diuretic to a patient hypersensitive or allergic to thiazides or sulfonamides or to a patient with severe renal dysfunction; the drug could further damage her kidneys. Also, don't give a thiazide diuretic to a pregnant woman or to a patient with severe hepatic dysfunction or hepatic coma.

Don't give a loop diuretic to a patient hypersensitive to sulfonurea compounds. Although a loop diuretic can be helpful for a patient with renal insufficiency, don't give it to a patient who's anuric. Also, don't give it to a patient with severe liver disease, hepatic coma, severe electrolyte depletion, or hypovolemia. If your patient is pregnant, give her a loop diuretic only when absolutely necessary because of its potential to harm the fetus.

Don't give a potassium sparing diuretic to a patient hypersensitive to it or to a patient with hyperkalemia, renal insufficiency, or anuria. Also, don't give this type of diuretic to a pregnant patient.

Nursing considerations
Ideally, give an oral diuretic early in the day, preferably after breakfast. If the patient needs more than one dose a day, give the last one no later than 6 P.M. to avoid nocturnal diuresis. To prevent nausea and gastrointestinal (GI) irritation, give the drug with food. Once the patient's condition has stabilized, she may be able to switch to alternate-day dosing and still achieve adequate diuresis.

Many physicians routinely order potassium supplements for patients taking thiazide or loop diuretics. If your patient's drug regimen doesn't include a potassium supplement, consider asking the physician about it.

If you're giving a diuretic I.V., remember that rapid administration can quickly cause hypotension. Keep the patient in a reclining position while giving the drug.

Monitoring tips
Before and during diuretic therapy, assess your patient's fluid status and note any signs or symptoms of dehydration or overload. Carefully record intake and output.

Weigh your patient at the start of diuretic therapy and every day thereafter, at least for the first few days, as ordered. Weigh the patient at the same time of day using the same scale. Make sure she wears similar clothing each time. If she gains or loses 2 pounds in a day or 5 pounds or more in a week, report it to a physician.

During diuretic therapy, carefully monitor the patient's serum electrolyte levels, including sodium, potassium, magnesium, calcium, and bicarbonate. Watch for signs and symptoms of electrolyte imbalance, including hypotension, tachycardia, changes in mental status, and oliguria. Also, remember that thiazide and loop diuretics can alter your patient's arterial blood gas values, blood pH, complete blood count, and blood glucose, uric acid, blood urea nitrogen (BUN), and creatinine levels.

Frequently monitor the patient's vital signs, especially her blood pressure. As you know, diuretics, especially I.V. diuretics, can cause a marked drop in blood pressure. To detect such a drop, monitor the patient for dizziness or light-headedness when she changes positions. Also, check for orthostatic hypotension with the patient in supine, sitting, and standing positions.

Be especially alert for hypotension if your patient takes central nervous system depressants, barbiturates, narcotics, or antihypertensives—drugs likely to cause hypotension early in diuretic therapy (see *Diuretics: Drug interactions at a glance,* page 176).

If your patient takes a loop diuretic, make sure she has no allergy to sulfonamides because loop diuretics are sulfonamide derivatives. Also, monitor her for signs and symptoms of ototoxicity, including tinnitus, reduced hearing, and vertigo. If she takes warfarin, check her anticoagulant levels carefully because she may develop excessive anticoagulation.

Patient teaching
Tell your patient to take her diuretic early in the day to avoid the need to urinate during the night. Also, suggest that she take the drug with food or milk to avoid stomach upset. If the patient will be taking a liquid preparation, urge her to measure it as precisely as possible and to always use a specially calibrated drug cup or spoon. Emphasize that diuretics are potent and should not be dosed carelessly.

Urge the patient to continue taking her diuretic exactly as prescribed even if her symptoms disappear. Make sure she understands that a diuretic will not cure her heart failure but rather will help to manage the symptoms it causes. Tell her to take a missed dose as soon as she realizes she missed it. If she only has a few hours to go until the next scheduled dose, however, tell her to skip the missed dose and continue with her regular schedule.

Teach the patient and a family member how to measure blood pressure and tell them how often to do so, based on the physician's order. Also, tell the patient to check her blood pressure and pulse any time she feels dizzy or light-headed. Urge her to change positions slowly and to lie down if she feels dizzy. Advise her to avoid exercising or standing for long periods in a hot environment because doing so could worsen her light-headedness.

Tell the patient to keep a daily record of her weight and to report a gain or loss of 2 pounds or more in a day or 5 pounds or more in a week. Reinforce the importance of following her prescribed diet regimen. If she uses a salt substitute,

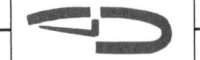

DANGEROUS COMPLICATIONS

Diuretics: Drug interactions at a glance

Drug	Effect of interaction
Thiazide diuretics	
antidiabetic drugs	• decreased antidiabetic effect
antihypertensives	• increased antihypertensive effect
digitalis glycosides	• toxic reaction
nitrates	• hypotension
nonsteroidal anti-inflammatory drugs	• decreased hypotensive effects
Loop diuretics	
adrenergic blockers	• increased diuretic effect
anticoagulants	• increased anticoagulant effect
antidiabetic drugs	• decreased antidiabetic effect
antihypertensives	• increased antihypertensive effect
digitalis glycosides	• hypokalemia and hypomagnesemia
Potassium sparing diuretics	
angiotensin-converting enzyme inhibitors	• hyperkalemia
antihypertensives	• increased antihypertensive effect
aspirin	• decreased diuretic effect
digitalis glycosides	• increased digitalis glycoside action
nonsteroidal anti-inflammatory drugs	• decreased antihypertensive effect

tell her not to change brands without first consulting her physician. Caution her against starting any new drugs (including nonprescription) or drinking alcoholic beverages without her physician's approval. Tell her that serious drug interactions could arise.

Especially if the patient takes a thiazide or a loop diuretic, instruct her to wear sunscreen, protective clothing, or both to prevent sunburn. If she takes a loop diuretic, tell her to report any signs or symptoms of ototoxicity, such as ringing or buzzing in her ears, reduced hearing, or vertigo.

If she has diabetes, diuretic therapy—especially thiazide therapy—may cause or aggravate hyperglycemia after 1 to 4 weeks. Tell her to monitor her blood glucose levels carefully and to report any evidence of hyperglycemia.

If your patient takes a potassium sparing diuretic, caution her about the risk of hyperkalemia. Warn her to avoid potassium supplements, salt substitutes that contain potassium, and foods high in potassium.

Inotropic drugs

Patients with heart failure receive positive inotropic drugs, which increase the strength of myocardial contractions, rather than negative inotropic drugs, which decrease the strength of these contractions. By increasing CO, positive inotropic drugs reduce venous pressure and increase blood flow to the kidneys, indirectly causing diuresis and reducing pulmonary and peripheral edema. However, because these drugs increase myocardial oxygen demand as they improve pump strength, use them cautiously in patients who have both a myocardial infarction (MI) and heart failure.

The three categories of positive inotropic drugs prescribed for patients with heart failure are digitalis glycosides, adrenergic agonists, and phosphodiesterase inhibitors.

Digitalis glycosides
Powerful inotropic drugs, digitalis glycosides have proven especially useful in treating left ventricular heart failure. Those prescribed most commonly for heart failure include digoxin and digitoxin.

By inhibiting the function of extracellular sodium and potassium-adenosinetriphosphatase, digitalis glycosides enhance the function of intracellular calcium, which activates the contractile proteins actin and myosin, thus increasing the force of contraction.

These drugs suppress activity at the sinoatrial node and prolong conduction velocity through the atrioventricular (AV) node. The resulting decrease in heart rate helps to reduce myocardial workload and improve perfusion of the coronary arteries during diastole.

Digoxin has a half-life of 36 to 48 hours; digitoxin has a half-life of 4 to 6 days.

Adrenergic agonists
Milder inotropic drugs, adrenergic agonists work by stimulating the adrenergic sites of the sympathetic nervous system. Drugs prescribed to treat heart failure include dopamine and dobutamine. Because they exert a more modest effect on the myocardium, they make a better choice for patients with both an MI and heart failure. However, because these drugs may increase the heart's workload, you need to monitor your patient closely to make sure the dosage is appropriate.

At low doses (up to 5 µg/kg/minute), dopamine maintains and improves renal and mesenteric blood flow by activating dopaminergic receptors. At higher doses (10 to 15 µg/kg/minute), it stimulates beta$_1$ receptors in the heart, increasing the heart rate, force of contraction, and systemic vascular resistance to increase blood pressure. Infusions of more than 20 µg/kg/minute begin to stimulate alpha receptors, which causes generalized vasoconstriction and may trigger arrhythmias, increase myocardial oxygen consumption, and worsen myocardial function.

Most physicians prefer dobutamine for acute heart failure because it doesn't increase heart rate or blood pressure and it has a vasodilating effect. Infusions of 2.5 to 10 µg/kg/minute directly activate beta$_1$-receptor and beta$_2$-receptor sites, causing mild vasodilation. At more than 10 µg/kg/minute, dobutamine may increase hypotension and tachycardia, worsening heart failure.

After a patient's condition stabilizes, dopamine can be given at doses below 5 µg/kg/minute in a medical-surgical or progressive care environment. However, dobutamine must be given in a critical care setting where hemodynamic monitoring can take place. No matter what the prescribed dosage, you'll need to adjust it to maximize hemodynamic readings and patient response, while avoiding alterations in mental status, tachycardia, arrhythmias, and oliguria.

Phosphodiesterase inhibitors
Amrinone, the most commonly prescribed phosphodiesterase inhibitor for heart failure, blocks the action of phosphodiesterase on the myocardium. As a result, the level of cyclic adenosine monophosphate increases along with the availability of calcium, improving pump efficiency and dilating arteries. The drug also improves CO by reducing preload and afterload through direct relaxation of vascular smooth muscle. Usually, you'll give amrinone on a short-term basis when other drugs—such as digitalis glycosides, diuretics, or vasodilators—have failed to ease your patient's heart failure.

Adverse effects and interactions
Because digitalis glycosides have a narrow therapeutic range, they cause toxic reactions in about 20% of patients treated with them. Vague signs and symptoms of a toxic reaction can mimic the heart failure itself (see *Digitalis glycosides: Signs and symptoms of a toxic reaction,* page 178).

Drug interactions arise with digoxin and digitoxin primarily when blood drug levels or serum electrolyte levels increase or decrease. Many drugs can affect blood levels of digitalis glycosides. For instance, concurrent use of a beta-blocker and a digitalis glycoside can quickly slow or stop conduction through the AV node, causing complete heart block. A diuretic can increase or decrease the toxic effects of a digitalis glycoside by causing hypokalemia or hyperkalemia. Closely monitor the serum potassium level of a patient taking a diuretic and a digitalis glycoside.

Don't give a digitalis glycoside to any patient with a known hypersensitivity to this type of drug or to anyone with severe bradycardia, previous episodes of ventricular tachycardia or fibrillation, hyperkalemia, myxedema, severe pulmonary disease, acute MI, or carditis. Give a digitalis glycoside cautiously to any patient who has had a previous toxic reaction.

Digitoxin may be a better choice for patients with impaired renal function because it's metabolized by the liver. Patients with hepatic failure should receive digoxin or low doses of digitoxin.

Dopamine and dobutamine can cause tachy-

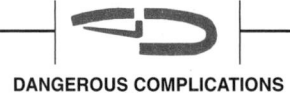

DANGEROUS COMPLICATIONS

Digitalis glycosides: Signs and symptoms of a toxic reaction

Because digitalis glycosides have a narrow therapeutic range, you'll need to assess your patient carefully for signs and symptoms of a toxic reaction.

Type of assessment	Signs and symptoms
Cardiovascular	• *common:* bradycardia, first-degree heart block, bigeminy, premature ventricular contractions • *less common:* hypotension; second-degree or third-degree heart block; wandering pacemaker; atrial, junctional, and ventricular tachycardias
Gastrointestinal	• *common:* anorexia, nausea, vomiting • *less common:* diarrhea, constipation, abdominal pain
Neurologic	• *common:* fatigue, headache, weakness, insomnia, malaise, vertigo, drowsiness • *less common:* neuralgias (especially trigeminal neuralgia), paresthesia, convulsions, disorientation, electroencephalogram abnormalities, seizures
Mental status	• *common:* confusion, depression, restlessness • *less common:* delirium, psychosis, hallucinations
Vision	• *common:* blurred vision, disturbances in color vision (especially green or yellow), colored halos around lights • *less common:* flashing lights, shimmering vision, scotomas, micropsia, macropsia, temporary or permanent amblyopia

cardia, headache, nausea, vomiting, and chest pain. Patients with these problems usually require a lower dose or discontinuation of the drug. Infiltration of dopamine at the I.V. site can cause severe tissue damage and requires prompt injections of phentolamine into the site to prevent necrosis.

The adverse effects of amrinone include cardiac arrhythmias, hypotension, thrombocytopenia, anorexia, nausea, vomiting, and abdominal pain.

Nursing considerations
Keep in mind that digoxin can be given orally or I.V., whereas digitoxin is only given orally. The quickest route to digitalization (the process of achieving therapeutic blood levels of digitalis glycoside) is I.V. administration, although you can use the oral route if the patient's condition is stable.

If a physician has ordered I.V. digoxin, start with a loading dose of 0.5 mg administered over 5 to 20 minutes, as specified. You can give the drug undiluted or you can dilute 1 mg of it in 4 ml of sterile water, D_5W, or normal saline solution. Use diluted solutions immediately.

After 3 hours, give another 0.25-mg or 0.125-mg dose until you reach a total dose of 1 mg to 1.25 mg, as prescribed. Remember that I.V. digoxin begins to act within 30 minutes and has a duration of action of 1½ to 3 hours. Throughout therapy, monitor your patient's vital signs and heart rhythm closely.

If a physician ordered oral digoxin, give a loading dose of 1 to 1.25 mg divided over 24 hours. Then give another 0.5 mg during the next 24 hours. Usually, patients who take oral digoxin require 0.5 mg daily for 3 days before they achieve therapeutic levels.

Daily doses of 0.125 to 0.25 mg I.V. or orally will typically maintain adequate drug levels.

Dopamine, dobutamine, and amrinone come premixed in D_5W at a concentration determined by your facility. Deliver them at a rate of 2 to 10 µg/kg/minute, as prescribed, and titrate the dosage to achieve the desired effects. To avoid the complications of dopamine infiltration, you can infuse it through a central venous line.

Monitoring tips

Watch for signs of improvement in your patient's CO and myocardial efficiency. These signs include reduced fluid retention, normalized hemodynamic status, improved respiratory pattern, and increased activity tolerance.

Also, watch carefully for signs and symptoms that your patient is having a toxic reaction to the digitalis glycoside, including bradycardia, anorexia, nausea, and vomiting. If you suspect a toxic reaction, withhold the drug, monitor your patient's vital signs, and notify a physician. In all likelihood, you'll need to check her blood digoxin level and obtain an electrocardiogram (ECG).

Monitor her serum electrolyte, BUN, and creatinine levels and liver function tests, especially if she's taking digitoxin. Keep in mind that impaired renal function can raise blood drug levels and that hypokalemia can prompt a toxic reaction.

If you find increased blood digoxin levels, you may be able to simply withhold the drug temporarily while you treat the patient's symptoms and allow drug levels to return to the therapeutic range. However, if the patient has a severe or life-threatening toxic reaction, you may need to administer digoxin immune FAB. It contains antibody fragments that bind with free digoxin in the bloodstream. One vial of the drug binds an equivalent of three 0.25-mg digoxin tablets; you may need to give up to three I.V. doses to bind all the free digoxin in the patient's vascular system. Before giving it, test your patient's skin for a hypersensitivity reaction.

After starting your patient on an inotropic drug, continue to assess her for signs of returning heart failure. Measure her weight every day and keep an accurate record of her intake and output. Notify the physician if she gains 2 pounds or more in a day or 5 pounds or more in a week.

Also, assess the patient for crackles, dyspnea at rest or with exertion, dependent edema, jugular vein distention, and increased abdominal girth. Monitor her for changes in vital signs or heart sounds (such as tachycardia or a third heart sound). Note any changes in her activity tolerance, skin color, or mental status. All of these signs suggest ineffective drug therapy and the need to reevaluate the treatment plan.

If you're giving dopamine, dobutamine, or amrinone, carefully follow the patient's vital signs, heart rate and rhythm, hemodynamic status, fluid and electrolyte levels, platelet count, intake and output, and body weight. If the patient has hypokalemia, correct it before giving amrinone.

Prolonged amrinone therapy commonly leads to thrombocytopenia, especially at higher doses. If your patient's platelet count drops below 150,000 mm^3, discontinue the drug, as ordered.

Patient teaching

Tell your patient about the digitalis glycoside prescribed for her, including its actions, adverse effects, and purpose. Emphasize that she should take the drug exactly as prescribed. Review the dosage schedule with her and make sure she understands it. Many patients find it difficult to alternate doses from day to day and need special help to manage the fluctuating regimen.

Remind the patient that the drug is absorbed more slowly when taken with food—especially food high in bran fiber. However, if she develops stomach upset, tell her to take the drug with a snack or meal. Urge her to take it at the same time every day.

Tell the patient to take a missed dose as soon as she remembers it if less than 12 hours have passed since the scheduled dose. Otherwise, tell her to wait until the next scheduled dose and continue on her usual schedule. Warn her never to double-dose to try to catch up. Tell her to call her physician for instructions if she fails to take the drug for 2 days or more.

Review the signs and symptoms of a toxic reaction with your patient and tell her to call her physician if any develop. If your patient is elderly, thus more prone to a toxic reaction, spend extra time making sure she understands and can identify these signs and symptoms.

Besides urging her to take her inotropic drug faithfully, tell the patient to continue following all aspects of her treatment plan, possibly including potassium supplements, diuretics, vasodilators, antihypertensive drugs, a low-sodium diet, and so on. Caution her to avoid using over-the-counter (OTC) drugs without her physician's consent.

Teach the patient to take and record her radial or carotid pulse. Especially during the first few weeks of therapy, she should take it every day, preferably at the same time of day and in the same position, either sitting or lying down. Also, tell her to take it any time she feels palpitations or doesn't feel well.

If the patient can't take her own pulse, teach a family member how and when to do it. Make sure the patient and her family members know her usual pulse rate so that they can call her physician if it varies more than 15 beats from normal.

Also, instruct her to weigh herself at the same time every day, using the same scale and wearing similar clothes. Suggest that she weigh herself in the morning, after urinating but before eating. And tell her to call her physician if she gains 2 pounds or more in a day or 5 pounds or more in a week.

Finally, urge the patient to carry or wear medical identification that lists the name of her inotropic drug, the dosage she takes, and the reason she takes it.

Angiotensin-converting enzyme inhibitors

By blocking the enzyme responsible for converting angiotensin I into angiotensin II, ACE inhibitors reduce the effects of the renin-angiotensin-aldosterone system. They also inhibit aldosterone secretion by interfering with the degradation of bradykinin, a potent vasodilator. Called balanced vasodilators, ACE inhibitors decrease both arterial and venous smooth-muscle tone to reduce both preload and afterload.

As a result, they reduce vascular resistance and blood volume, improve renal blood flow, promote excretion of sodium and water, and help control the elevated blood pressure caused by excess intravascular volume. What's more, because ACE inhibitors help correct hyponatremia and hypokalemia, they reduce the risk of cardiac arrhythmias.

The most commonly prescribed ACE inhibitors for patients with heart failure include captopril, the first ACE inhibitor, and enalapril. Sometimes, these ACE inhibitors are given in combination with the diuretic hydrochlorothiazide.

Adverse effects and interactions

Because ACE inhibitors produce widespread vasodilation, they tend to cause marked hypotension early in therapy, especially among hypovolemic patients and those who drink too much al-cohol or take diuretics, phenothiazines, monoamine oxidase inhibitors, or benzodiazepines. If your patient already takes a diuretic or a vasodilator, withhold it for 24 hours or more, as ordered, before starting the ACE inhibitor. You can also help minimize hypotension by starting therapy with a reduced dose and by giving captopril, which has a short half-life.

Other adverse effects include headache, loss of taste sensation, nausea, diarrhea, a chronic dry cough (especially in women), and a skin rash that may be itchy. Patients with renal disease face a high risk of neutropenia and proteinuria at the start of therapy with ACE inhibitors; monitor them for protein in their urine and for signs of infection.

When aldosterone secretion is inhibited by reduced production of angiotensin II, serum potassium levels may increase, especially if the patient has impaired renal function. This change places the patient at risk for hyperkalemia. Concurrent use of drugs that elevate potassium levels or transfusion of banked blood only increases that risk. Likewise, consumption of high-potassium foods or salt substitutes can raise the risk. Follow your patient's potassium level closely.

Angioedema is a rare but life-threatening adverse effect of ACE inhibitors. If a patient complains of throat discomfort or difficulty swallowing or breathing after she starts taking an ACE inhibitor, withhold the drug and consult with a physician.

Remember that concurrent use of an ACE inhibitor and lithium may increase blood lithium levels. Concurrent use of tetracycline and an ACE inhibitor may impair tetracycline absorption.

Don't give an ACE inhibitor to a patient hypersensitive to this type of drug or to a patient with heart block, bilateral renal stenosis, or liver insufficiency. Usually, you won't give an ACE inhibitor to a patient who takes a potassium sparing diuretic either. If the patient has renal insufficiency, you'll most likely start with a reduced dose.

Nursing considerations

All ACE inhibitors can be given orally, but enalapril also can be given I.V. Following oral administration, captopril is rapidly absorbed into the bloodstream. The liver metabolizes about half the drug; the kidneys excrete the rest unchanged.

Give captopril an hour before the patient eats because food alters absorption of the drug.

Because captopril has a half-life of $1\frac{1}{2}$ to 2 hours, multiple dosing is required for effective therapeutic use. Oral enalapril has a half-life of about 11 hours and can be given once daily.

Monitoring tips

Before starting the patient on an ACE inhibitor, obtain kidney and liver function tests, as ordered. Also, obtain a baseline blood pressure so that you can track the development and severity of hypotension caused by the drug. Remember that captopril reaches its peak effect 30 to 90 minutes after administration because of its short half-life. You may need to withhold the drug, as ordered, if the patient's systolic pressure drops below a specified level.

If the patient develops hypotension, notify the physician and encourage the patient to lie down. If she has marked hypotension, you may need place her in a modified Trendelenburg position or give her fluids I.V., preferably normal saline solution.

Watch for signs and symptoms of the drug's effectiveness, such as improved activity tolerance and decreased dyspnea, crackles, cyanosis, jugular vein distention, and edema.

Assess the patient's serum sodium and potassium levels as ordered, and anticipate reducing the ACE inhibitor's dosage if necessary.

Patient teaching

Teach your patient how to take her ACE inhibitor correctly. For example, explain that she should take captopril an hour before eating because food significantly alters absorption of the drug. Food intake doesn't affect enalapril's action. Mention that coffee, tea, cola, chocolate, and other xanthine-containing substances may inhibit the action of ACE inhibitors. Also, encourage her to avoid salt substitutes because they can be high in potassium.

If your patient misses a dose of captopril, tell her to take the missed dose as soon as she remembers it, unless the next scheduled dose is within 4 hours. The same goes for enalapril, unless the next scheduled dose is within 8 hours. Urge the patient not to double-dose to catch up and not to stop ACE-inhibitor therapy abruptly.

Explain the causes and the symptoms of orthostatic hypotension, and encourage the patient to change positions slowly and to rise slowly from a sitting or reclining position. Tell her to

sit or lie down if she feels dizzy or light-headed and to avoid driving or performing hazardous activities if she feels dizzy.

Caution the patient not to use overly hot water for baths or showers because it increases vasodilation and hypotension. Also, warn the patient to avoid alcohol unless her physician has approved its use. Tell the patient to expect to feel tired during the first few weeks of therapy.

Urge the patient to call her physician if she develops mouth sores, nausea and vomiting, a rash, fever, sore throat, swollen hands or feet, a cough, difficulty breathing, palpitations, or chest discomfort. Also, tell her to report excessive perspiration or diarrhea because dehydration worsens hypotension. Warn the patient not to exercise in hot weather, and to stay well hydrated within the limits of her prescribed fluid intake.

Instruct the patient to avoid any drugs not specifically approved by her physician, especially OTC cough and cold drugs. Urge her to avoid using nonsteroidal anti-inflammatory drugs, especially if she has diabetes because they can induce acute renal failure.

Beta-blockers

Beta-blockers reduce myocardial oxygen demand and workload by reducing heart rate, the force of contractions, and conduction velocity. Reducing heart rate and myocardial contractility in a failing myocardium may actually worsen heart failure briefly before improving it. Beta-blockers exert the following effects:
• They reduce the effect of excess circulating catecholamines on the sympathetic nervous system.
• They reduce the risk of hypokalemia and thus increase the threshold for ventricular fibrillation.
• They normalize beta-receptor sensitivity to sympathetic stimulation.
• They increase filling time and stroke volume by reducing the heart rate, thus improving CO.

Physicians who prescribe beta-blockers for heart failure tend to use cardioselective metoprolol or nonselective carvedilol. Metoprolol undergoes significant metabolism on its first pass through the liver, which makes about 40% of the oral dose rapidly available in systemic circulation. Food enhances its bioavailability. The drug is eliminated by hepatic metabolism and renal excretion.

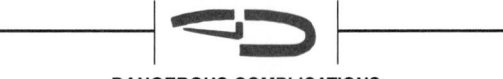

DANGEROUS COMPLICATIONS

Metoprolol: Drug interactions at a glance

Drug	Effect of interaction
alcohol	• hypotension
amphetamines	• hypertension and bradycardia
antihypertensives	• hypotension
digitalis glycosides	• bradycardia
epinephrine	• stimulation of alpha-adrenergic receptors
histamine$_2$-receptor antagonists	• increased effects of metoprolol
hydralazine	• increased effects of metoprolol and hydralazine
indomethacin	• decreased effect of metoprolol
methyldopa	• hypotension and bradycardia
monoamine oxidase inhibitors	• bradycardia
nitrates	• hypotension
I.V. phenytoin	• myocardial depression
prazosin	• hypotension and bradycardia
reserpine	• hypotension and bradycardia
theophylline	• decreased bronchodilation
thyroid hormone	• decreased effectiveness of thyroid hormone
verapamil	• myocardial depression

Adverse effects and interactions

Metoprolol's adverse effects tend to be transient and rarely require withdrawal of therapy. Some patients may develop insomnia and dizziness. A few may develop GI problems, such as hiccups, nausea, vomiting, and diarrhea. And a few develop hematologic effects, such as agranulocytosis, eosinophilia, and thrombocytopenic purpura.

Because metoprolol's selectivity isn't absolute, monitor your patient for shortness of breath with exertion and rest. Also, check for bronchospasm caused by beta$_2$-receptor blockade.

A patient with heart failure requires a certain amount of sympathetic stimulation to support circulation. Consequently, using beta-blockers can worsen her heart failure by depressing cardiac motility, slowing AV conduction, and decreasing CO. However, excessive sympathetic stimulation can be harmful as well. So you'll need to find that critical balance between therapeutic and detrimental effects when administering a beta-blocker to a patient with heart failure. Usually, you'll start with a very low dose and increase it slowly until the patient's signs and symptoms improve, as ordered.

Keep in mind that concurrent use of a beta-blocker and a digitalis glycoside can raise the patient's risk of depressed AV-node conduction even more than with a beta-blocker alone. Many more drugs interact with beta-blockers as well (see *Metoprolol: Drug interactions at a glance*).

Don't give metoprolol to a patient hypersensitive to it. Also, don't give the drug to a patient with moderate to severe heart failure, cardiogenic shock, a heart rate below 50 beats per minute (bpm), or second-degree or third-degree heart block. And because some nonselective beta-blockers affect beta$_2$ receptors, don't give these drugs to a patient with bronchospasm or asthma.

Nursing considerations

If you're giving metoprolol I.V., do so over 2 minutes or more and keep the patient in a recumbent position for at least 3 hours afterward to prevent hypotension. Monitor the patient carefully in case she has a rapid drop in blood pressure or heart rate.

If you're giving the drug orally, do so in a consistent manner, with or without food at the same time each day.

Don't discontinue metoprolol—or any beta-blocker for that matter—abruptly. Doing so could cause or worsen angina, especially in patients with coronary artery disease. Store the drug at room temperature and protect it from light.

Monitoring tips

Before starting beta-blocker therapy, assess the patient's apical and radial pulse rates to detect signs of heart block. Note the rate, rhythm, and quality of her pulses. Notify a physician if her pulse is less than 50 bpm or she experiences any signs or symptoms of respiratory distress.

Also, assess your patient for signs and symptoms of fluid retention. Monitor her intake and output and her daily weights, noting any significant changes.

Laboratory work for renal and liver function should be performed before starting therapy; check it periodically throughout drug therapy.

If your patient has diabetes, monitor her blood glucose levels closely. Remember, beta-blockers can suppress the signs and symptoms of hypoglycemia or prolong a hypoglycemic episode.

Patient teaching

Teach your patient to take her drug at the same time of day and in the same relation to food. If she misses a dose, tell her to take it as soon as she remembers, within 4 hours after the scheduled time. Warn her not to double-dose or to stop taking the drug abruptly. Urge her to avoid taking OTC drugs while taking a beta-blocker unless she first consults her physician.

Show the patient how to check her pulse and blood pressure. Tell her to notify the physician if her pulse goes below 50 bpm or if her systolic blood pressure differs by more than 20 points from her last reading. Determine her normal pulse and blood pressure range, then base her personal guidelines on those readings.

Because beta-blockers can cause drowsiness or dizziness, caution the patient to avoid driving or engaging in other hazardous activities until she's accustomed to the drug's effects. Also, tell her to report feelings of depression and nightmares, also common adverse effects.

Warn the patient not to drink alcoholic beverages or to smoke while on taking a beta-blocker. Alcohol can increase the drug's hypotensive effects and nicotine can raise her heart rate.

Tell the patient to weigh herself daily, especially at the start of therapy. Afterward, she can weigh herself every few days. Make sure she knows to tell her physician about a weight gain of 2 pounds or more in a day or 5 pounds or more in a week. Also, tell her to notify her physician about increasing signs and symptoms of heart failure, such as difficulty breathing (especially with exertion or in a reclining position), distended jugular veins, increased swelling in her limbs, increased abdominal girth, or increased weight gain.

Remind the patient to store the drug in a cool place, away from direct light. Also, encourage her to carry or wear identification that lists the drugs she takes and any allergies she may have.

Because beta-blockers can cause triglyceride levels to rise and high-density lipoprotein levels to fall, tell the patient to have her lioprotein levels monitored often after discharge.

Diet

Despite the appearance of being puffy or overweight, most patients with heart failure are actually nutritionally depleted or, worse, cachectic; they may also be hypovolemic or dehydrated. They look overweight because they have too much fluid in their interstitial space, a condition called third spacing, or fluid shifting.

What happens is that a poor diet causes serum protein and albumin levels to decrease. Fluid then shifts out of the bloodstream and into the interstitial space, an area of higher protein concentration. Up to 5 pounds of fluid can enter the interstitial space before the patient develops pitting edema. The most common treatment for this imbalance is diet management.

Assessment

First, perform a detailed assessment to determine whether the patient is obese or retaining fluid. When beginning your examination, look for signs of poor oxygenation, such as pale, cool skin or cyanosis of the lips, fingers, or toes. After obtaining the patient's weight and vital signs, look for places where fluid may be hidden. Check for obvious signs of fluid retention, such as dependent edema, jugular vein distention, a productive cough, and dyspnea with minimal activity. Auscultate her lungs for fine or coarse crackles that don't clear with coughing. Listen for a third heart sound. And check her abdomen for distention or a fluid wave.

If your patient has mild heart failure, she may show no signs of distress. More commonly, however, you'll encounter a typical set of signs and symptoms produced by the combination of muscle wasting and fluid retention. The patient may appear frail, weak, and dyspneic, with abdominal distention, puffy legs and ankles, and distended neck veins.

In severe heart failure, the patient has a persistently inadequate oxygen supply in the peripheral tissues. A generalized catabolic state results, with a loss of body mass and the development of cardiac cachexia. Characterized by a negative energy balance, weight loss, and systemic wasting, this condition is common in patients with end-stage heart failure. As the amount of energy required for normal breathing, cardiac activity, and other body functions grows, these patients develop a higher resting metabolic rate. It probably results from sympathetic overactivity and circulating catecholamines.

Based on your impressions of the patient's physical condition, ask her about her diet and lifestyle habits. Have her describe her typical daily eating pattern, including what and when she eats (including snacks), how she uses salt or salt substitutes, how often she eats out or eats fast food, and which vitamins, supplements, and OTC drugs she takes.

To determine her physical conditioning and exercise tolerance, have her describe her activity level. Assess her ability to perform daily activities, including caring for herself, grooming, cooking, particpating in recreational activities, working around the house, and so on.

Also, ask her to tell you what she knows about the relationship between foods and heart failure. This baseline information will help you to determine realistic diet, fluid management, and teaching goals to be included in your patient's diet plan.

Diet plan

Together with the patient's physician and, if possible, a dietitian or nutritional counselor, develop a diet plan for your patient. This plan should include sodium reduction, fluid restriction, and any other steps needed to minimize the effect of fluid retention on your patient's condition.

Sodium

Although the body requires only about 500 mg of sodium each day, most Americans consume between 3 and 6 grams daily—enough to aggravate the tendency toward salt and water retention in a patient with heart failure. That's why, if your patient has mild symptoms, you should discourage her from adding salt to her foods at the dining table. She should also eliminate highly salted foods from her diet, such as potato chips, pretzels, candy bars, canned foods (including soup), deli meats, and condiments, such as pickles and olives. Taking these steps should reduce her daily sodium intake to between 1.5 and 3 g daily.

Patients with more pronounced symptoms should reduce their daily sodium intake to between 1.0 and 1.5 g by eliminating salt from cooking. Many patients use salt substitutes to improve the flavor of low-salt foods. Some substitutes are herb based; others contain high levels of potassium—an important difference that patients should understand.

Sodium can be hidden in beverages as well as foods, so encourage your patient to read the nutrition information on all labels. Urge her to avoid alcohol or consume it only in small amounts. Emphasize that it may contain significant amounts of sodium and that it may cause myocardial depression. Also, mention that many carbonated beverages are high in either sodium or potassium; help the patient determine which carbonated beverages she can safely consume. Finally, tell her that some OTC and prescription drugs contain high levels of sodium. Suggest that she ask a pharmacist about the sodium content of all her drugs.

Fluids

Most patients with heart failure must follow fluid restrictions, although not as strictly as physicians once advised. Research has shown that total extracellular fluid volume is controlled primarily by sodium content and that aggressive fluid intake doesn't help to flush sodium from the body. Consequently, you'll want to instruct your patient to drink fluids in moderation.

However, patients with severe heart failure may need to follow more rigid fluid restriction. That's because these patients have an increased concentration of circulating antidiuretic hormone (ADH), which is released by the kidneys. Increased ADH impairs the body's ability to excrete water, which causes dilutional hyponatremia. Restricting water intake to less than 2 quarts daily will help relieve fluid retention and prevent complications.

Fats, proteins, and carbohydrates

Although fat reduction forms a cardinal diet goal for most patients with heart disease, overzealous fat reduction can be detrimental for those with heart failure. That's because patients with heart failure have higher metabolic rates during rest and exercise; consuming some fat can help to meet their increased calorie needs, maintain tissue structure, and prevent deconditioning.

In fact, these patients need a higher daily intake of calories, protein, and other essential nutrients to maintain a normal weight and body functions. An inadequate or improper diet can lead to a catabolic state, fluid retention, electrolyte imbalances, worsening of heart failure, and an increased risk of dangerous complications. The combined effect of impaired myocardial function and muscle wasting from malnutrition further increases the risk of death.

Because carbohydrates require less energy to break down, the body metabolizes them quickly into simple sugars. Although they provide energy to fill immediate metabolic needs, they don't provide energy to fill long-term needs, and they don't provide energy or protein to build muscle mass or prevent muscle wasting. Any carbohydrates not used are stored as fat. Therefore, your patient needs a diet plan that not only incorporates healthy heart principles but also is properly balanced to help her maintain a normal body weight, build muscle mass, and prevent a catabolic or ketotic state.

Finally, when developing your diet plan, consider the patient's other medical conditions, such as renal or hepatic insufficiency, diabetes, malabsorptive conditions, or any conditions that affect her GI tract. Also, you'll need to consider her activity level, any drugs that affect her metabolism, and any allergies she has to foods.

Patient teaching

As you know, creating an appropriate diet plan isn't enough to ensure compliance. That's why, in addition to designing the plan, you'll need to teach the patient and her family how to succeed with it.

One of the keys to success may lie with the patient's family. As you teach the patient about her food requirements, try to include appropriate family members in the discussion. Find out whether the patient will be preparing her own meals or whether a family member or someone else will be preparing them for her. If the latter, make sure the person understands the patient's diet plan and the reasons behind it.

Also, as you devise the patient's diet plan, solicit suggestions and input from the patient and her family. Giving them a heightened sense of control and participation commonly leads to increased compliance with the plan.

Consider the patient's financial status, as well. Maintaining a sodium restriction may prove difficult for poorer families because the least expensive foods tend to be highest in sodium. Naturally, a meal plan that your patient can't afford or that won't fit into her family's lifestyle is doomed to failure.

Don't assume that every patient of a certain ethnic background follows a similar diet. Consider each patient's individual diet preferences. To devise a truly helpful diet plan, you'll need to understand the patient's values, beliefs, preferences, socioeconomic status, and living arrangements.

Take time to review practical ways to reduce sodium in the patient's diet (see *Low-sodium diet: Teaching tips,* page 186). Remember that most patients find a low-sodium diet highly unpalatable. Thus, your patient may not comply with the diet, or she may not consume as many calories as she should. Emphasize that eliminating as much sodium from the diet as possible will reduce her symptoms, improve her quality of life, and may help her avoid life-threatening complications.

If your patient must restrict fluids, tell her to start the day by measuring her fluid allowance into a clean pitcher or bottle. Then, when she wants a drink of water, she can simply pour it from the pitcher. If she wants to drink a different beverage, such as juice, tell her to pour a volume of water out of the pitcher that's equal to the volume of juice she wants to drink. Likewise, if she eats soup or a fluid-based dessert, such as flavored gelatin, tell her to pour a volume of water from the pitcher that's roughly equal to what she ate. Remind her that once she empties the pitcher she has consumed the day's fluid allotment.

Tell your patient that frequent small meals may be easier to manage than two or three large meals. If you find, over time, that she can't consume enough calories orally, she may need tube feedings or total parenteral nutrition to help prevent progressive nutritional deterioration.

Nutritional counseling, community support, and home follow-up may be essential for pa-

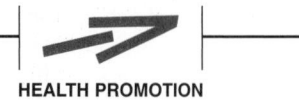

Low-sodium diet: Teaching tips

When teaching your patient how to adopt a low-sodium diet, be sure to cover these points:
- Explain how to read food labels so that your patient and her family can determine how much sodium their food contains. Remind them that 200 mg of salt equals 200 mg of sodium chloride.
- Emphasize the need to avoid adding salt while cooking or eating.
- Tell your patient to stay away from overly salty foods, such as pretzels, potato chips, candy bars, canned foods, frozen dinners, deli meats and cheeses, and foods preserved in brine.
- Urge your patient to avoid horseradish and monosodium glutamate because they contain high amounts of sodium.
- Emphasize the importance of avoiding over-the-counter drugs that are high in sodium, such as antacids, unless they're recommended by a physician.
- Remind your patient that many soft drinks contain sodium, especially low-calorie ones.
- Tell the patient to include unsalted meat, broth, soup, and butter in her diet plan.
- Inform your patient and her family about the availability of low-salt canned vegetables, canned soups, and baking powder.
- Encourage the use of herbs—especially fresh herbs—and spices to enhance food flavors.
- Tell the patient that when eating out she should order foods that are baked, broiled, or roasted and avoid gravies, soups, cheese sauces, and fast foods.
- Remind the patient to consult her physician before using a salt substitute, especially if she takes a potassium sparing diuretic.

tients who have trouble preparing or eating appropriate foods in appropriate quantities. For example, elderly patients who live alone tend to make simple, easy-to-prepare meals, such as soup or toast. They may have trouble hearing, seeing, chewing, or swallowing, or they may dis-

like the taste of unsalted foods. As a result, they may not receive calories or nutrients adequate to sustain body weight or to prevent muscle wasting. Community services can help avoid such problems and minimize progression of the patient's heart failure.

Invasive therapies

If a patient's heart failure progresses despite drug and diet therapy, she may need an invasive form of cardiac support. A physician may choose such a treatment for a number of reasons:
- to partially or completely take over the heart's function until an acute episode of heart failure has passed
- to keep the patient alive until she can undergo heart transplantation
- to improve the quality of life for a patient who isn't a candidate for heart transplantation
- to relieve unremitting symptoms of heart failure.

Invasive therapies for patients with heart failure include dynamic cardiomyoplasty, insertion of a ventricular assist device (VAD), and heart transplantation.

Dynamic cardiomyoplasty

In this procedure, a surgeon wraps a flap of skeletal muscle (usually the left latissimus dorsi) around the patient's heart and then conditions it to perform as cardiac muscle (see *Understanding dynamic cardiomyoplasty*). Contractions provided by the healthier skeletal muscle support and enhance the patient's ventricular function.

During the first 2 weeks after surgery, the patient recovers and collateral circulation begins to develop. After about 2 weeks, a cardiac surgeon or cardiologist begins to train the latissimus dorsi muscle by stimulating it with an electrode. This lengthy training process proceeds gradually, starting with one impulse for every other cardiac cycle. Electrical stimulation is timed to coincide with closure of the mitral valve. Gradually, over about 7 weeks, the amplitude and number of impulses increase until the skeletal muscle contracts forcefully.

Because the muscle must be trained to function in its cardiac support role, most patients

Understanding dynamic cardiomyoplasty

In this procedure, a surgeon frees a flap of skeletal muscle and wraps it around the failing myocardium. The first illustration shows the left latissimus dorsi muscle in its normal position. Strong and flat, it has a robust nerve and blood supply.

In the next illustration, the free end of the muscle has been curled around the heart and connected to a muscle stimulating device implanted in the abdominal wall.

Posterior view

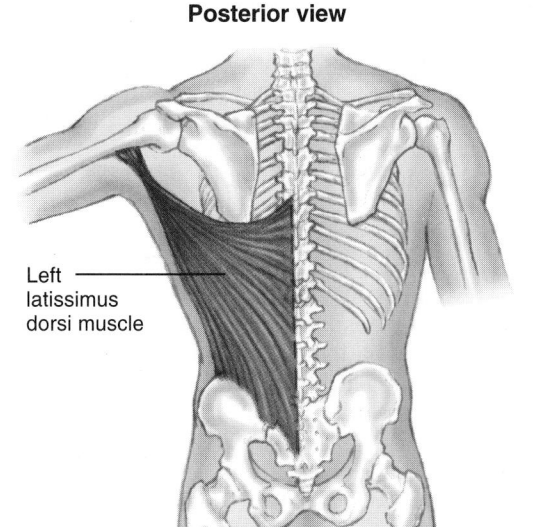

Left latissimus dorsi muscle

Anterior view

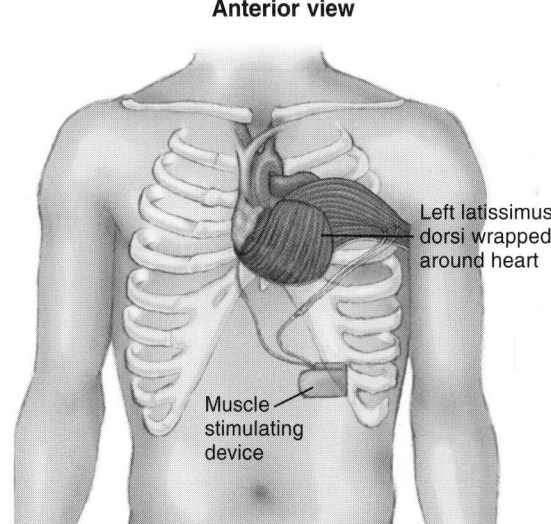

Left latissimus dorsi wrapped around heart

Muscle stimulating device

don't begin to feel an improvement in left ventricular function until about 6 months after surgery. These patients will rely on the muscle flap for the rest of their lives and will need continual close follow-up.

Patients selected for dynamic cardiomyoplasty have severe end-stage heart failure and aren't candidates for heart transplantation because of their age, previous open-heart surgery, or other problems. Hemodynamically unstable patients (those receiving inotropic drugs I.V. and intra-aortic balloon counterpulsation therapy) make poor candidates because of the time it takes for benefits to begin.

Keep in mind that the procedure itself doesn't improve heart function. Consequently, patients typically get worse after surgery before they get better. You'll need to be somewhat more as- sertive than usual to prevent complications and minimize signs and symptoms of heart failure. You'll also need to provide emotional support and encouragement until the patient begins to see the benefits of surgery.

Ventricular assist devices

If your patient's left ventricle can no longer pump enough blood to adequately perfuse her body, she may be a candidate for a VAD (see *Ventricular assist device: Added pumping power,* page 188). The VAD may be placed outside the patient's body or implanted in her chest or abdominal cavity. A surgeon connects the device to the patient's left ventricle and synchronizes its pumping action with her ECG.

Ventricular assist device: Added pumping power

Used to enhance the heart's pumping ability, a ventricular assist device receives blood from a failing left ventricle and pumps it into the ascending aorta. The device can be powered by a battery pack or by a pneumatic power source.

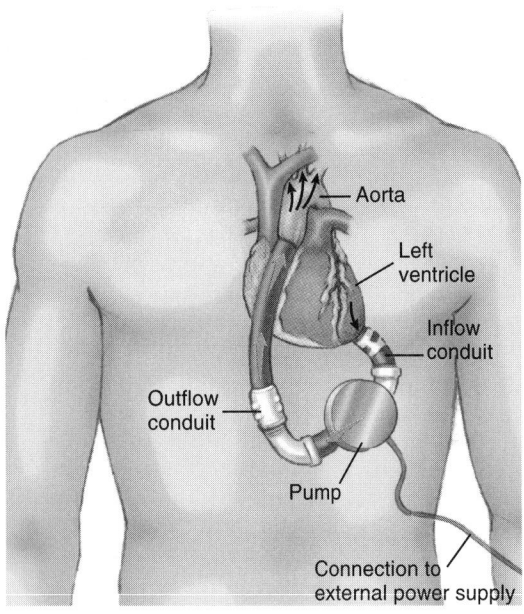

Once the patient receives a VAD, she won't be weaned from it unless the underlying cause of her heart failure can be reversed or until she undergoes heart transplantation.

Heart transplantation

Now a standard treatment option for selected patients with intractable heart failure, heart transplantation takes place about 2,500 times each year at 230 transplant centers across the United States.

Patients waiting for transplantation are categorized as status 1 or status 2. Status 1 patients depend on VADs, inotropic drugs, or both. They have first priority. Status 2 patients need a transplant but aren't as sick and can afford to wait longer, possibly at home.

Patients who need continuous telemetry and hemodynamic monitoring may be admitted to a heart failure unit while waiting for transplantation. Besides receiving drugs or assistance from a VAD, these patients undergo strength training with exercises and weights. They also receive nutritional and emotional support. And they develop long-term relationships with nurses and physicians.

Complications of heart transplantation include infections, hypertension, renal dysfunction caused by cyclosporine, rapid development of coronary arteriosclerosis, and immunosuppressant-related cancers.

11

HEART FAILURE

Complications

Caring for a patient with heart failure means staying alert for the inevitable complications. Over the course of this disease, a patient will surely develop one or more of its acute or chronic complications.

Some of the most serious acute complications you're likely to face include pulmonary edema, acute renal failure, and arrhythmias. Common chronic complications include activity intolerance, renal impairment, gastrointestinal (GI) impairment, metabolic impairment, and thromboembolism. In this chapter, you'll find in-depth reviews of these complications of heart failure and thorough explanations of treatment strategies and nursing considerations.

Pulmonary edema

When the left ventricle doesn't pump effectively, blood backs up into the left atrium. Atrial pressure rises, which causes blood to continue backing up into the pulmonary vasculature, where pressure rises in the pulmonary capillaries. For a time, the heart and lymphatic system compensate for this increased pressure and the leaking fluids it creates. Eventually, however, these compensatory mechanisms fail, and pulmonary edema develops.

The disorder develops in three stages, starting with pulmonary vascular congestion and moving on to interstitial edema and finally to alveolar edema (see *Three stages of pulmonary edema,* page 190). Pulmonary vascular congestion begins as increased hydrostatic pressure shifts fluids out of the pulmonary vasculature and into the interstitial spaces of the lungs. The lymphatic system removes this excess fluid, preventing a net increase in interstitial volume.

Eventually, however, fluids may exit the pulmonary capillaries in a larger volume than the lymphatic system can drain. Consequently, blood and colloids accumulate in the interstitial space surrounding the bronchioles, arterioles, and venules. The patient now has interstitial edema.

Over time, as fluids continue to accumulate, they move into the alveoli, reducing the surface area available for gas exchange and creating the signs and symptoms of acute pulmonary edema. The faster this condition develops, the more ominous the prognosis becomes because the patient's pulmonary lymphatic system is less conditioned to handle the excess fluids. If the condition continues, pulmonary vascular resistance will continue to rise, hampering the right ventricle as well as the left.

Signs and symptoms

A patient with stage 1 pulmonary edema typically has mild or barely noticeable signs and symptoms. She may report some shortness of breath on exertion and a dry cough. You may note mild inspiratory crackles when you auscultate her lungs.

As she progresses to stage 2, her signs and symptoms will worsen, and she may become tachypneic. By stage 3, she'll be severely hypoxemic and in obvious respiratory distress. The volume of air in her lungs will be drastically reduced, her respiratory rate will increase, and she'll be severely breathless.

Three stages of pulmonary edema

In the first stage of pulmonary edema, increased hydrostatic pressure in the pulmonary capillaries forces fluid to move out of the capillaries and into the interstitial space.

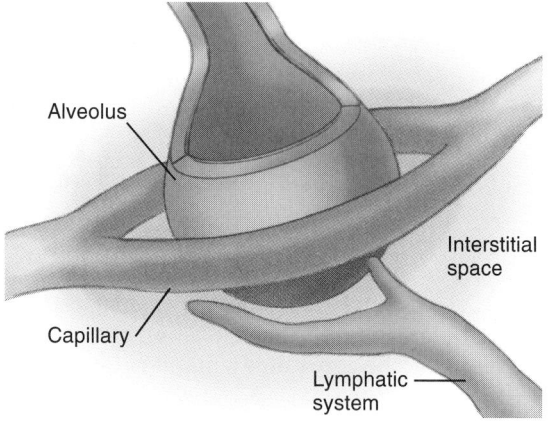

In the second stage, the lymphatic system compensates by drawing fluid out of the interstitial space.

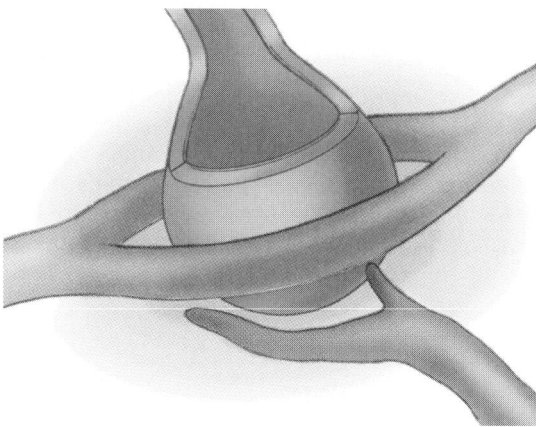

In the third stage, the lymphatic system becomes overwhelmed and is unable to draw out all of the fluid. The resulting fluid accumulation increases hydrostatic pressure in the interstitial space. This increased pressure, in turn, forces fluid into the alveoli, causing alveolar edema and hampering gas exchange.

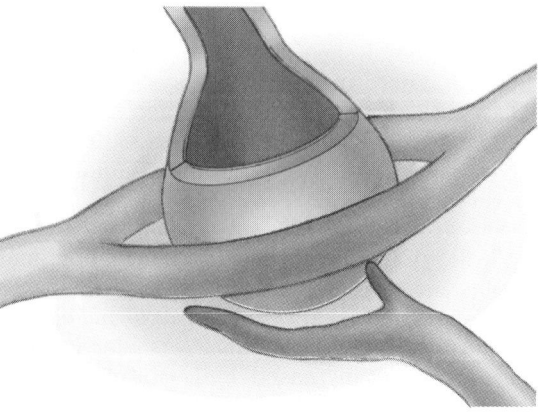

Acute pulmonary edema can be terrifying. Your patient may feel as though she's suffocating or drowning, and she may expectorate blood-tinged sputum. She may thrash about or sit upright in bed with her nostrils flared, using accessory muscles in her neck and shoulders to help her breathe. Her intercostal and sternal muscles may retract inward when she inspires. She may sweat profusely, and her skin may be pale, ashen, or cyanotic; it may be cool and clammy to the touch.

Even without a stethoscope, you may be able to hear inspiratory and expiratory gurgling. On auscultation, you'll hear bilateral moist crackles starting at the lung bases and rising in the lung fields as pulmonary edema worsens. You may have trouble hearing the patient's heart sounds over her noisy respirations, but try to listen for a third heart sound—common in heart failure. You probably also will find tachycardia and an elevated blood pressure.

Early in pulmonary edema, arterial blood gas (ABG) measurements may show respiratory alkalosis caused by hyperventilation. Later, they'll probably reveal respiratory acidosis and hypoxemia, although metabolic acidosis may occur as well.

A chest X-ray usually will show sharp pulmonary vascular markings and haziness, a result that suggests pulmonary congestion and interstitial edema.

Treatment

For a patient with pulmonary edema, your treatment goals are twofold: to decrease preload or blood volume and to provide adequate oxygenation. Interventions can include administering vasodilators, positive inotropic drugs, diuretics, supplemental oxygen, and bronchodilators.

Commonly, treatment starts with I.V. morphine to dilate pulmonary and systemic blood vessels, thus reducing left atrial pressure, pulmonary vascular resistance, preload, and afterload. Morphine also reduces the patient's oxygen demand, anxiety, and dyspnea.

You also may give nitroglycerin I.V. to decrease preload and, to a lesser extent, afterload. Or you might give sodium nitroprusside I.V. to reduce preload and afterload. Use great caution when giving any vasodilator to a patient who's hypotensive or bordering on cardiogenic shock.

Positive inotropic drugs—such as dobuta-mine, dopamine, milrinone, and amrinone—may be administered by continuous I.V. infusion to increase the force of myocardial contractions. In less severe pulmonary edema, give a digitalis glycoside, as prescribed.

Diuretics reduce preload by decreasing the patient's blood volume, thereby reducing the left ventricle's workload. Your patient will begin to breathe easier as pulmonary vascular pressures decline and gas exchange in the alveoli improves. Loop diuretics, such as bumetanide, furosemide, and ethacrynic acid, work quickly and may be given either by I.V. bolus or continuous infusion.

Administer oxygen by nasal cannula or mask, as ordered. Also, give aminophylline I.V. to ease the bronchospasm that results from congestion in the bronchioles. Besides producing bronchodilation, the drug also dilates veins and improves cardiac output (CO) and urinary diuresis.

If your patient is acutely ill, she may need endotracheal intubation and mechanical ventilation in a critical care setting. She may benefit from positive end-expiratory pressure because the positive pressure in her airways can help to reduce venous return. She also may need a pulmonary artery catheter, which allows you to monitor her CO and pulmonary artery wedge pressure. If she has profound heart failure, a physician may order intra-aortic balloon counterpulsation to mechanically reduce afterload and increase coronary blood flow. Or the patient may undergo coronary artery bypass grafting to restore blood flow to her myocardium.

Nursing considerations

Because of your patient's pulmonary congestion, you'll need to assess her airway and breathing frequently. Listen for rhonchi, crackles, wheezes, and gurgling. Consider her respiratory rate and effort. As pulmonary congestion improves, her respiratory rate and work of breathing will decline.

If you're giving the patient morphine, assess her respiratory rate and depth frequently for respiratory depression. Watch for cyanosis and monitor your patient's ABG levels, pulse oximetry readings, or both. Report abnormal ABG results—such as respiratory acidosis or hypoxemia—to a physician.

To help ease the work of breathing and lower your patient's oxygen demand, encourage her to

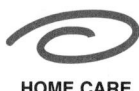

HOME CARE

Dobutamine therapy at home

Because dobutamine increases myocardial contractility, it can improve cardiac output and thus a patient's functional ability. After receiving dobutamine I.V., a patient should achieve a more stable weight, lose fluid, breathe easier, and have an increased activity tolerance. Today, many patients receive dobutamine I.V. at home.

Typically, the patient is discharged with a permanent venous access device, such as a peripherally inserted central catheter (PICC) or an implanted vascular access port.

A PICC is inserted into a vein in the antecubital fossa and extends into the central venous system. An implanted vascular access port, which is connected to a central venous catheter, is usually placed in the subcutaneous tissue of the patient's abdomen or chest, depending on the catheter insertion site. To give the drug, a home care nurse uses a special noncoring needle that pierces the self-sealing septum.

Infusing the drug

The home care nurse prepares the infusion and uses an infusion pump to regulate the flow. During the infusion, the nurse monitors the patient for an increase in heart rate of more than 15 beats per minute, a change in systolic or diastolic blood pressure of 15 mm Hg or more, and chest pain, palpitations, shortness of breath, nausea, vomiting, and extreme anxiety. The nurse also assesses the patient's heart sounds, breath sounds, level of consciousness, and activity tolerance and checks for jugular vein distention and edema.

Peripherally inserted central catheter

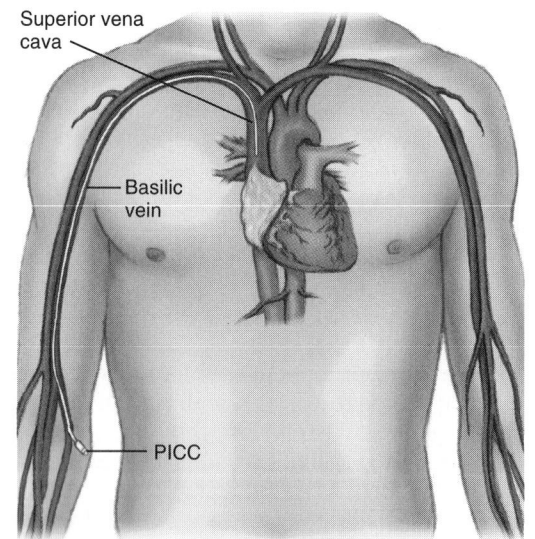

Superior vena cava

Basilic vein

PICC

Implanted vascular access port

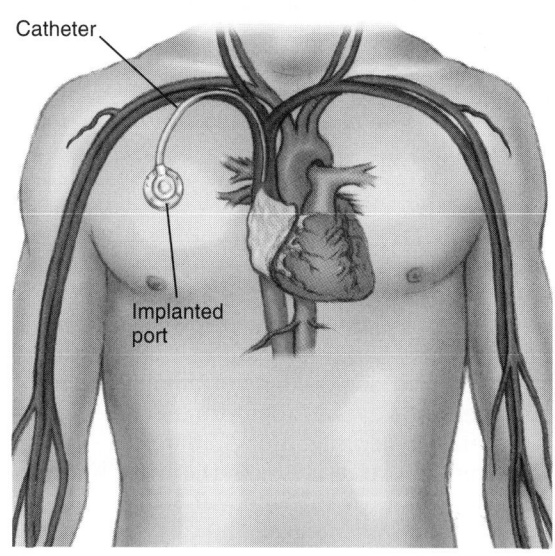

Catheter

Implanted port

---

rest. Help her into a comfortable position. Most people with pulmonary edema feel best when positioned upright with feet dependent, possibly hanging over the side of the bed. That position increases lung expansion and reduces venous return by pooling blood in the legs. Support the patient's head, arms, and torso on a pillow placed over the bedside table. If your patient can't maintain this position, try the high Fowler position instead.

Carefully monitor your patient's response to oxygen therapy by assessing her respiratory rate and effort, skin color, and ABG or pulse oximetry values. If the patient becomes apprehensive about using an oxygen mask, explain its purpose in simple terms and a calm voice, reassuring her that oxygen is flowing into it.

Because anxiety increases the work of breathing, be sure to provide for your patient's emotional needs. Stay with your patient as much as possible, speak calmly, and provide emotional support as appropriate. This effort becomes even more important if the patient's respiratory function declines and she must move to a critical care setting.

If you're administering aminophylline, watch closely for tachycardia, arrhythmias, and hypotension. Also, stay alert for possible adverse effects or interactions caused by any of the patient's drugs.

Patient teaching

Pulmonary edema is terrifying not only for the patient but also for those around her. Provide support and encouragement for family members as well as the patient herself.

After the crisis passes, focus your teaching on preventing a relapse. Review the process of heart failure and its causes, contributing factors, and effects. Review lifestyle changes that the patient will need to make, including eating a low-sodium diet, restricting fluids, and monitoring daily weights. Tell the patient to report any increased shortness of breath, increased anxiety, coughing up of frothy pink-tinged sputum, and feelings of drowning or suffocation.

Review the patient's drug regimen and make sure she understands which drugs to take, why to take them, and how to take them. Tell her about adverse effects she should watch for and report.

Home care

A growing number of patients with heart failure now receive ongoing nursing care in their homes to help prevent acute complications, such as pulmonary edema. Some even receive dobutamine at home for treating mild episodes of acute pulmonary edema and heart failure (see *Dobutamine therapy at home*).

Acute renal failure

Acute renal failure can be divided into three categories, depending on where the problem occurs:
- prerenal, in which causes outside the kidneys—such shock or reduced intravascular volume—diminish renal blood flow
- intrarenal, in which the renal tissue sustains damage—from nephrotoxic drugs, inflammation, or injury, for instance
- postrenal, in which urine flow becomes obstructed—from prostatic hypertrophy, kidney stones, or a bladder tumor, for example.

Heart failure is a prenal cause of acute renal failure because reduced CO greatly reduces blood flow to the kidneys, reducing the glomerular filtration rate (GFR) and causing the patient to retain metabolic waste (see *Reviewing glomerular filtration,* page 194). Because nephrons aren't damaged, however, kidney function returns to normal as CO rises.

In mild heart failure, angiotensin II can cause the efferent arteriole to constrict, and atrial natriuretic factor and prostaglandins can dilate the afferent arteriole, thus compensating for the reduced CO and supporting the GFR.

In severe heart failure, these compensatory mechanisms are overwhelmed by the vasoconstricting effects of the sympathetic nervous system, the renin-angiotensin-aldosterone system, and arginine vasopressin. The afferent arteriole constricts, resulting in fluid retention and reduced urine output.

What's more, the kidneys become less responsive to atrial natriuretic factor as the endothelium of the renal blood vessels becomes less able to dilate. Endothelial cells produce endothelin, a strong vasoconstrictor that supports the actions of angiotensin II and norepinephrine, thus reducing GFR.

Intrarenal failure can result from nephrotoxic drugs, such as angiotensin-converting enzyme (ACE) inhibitors. In a patient with reduced renal perfusion, angiotensin helps to maintain the GFR by constricting the efferent arteriole. Thus, by inhibiting the conversion of angiotensin I to angiotensin II, ACE inhibitors may allow the GFR to drop and metabolic waste products to accumulate. Prolonged use of ACE inhibitors can damage the nephrons' tubules, leading to acute tubular necrosis.

Reviewing glomerular filtration

Large amounts of water and sodium filter out of the blood as it passes through the high-pressure glomerulus. Urea, urate, uric acid, creatinine, potassium, chloride, glucose, hydrogen, proteins, amino acids, bicarbonate, and phosphate filter out of the blood as well. A normal glomerulus filters about 125 ml of blood each minute.

At the proximal convoluted tubule, most of the water and electrolytes pass back into the vasculature along with glucose, amino acids, and bicarbonate. In the descending loop of Henle, the filtrate becomes hypertonic when sodium diffuses into the tubule and water moves into the vasculature. Then, in the ascending loop of Henle, it becomes hypotonic as sodium is reabsorbed into the vasculature.

At the distal convoluted tubule and collecting duct, water, bicarbonate, calcium, phosphate, sodium, and potassium move back into the vasculature, although potassium, uric acid, and hydrogen can be secreted from plasma into the collecting duct, as needed. The fluid remaining in the collecting duct is urine.

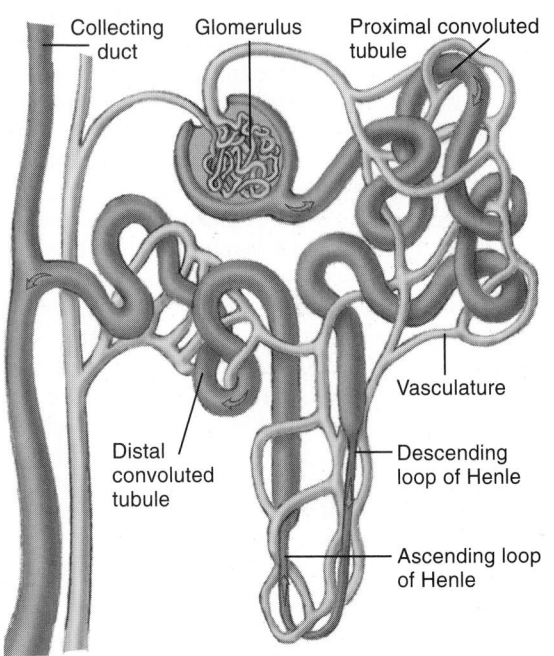

Signs and symptoms

Initially, your patient's urine output may decrease to less than 400 ml in 24 hours. Fluid retention results in edema that may be unresponsive to diuretics. You may observe distended neck veins and auscultate crackles in the patient's lungs.

Uremia develops when azotemia progresses to the point where your patient begins to develop signs and symptoms that affect all body systems. She may develop problems with her central nervous system, such as lethargy, confusion, and seizures. She may develop GI bleeding from uremic gastritis or colitis, and she may report nausea, vomiting, and a lack of appetite. If your patient's hematologic system is involved, she'll be prone to infection, bruising, and bleeding.

Accumulated metabolic wastes also may irritate the pericardial sac, resulting in pericarditis and pericardial effusions. You may hear a pericardial friction rub when auscultating your patient's heart. Respiratory involvement may include pulmonary edema, Kussmaul's respirations, and pleural effusions.

Diagnostic tests

Your patient's history provides important clues about whether her acute renal failure stems from prerenal, intrarenal, or postrenal causes. Carefully review her recent clinical course for acute events, such as hypotension or reduced CO. Also, look at her drug regimen for possible causes of nephrotoxicity.

Patients with heart failure may have a blood urea nitrogen (BUN) level between 30 and 100 mg/dl, which reflects the kidneys' declining ability to clear metabolic wastes. Elevated serum creatinine levels suggest volume overload from renal failure, although creatinine levels typically stay below 4 mg/dl. Creatinine clearance reflects the patient's GFR; it will be reduced in a patient with acute renal failure caused by heart failure.

Urinalysis provides helpful diagnostic data as well. Normally, protein molecules can't pass through the glomerulus because of their large size. However, proteinuria can occur intermittently in heart failure. The presence of cells, casts, or proteins may indicate an intrarenal cause of acute renal failure. Urine sodium levels may be decreased to less than 20 mEq/L/day from prerenal causes because the body retains sodium in an attempt to improve renal perfusion.

Electrolyte levels are also affected by acute renal failure. Typically, serum potassium, magnesium, and phosphate levels increase. Despite the increased sodium retention, you probably won't see hypernatremia because of the increased volume of fluid in the patient's body.

If the cause of your patient's acute renal failure can't be easily determined or your patient may have severe damage, then further diagnostic tests may be needed. They may include renal ultrasound, excretory urography, computed tomography (CT) scanning, renal arteriography, and X-rays of the kidneys, ureters, and bladder.

Treatment

Therapy aims to increase the patient's GFR by improving her CO. It also focuses on preventing complications by reducing fluid overload, dilating the renal artery, normalizing electrolyte levels, and if necessary, providing continuous renal replacement therapy.

Diuretics given I.V. can help to support renal blood flow and GFR. Commonly, patients receive a combination of loop and thiazide diuretics, such as furosemide and hydrochlorothiazide. Low doses of dopamine, 5 µg/kg/minute or less, can be given I.V. to stimulate dilation of the renal artery and thereby improve renal blood flow.

If your patient's acute renal failure stems from an ACE inhibitor, it probably will be discontinued. Doses of drugs excreted by the renal system—such as digoxin and some antiarrhythmics and antibiotics—may need to be lowered as well.

Electrolyte replacement or restriction may be necessary based on the patient's laboratory values. Her fluid consumption may be restricted to an amount that equals slightly more than the sum of her output and insensible losses—commonly about 600 ml/day.

If conservative therapy doesn't resolve your patient's acute renal failure, she may need peritoneal dialysis, hemodialysis, or continuous renal replacement therapy (see *Continuous renal replacement therapy,* page 196). The advantage of continuous replacement lies in its slow filtration of water and electrolytes, a rate that mirrors normal kidney function and makes the procedure easier for a hemodynamically compromised patient to tolerate.

Nursing considerations

Monitor your patient's fluid volume carefully. Weigh her daily and maintain precise intake and output records. Report any increase or decrease in urine output to her physician. If your patient has received a diuretic, also monitor her for diuresis.

Auscultate your patient's lungs for crackles and assess her respiratory rate and effort, heart rate, and blood pressure. Also, auscultate for a third heart sound, which suggests fluid volume overload. Examine the patient's skin for turgor and edema, and observe her neck veins for distention.

Help your patient cope with fluid restrictions by offering ice chips, if permitted, hard candy, and breath spray to moisten her mouth. Also, try having her rinse her mouth with cold water or allowing ice chips to melt in her mouth before spitting out the water. Give drugs with meals so that the patient can drink her allowed fluids when she's thirsty.

The patient probably will need a low-sodium, low-protein, low-potassium diet. Replacement or restriction of electrolytes will depend on daily serum levels. So monitor tests of her electrolyte, BUN, and creatinine levels and notify a physician of any changes. Also, make sure you can spot the signs and symptoms of specific electrolyte abnormalities. For instance, hyperkalemia can cause neuromuscular abnormalities, such as weakness, abdominal cramps, and loss of deep tendon reflexes. If your patient has a cardiac monitor, look for prolonged PR and QRS intervals, peaked T waves, and depressed ST segments.

Also, watch for evidence of uremia, particularly pruritus. If your patient develops pruritus, apply moisturizing creams liberally and administer oral antihistamines, as prescribed. To prevent skin breakdown and infection, urge her not to scratch. As needed, trim and clean her fingernails.

Continuous renal replacement therapy

If your patient has heart failure and acute renal failure, she may undergo continuous renal replacement therapy because, unlike standard hemodialysis, it removes fluids, urea, creatinine, and electrolytes slowly, as a normal kidney does. Because this therapy avoids rapid changes in fluid and electrolyte levels, patients with severe cardiac disease can tolerate it more easily.

The procedure may last 12 hours or longer and uses a patient's own blood pressure to move blood through the filter. Usually, the patient must have a mean arterial pressure of at least 60 mm Hg.

Your patient may undergo continuous arteriovenous (AV) therapy or, if she has poor arterial access, a low platelet count, or clotting problems, continuous venovenous therapy. The most common forms of AV therapy for patients with heart failure are slow continuous ultrafiltration and continuous AV hemofiltration.

Slow continuous ultrafiltration removes fluids at a rate of 100 to 300 ml/hour. Continuous AV hemofiltration removes them at 500 to 800 ml/hour, but the volume lost is continuously replaced by I.V. infusion based on the patient's fluid status. In both procedures, solutes are removed by convection rather than by osmosis or diffusion, making a dialysate unnecessary.

Edema also raises your patient's risk of skin breakdown. If your patient is on bed rest, turn and reposition her at least every 2 hours and look for signs of breakdown. If her condition allows it, help your patient get out of bed and walk or sit in a chair.

Carefully assess the patient for signs and symptoms of infection, and take measures to reduce the risk, such as avoiding the use of an indwelling urinary catheter whenever possible.

Patient teaching

Clear, comprehensive teaching about heart failure and its risks can help your patient avoid acute renal failure. So make sure she understands heart failure and its causes and contributing factors. Also, explain the purpose, dosage, and adverse effects of her drug regimen. Take time to discuss over-the-counter drugs that may be nephrotoxic, such as nonsteroidal anti-inflammatory drugs.

Carefully explain the need for any fluid restrictions to help gain the patient's cooperation. Also, discuss the signs and symptoms of electrolyte imbalances, such as muscle cramps, and explain that they should be reported to a physician right away. Emphasize the importance of follow-up examinations and ongoing laboratory tests, especially the 24-hour urine test to measure creatinine clearance.

As needed, ask a dietitian or nutrition counselor to help your patient understand her diet plan. Urge her to stay away from sick people to reduce her risk of infection. And list the signs and symptoms that should prompt a call to a physician, including a reduced or absent urine output, rapid weight gain, increasing swelling, excessive bruising or bleeding, signs or symptoms of infection, an irregular pulse, increasing shortness of breath, lethargy, and a loss of appetite.

Arrhythmias

Patients with heart failure may develop arrhythmias for several reasons, some related to their cardiac condition and some related to its treatment. What's more, arrhythmias can cause or worsen heart failure.

In some patients with heart failure, arrhythmias result from diuretics, vasodilators, ACE inhibitors, aminophylline, or digoxin. Hemodynamic changes—such as increased pressure in the ventricles—can cause arrhythmias as well.

Ischemia and stimulation of the sympathetic nervous system can also trigger arrhythmias, as can electrolyte disturbances. Many patients with heart failure take a potassium-wasting diuretic, such as a loop or thiazide diuretic. And low potassium levels make the heart muscle more excitable, which increases its chance of being depolarized by a stimulus that can trigger an atrial or ventricular arrhythmia. Hypokalemia also raises the risk of a toxic reaction to a digitalis glycoside, which can provoke either atrial and ventricular arrhythmias. Patients who are taking a potassium sparing diuretic face a risk of arrhythmias resuling from hyperkalemia.

Ventricular arrhythmias are common among patients with heart failure. In fact, the more impaired the left ventricle, the more likely the patient will develop a lethal ventricular arrhythmia, including sudden cardiac death. More than half the patients who die of heart failure do so after experiencing sudden cardiac death.

Atrial arrhythmias develop in up to half of patients with advanced heart failure, typically because increased pressures damage the left atrium. Scarring can result, causing ineffective pumping. Sympathetic stimulation can cause atrial arrhythmias as well.

Naturally, an atrial arrhythmia can worsen your patient's heart failure by reducing the effectiveness of atrial contractions and further reducing CO. Atrial fibrillation raises the risk of thromboembolism as well.

Signs and symptoms

Cardiac arrhythmias may produce varied signs and symptoms or none at all. Your patient may complain of palpitations, weakness, dizziness, shortness of breath, and chest pain. Serious ventricular arrhythmias or bradycardia may make her feel faint.

An electrocardiogram can confirm your patient's arrhythmia. Also, check her serum electrolyte levels for problems that can promote arrhythmias, such as hypokalemia or hyperkalemia. If your patient is receiving a digitalis glycoside, check for evidence of a toxic reaction. And because hyperthyroidism can cause atrial fibrillation, check the patient's thyroid-stimulating hormone and thyroxine levels if she has this arrhythmia.

Treatment

If your patient develops an arrhythmia, treatment will aim to determine its cause and treat it through drug therapy or electrical cardioversion. If these interventions fail, the patient may need surgical treatment, possibly including endocardial resection, radiofrequency catheter-induced ablation therapy, or insertion of an implantable cardioverter-defibrillator.

If the arrhythmia stems from an electrolyte imbalance, the first step will be to correct the imbalance. If it stems from a drug given to treat the patient's heart failure, such as aminophylline or a bronchodilator, a physician may discontinue the offending drug.

If the arrhythmia continues, the patient may undergo electrical cardioversion or receive an implantable cardioverter-defibrillator to control arrhythmias through pacing or electric shocks. Before cardioversion, the patient probably will receive an anticoagulant to reduce the risk of embolism. Afterward, she may take an oral anticoagulant, such as warfarin, for 6 to 12 months. If the fibrillation resumes, she may undergo a second cardioversion or, still in fibrillation, she may continue taking the anticoagulant indefinitely.

Because antiarrhythmic drugs can worsen arrhythmias in patients with heart failure, give them only in the most severe cases. Amiodarone is the antiarrhythmic drug of choice for patients with heart failure. Keep in mind that although amiodarone can reduce ventricular arrhythmias and improve ventricular function, it may not reduce the risk of sudden cardiac death.

Patients who don't respond to standard therapy may need surgical treatment. First, electrophysiology studies locate and map the sites where arrhythmias originate. Afterward, the patient may undergo endocardial resection to remove the portion of endocardium responsible for the arrhythmia. Or she may undergo radiofrequency catheter-induced ablation therapy, in which a catheter with an electrode at its tip dispenses radiofrequency energy to destroy arrhythmia-causing cells. These procedures may be combined with drug therapy and sometimes with an implantable cardioverter-defibrillator.

Nursing considerations

Detailed nursing assessments provide crucial information for detecting and responding to arrhythmias in a patient with heart failure. Monitor your patient's heart rate and rhythm frequently. Also, watch for increasing signs and symptoms of reduced CO, such as hypotension, syncope, dizziness, confusion, decreased urine output, and chest pain. Report these changes to a physician immediately.

Because hypoxia can worsen arrhythmias, you may need to administer supplemental oxygen by mask or nasal cannula, as prescribed. Monitor the

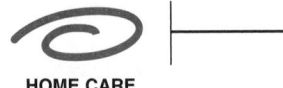

HOME CARE

Teaching your patient to take her pulse

If your patient with heart failure has an arrhythmia or takes a digitalis glycoside or an antiarrhythmic drug, you'll need to teach her how to take her pulse, when to take her pulse, and how to record and report the results.

When to check
Start by explaining the implications of changes in her heart rate and rhythm. Then tell her that taking a pulse offers an easy way to detect these changes. Urge her to check her pulse routinely each day. She also should check it before, during, and after exercising. And she should check it any time she feels symptoms, such as palpitations or dizziness.

What to do
Next, teach her and her family how to check her pulse. Demonstrate each step as you teach it, allow time for the patient to practice, and then verify that she can perform the procedure correctly. Tell your patient to follow these steps:
• To take your peripheral pulse, rest the tips of your index and middle fingers against the bony prominence on the thumb side of your opposing wrist.
• Slide your fingers inward toward the midline of your wrist until you feel pulsations.
• Press lightly but firmly on the artery.
• To take your carotid pulse, place your fingertips on your Adam's apple.
• Slide them to the right or left until you feel pulsations in the groove formed by your throat and neck muscles.
• Press lightly and keep your fingertips low on your neck; massaging higher up on your neck can cause your heart rate to drop.
• For either pulse, count the pulsations for 30 seconds and then multiply by two. (If you take digoxin, count for a full minute.)
• Report irregular beats or a change of 10 beats per minute or more to your physician.
• Record your pulse in a diary, noting the date, time, and any activities you performed or symptoms you felt. Take your pulse diary to all physician visits.

patient's response by pulse oximetry or ABG measurements. Also, assess her respiratory rate and effort, skin color, and capillary refill.

Monitor your patient's serum electrolyte levels and assess her for signs and symptoms of electrolyte imbalances. Report abnormal laboratory values or other evidence of imbalance right away. Anticipate giving electrolyte supplements either orally or I.V. or restricting the intake of certain electrolytes.

If your patient has atrial fibrillation or has had electrical cardioversion, stay alert for evidence of systemic or pulmonary embolism. A cerebral embolus may cause an altered level of consciousness, slurred speech, and weakness or paralysis on one side of the body. A pulmonary embolus may cause abrupt apprehension, dyspnea, pleuritic pain, hemoptysis, tachycardia, crackles, tachypnea, a cough, and possibly an altered level of consciousness. An embolus in a limb may cause sudden pain, weakness, paralysis, pulselessness, pallor, or coldness in the affected limb.

If your patient takes an oral anticoagulant, maintain her prothrombin time (PT) at 1.5 to 2.0 times the control or her international normalized ratio (INR) at 2.0 to 3.0 times the control. Assess her for evidence of bleeding, such as bleeding gums or tarry stools. Protect the patient from accidents and injuries.

Watch your patient closely for signs and symptoms of a toxic reaction to a digitalis glycoside and monitor her blood digoxin levels. If your patient is also receiving amiodarone, be aware of her increased risk of a toxic reaction. If she's taking amiodarone and warfarin, she's at increased risk for bleeding.

If your patient is scheduled for electrophysiology testing, have her fast for 6 to 8 hours before the procedure. Withhold her antiarrhythmic and any other drugs that could interfere with the test, as ordered. Afterward, watch for adverse effects from antiarrhythmic drugs that your patient may have received during the test. Keep her attached to a cardiac monitor and watch for arrhythmias. Enforce bed rest for 6 to 8 hours and assess the insertion site for bleeding.

Patient teaching

If your patient will be taking an antiarrhythmic drug, teach her how to take it properly. Urge her to report adverse effects right away, including weakness, dizziness, faintness, and chest discomfort. Review the signs and symptoms of a toxic reaction if she takes digoxin. Also, teach her how to monitor her heart rate and rhythm by taking her pulse at home (see *Teaching your patient to take her pulse*).

If the patient takes amiodarone, tell her to apply sunscreen and wear sunglasses when she goes outside to avoid skin reactions caused by increased photosensitivity. Warn her that the drug may cause her skin to turn blue-gray. Explain that she'll need regular follow-up appointments to check for a toxic reaction.

If the patient takes warfarin, review the precautions she should take to reduce her risk of bleeding. Caution her that taking amiodarone with warfarin can increase the toxic potential of each drug.

As indicated, help family members learn how to activate the emergency medical system in their area. And help interested family members find out where to learn cardiopulmonary resuscitation.

If your patient will be undergoing electrophysiology studies, tell her that the test may take up to 4 hours, during which time she'll need to lie still. Explain that the test induces arrhythmias in a controlled setting to help determine which drugs are most effective at stopping them. Tell her to notify the physician if she feels palpitations, light-headedness, or dizziness during the procedure. As ordered, give the patient a sedative to relax her before the test.

Home care

Because many patients with heart failure and arrhythmias have experienced frightening symptoms, they may resist leaving the safe hospital environment. A home health nurse can help ease the transition to home by continuing the teaching plan begun in the hospital, enhancing the patient's ability to take her own pulse, and—if she has an implantable cardioverter-defibrillator—reviewing the log to make sure the device is functioning properly.

During visits, the home care nurse will also assess how well the patient and family are coping and note whether family members are overprotective. Some families may benefit from a referral to a counselor or support group.

Activity intolerance

When your patient's CO can no longer supply her tissues with adequate oxygen, she'll develop an intolerance to activity that can sharply decrease her functional abilities along with her quality of life. Among heart failure patients, activity intolerance offers a fairly reliable predictor of early death.

Activity intolerance results when the patient's skeletal muscles exist in an oxygen-deprived state for so long that they become unable to take up and use oxygen efficiently. As the patient reduces her activity level in response to increasing weakness and dyspnea, her muscles become even more deconditioned. Poor nutrition caused by dyspnea, fatigue, and adverse drug effects may contribute to her activity intolerance as well.

Signs and symptoms

Typically, a patient with activity intolerance will complain that she becomes short of breath with minimal exertion. She'll probably also report weakness, fatigue, poor concentration, listlessness, and a general lack of energy. As her heart failure worsens, she may report feeling these symptoms even at rest.

Diagnostic tests

To quantify a patient's limitations, a physician may have her undergo graded exercise testing, in which she walks on a treadmill at increasing levels of exertion. This type of testing estimates her oxygen consumption based on the intensity she achieves during exercise.

An alternative for determining the patient's exercise tolerance is the self-paced or timed walking test. This test may be used when a patient can't or won't walk on a treadmill. In this test, the patient walks as far as she can for 6 to 12 minutes. She receives instructions to stop any time she feels breathless and then to continue when she feels able to do so. Changes in her total walking distance can be used to track the progress of her heart failure over time and to track the success of interventions, such as an exercise program.

RESEARCH UPDATE

Severe heart failure and the benefits of exercise

Not too long ago, physicians and nurses discouraged patients with severe heart failure from engaging in exercise. But recent research is beginning to cast doubt on that advice. In fact, study results suggest that exercise of low to moderate intensity can benefit these patients, even those sick enough to be awaiting heart transplantation.

In one study, patients hospitalized with severe heart failure followed a 3-week program of low-intensity to moderate-intensity exercise that included these activities:
- riding a stationary bike for 30 seconds, then resting for 60 seconds, for a total of 15 minutes five times a week
- walking on a treadmill for 10 minutes, alternating fast and slow paces, three times a week
- performing muscle-strengthening exercises for 20 minutes three times a week.

Other patients hospitalized with similarly severe heart failure followed traditional activity restrictions. They did no more than walk outside the hospital and climb one flight of stairs a day.

The results: Patients who exercised improved both their aerobic and ventilatory capacities and reduced the severity of their symptoms. Patients who observed activity restrictions showed no such improvements.

If these early results hold true in larger, longer-term studies, patients with severe heart failure may be adding some exercise to their regimen. For patients awaiting heart transplantation, the improvements to overall conditioning may translate into an easier, more successful postoperative course. And for a few patients, low-intensity to moderate-intensity exercise might mean being taken off the transplant list altogether.

Treatment

For a patient with activity intolerance, treatment aims to help improve her tolerance. In fact, the Food and Drug Administration includes this goal as a required outcome for many drugs used to treat heart failure. A number of drugs with differing actions can help to improve the patient's activity tolerance by improving CO, reducing myocardial workload, and easing some of the signs and symptoms brought on by activity.

For example, digoxin improves CO by increasing myocardial contractility, ACE inhibitors improve CO by reducing preload and afterload, and diuretics can reduce exertional dyspnea and edema.

Indeed, exercise itself can help to improve CO as well as the patient's perception of her energy level and well-being (see *Severe heart failure and the benefits of exercise*). Naturally, exercise must be prescribed to match the level of the patient's current functional ability.

When aggressive drug therapy and exercise can no longer control severe activity intolerance, a physician may consider heart transplantation as one of the few remaining treatment options.

Nursing considerations

A decreasing activity tolerance should alert you to the possibility that your patient's heart failure is worsening. Question your patient about her signs and symptoms and about the type and amount of activity that produces them. Find out to what degree her activities of daily living have been altered or reduced. Several assessment tools are available to help you collect information about your patient's activity intolerance, evaluate your interventions, track the patient's clinical progress, and assess her quality of life.

As you provide nursing care, pay attention to your patient's tolerance level and allow her to rest if she becomes short of breath. Monitor her for dyspnea while she performs self-care as well. Give her as much help as she needs while allowing her as much independence as possible. Plan your patient's care to allow rest periods and uninterrupted sleep at night.

Patient teaching

Your patient will need her family's support and understanding as she adapts her lifestyle to her decreased activity tolerance. Make sure to include her family in your teaching sessions so that they'll be able to help her appropriately and reinforce her lifestyle changes.

Tell your patient about the benefits of regular exercise, including increased exercise tolerance, improved muscle tone (which reduces oxygen demand), and an improved sense of well-being. Discuss the need to balance rest with activity, and encourage her to pace her activities. Teach energy-saving techniques, such as performing activities while sitting rather than standing.

Your patient may find it useful to track the pattern and intensity of her signs and symptoms in a daily log. Doing so will reinforce her self-awareness and self-care as well as provide a record for you and her physician. Show the patient how to use a perceived exertion scale to record her signs and symptoms and to manage her prescribed exercise level.

Together with the patient, cardiologist, and exercise physiologist or physical therapist, help your patient develop a comfortable, safe exercise program.

Renal impairment

In heart failure, chronically poor perfusion eventually can damage the patient's kidneys and lead to a permanent, irreversible reduction of function. Renal impairment threatens a patient with heart failure in more than one way. For example, preload becomes more difficult to manage because the kidneys can't produce enough urine to drain excess fluids. Also, impaired electrolyte reabsorption and excretion leads to an increased risk of electrolyte imbalance.

Signs and symptoms

If your patient has chronic renal failure and heart failure, evidence of uremia will develop in almost all her body systems as waste products accumulate. Evidence may include arrhythmias, edema, dyspnea, pruritus, anorexia, nausea, vomiting, weight loss, apathy, and confusion.

The patient may have a reduced serum sodium level from the increase in total body water that occurs in chronic heart failure. Hypokalemia and hypomagnesemia may result from thiazide and loop diuretics. Hyperkalemia may result from reduced renal blood flow, renal failure, or the use of certain ACE inhibitors. Typically, as the GFR declines, BUN and creatinine levels rise.

Urinalysis may show protein in the patient's urine. Red blood cell production may be altered because of the kidneys' decreased ability to produce erythropoietin. The anemia that results can put added stress on the failing heart muscle, aggravating the patient's heart failure.

Treatment

Treatment focuses on preventing and correcting fluid and electrolyte imbalances. If your patient takes a loop or thiazide diuretic, she may need potassium or magnesium supplements to replace electrolytes lost in her urine. If she takes an ACE inhibitor, she may need potassium restrictions to offset an elevated serum potassium level.

To reduce fluid volume, she may need to take a diuretic. She also may need to restrict fluids, a tactic that may help but also may raise her discomfort level and reduce her quality of life. Moderate water restriction, to about 1,500 ml a day, may offer a reasonable compromise for some patients. Severe restrictions rarely succeed and, fortunately, rarely become necessary because of the success of current drug therapies.

The patient also may need to restrict protein. Eventually, she may require peritoneal dialysis or hemodialysis to accomplish what her kidneys can no longer do.

Nursing considerations

To minimize the effect of renal impairment for your patient with chronic heart failure, assess her fluid and electrolyte levels carefully and frequently. To do so, weigh the patient each day, at the same time of day, on the same scale, with the patient in similar clothing. Monitor her intake and output, neck veins, heart sounds, breath sounds, and degree of dyspnea. Also, assess the location and severity of her edema. Check for sacral edema if she's confined to bed.

Track the results of laboratory tests and report any abnormal values to a physician. Make sure you know which electrolyte imbalances are most common with the diuretic your patient takes. Anticipate giving electrolyte supplements or applying diet restrictions, as ordered.

Because your patient's edematous skin is fragile and prone to breakdown, take measures to keep it intact. Encourage her and help her to change positions at least every 2 hours. While repositioning, check the patient's skin for areas of redness or breakdown, especially over bony prominences. Pad prominences well to protect them.

If your patient has trouble adapting to diet limitations or fluid restrictions, ask a dietitian to help with meal planning and food choices.

Because dialysis causes dramatic fluid shifts, patients who need this procedure require close monitoring, especially when they already have the hemodynamic instability created by chronic heart failure. Keep in mind that the buildup of abdominal fluid in peritoneal dialysis may make breathing difficult, increasing the heart's workload. In hemodialysis, fluid removal typically amounts to several pounds over a few hours and may make your patient hemodynamically unstable.

A low blood pressure from hypovolemia following dialysis can threaten an already weakened myocardium. What's more, some drugs used to treat heart failure are metabolized and excreted by the kidney and may be dialyzed out during treatment. For example, vasodilators should be withheld before and during dialysis and administered when dialysis is complete.

The emotional impact of end-stage heart failure and kidney failure can be devastating. Provide support to the patient, family, and caregivers as they make decisions about treatment plans and advance directives.

Patient teaching

Teach your patient to be alert for early signs and symptoms of fluid retention—such as edema, a persistent cough, and weight gain—and to seek prompt treatment if they arise. Suggest that she weigh herself each morning before breakfast, and that she keep a log of her daily weights. Tell her to contact her physician if she gains more than 2 pounds in a day or 5 pounds in a week. Also, tell her to report any decrease in her urine output.

Because taking daily diuretics is a way of life for most people with chronic heart failure, teach your patient how her diuretic works, the proper dosage, and the possible adverse effects. If she takes a potassium-wasting diuretic, stress the importance of eating foods high in potassium. Tell her to contact her physician if she develops muscle weakness, cramps, dizziness, or nausea because these problems may reflect a low potassium level.

To aid compliance, talk with the patient about the best time for her to take her diuretic. For many patients, the best time is early in the morning, just after breakfast. If the patient has a long commute in the morning, however, she may prefer to take the drug after she arrives at work.

Advise the patient to limit her salt intake to 2 to 3 g daily, as ordered. If her physician prescribed fluid restrictions, help her plan her daily fluid intake. As the patient's renal impairment proceeds, you'll probably need to help her adopt a low-potassium, low-protein diet.

If your patient will be undergoing peritoneal dialysis or hemodialysis, carefully explain these procedures to her and her family. Provide support and encourage them to air their feelings and concerns.

Home care

A home care nurse will assess the patient's compliance with potassium and protein restrictions and provide ongoing instruction as needed. If the patient receives dialysis at home, she'll need considerable support and teaching about the procedure. Depending on the procedure involved and the patient's condition, dialysis may be performed at home by a nurse, the patient, or a family member. Or it may be performed at an outpatient clinic.

Early recognition and prompt treatment of fluid and electrolyte imbalances can help keep the patient out of the hospital. Therefore, the home care nurse will assess the patient's fluid status and monitor her response to drug and diet therapies by weighing her, checking for edema, taking her vital signs, assessing urine output, and listening to breath sounds. The nurse also will review the patient's laboratory tests and signs and symptoms for evidence of electrolyte imbalances.

Gastrointestinal and metabolic impairment

Venous congestion that results from right ventricular heart failure causes numerous complications, such as hepatomegaly, ascites, and splenomegaly. In fact, the impact of chronic fluid retention on your patient's quality of life can be substantial, ranging from minor discomfort and a change in body image to profound malnutrition.

Specifically, heart failure may interfere with adequate nutrition by affecting the digestion, absorption, and metabolism of nutrients. In the later stages of heart failure, the patient may have a mild to moderate loss of lean body mass or cachexia.

Many factors can lead to cardiac cachexia. For example, hypoxia of the GI tract can lead to malabsorption of nutrients. Reduced perfusion can reduce delivery of nutrients to the tissues. Reduced blood flow to the liver and kidneys can impair the clearance of metabolites. And venous congestion can impair liver function.

What's more, dyspnea, fatigue, or ascites can cause anorexia and inadequate calorie intake. A toxic digoxin reaction can cause nausea and vomiting. And other drugs, such as the ACE inhibitor enalapril, can cause GI signs and symptoms that interfere with nutrition.

Signs and symptoms

A patient with chronic heart failure may complain of nausea, vomiting, and loss of appetite without looking as though she has lost much weight. That's because her edema may be masking her weight loss with fluid retention.

Your examination of such a patient may reveal an enlarged, tender liver. Liver function studies may show elevated levels of bilirubin, aspartate aminotransferase, and alanine aminotransferase caused by hepatomegaly. Her abdomen may show signs of ascites, such as distention and a fluid wave (see *Eliciting a fluid wave*). You may also notice petechiae or ecchymosis if your patient has a coagulopathy caused by hepatic congestion.

Other signs of inadequate nutrition include muscle wasting, loss of subcutaneous fat, hair loss, dry or brittle hair, gingivitis, spoon-shaped nails, and dry, scaly skin.

If your patient is malnourished, her protein levels (such as her serum albumin level) will be reduced. Keep in mind, however, that serum albumin levels may be falsely low in a patient with fluid overload. Look for reductions in the total protein level and total lymphocyte count to confirm a protein deficiency.

Typically, a malnourished person will have reduced BUN and creatinine levels because of her negative nitrogen balance, in which she excretes

Eliciting a fluid wave

One way to determine if a patient's abdominal distention results from fluid buildup is by testing for a fluid wave. To do so, you'll need to ask for help from a colleague. With the patient in the supine position, have your colleague rest the ulnar side of her arm and hand firmly against the midline of the patient's abdomen, as shown.

Now, while resting your nondominant hand against one side of the patient's lower abdomen, sharply percuss the other side of her lower abdomen with your dominant hand. If you feel a pronounced fluid wave against your nondominant hand, your patient probably has ascites. If the distention results from air or fat, you won't feel a fluid wave.

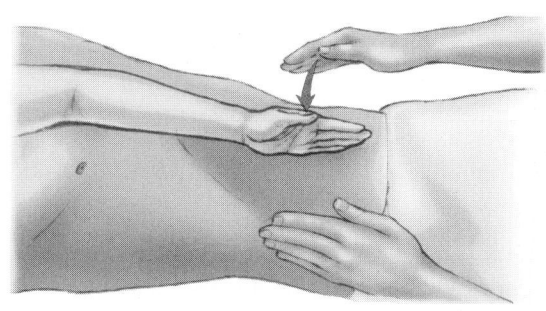

more nitrogen than she consumes. However, these values may vary if your patient has renal failure.

Hemoglobin levels and hematocrit will be reduced as well, although they'll be reduced in any patient with fluid overload. X-rays, CT scans, and ultrasound of the patient's abdomen can confirm suspected hepatomegaly and splenomegaly.

Anthropometric data can provide important indications of your patient's nutritional status as well, including her height, weight, build, and body-fat level. In cardiac cachexia, body fat falls below the 10th percentile.

Treatment

Treatment aims to identify and correct the cause of the patient's poor nutrition. For instance, if blood digoxin levels are in the toxic range, you should withhold the drug or reduce the dose, as prescribed, until they return to therapeutic levels. If fatigue is contributing to the patient's anorexia, the physician may review her drug regimen and alter it to improve her CO.

If possible, the patient's treatment program should include an exercise regimen. Even low-intensity exercise can increase your patient's appetite, improve her metabolism of carbohydrates, and build muscle mass. If she's severely malnourished, she may need enteral feedings or total parenteral nutrition (TPN).

Nursing considerations

A high priority for a malnourished patient with heart failure is to increase her calorie consumption. Administer an antiemetic, as ordered, if she battles nausea and vomiting. If she has trouble tolerating large meals, try giving her frequent, small meals high in nutrients. Also, offer her high-calorie supplements, such as puddings and commercial supplement drinks.

To help stimulate your patient's appetite, provide mouth care before meals and tidy the bedside area to make it pleasant for eating. Encourage your patient to sit in a chair to eat rather than lying in bed. Ask family members to bring some of the patient's favorite foods from home—as long as they comply with her diet restrictions. Provide rest periods before and after meals if she's fatigued.

If necessary, administer enteral feedings or TPN to provide the patient with adequate calories. Keep in mind that a patient on fluid restriction may need a high-calorie formula. She also may need to avoid formulas high in sodium. If she's receiving a high-osmolarity formula, watch for evidence of dumping syndrome, including diarrhea, nausea, tachycardia, dizziness, cold sweats, and weakness. Report any problems to the physician and provide the nursing care required for any patient receiving TPN.

Monitor the patient's laboratory test results for abnormal blood glucose levels and electrolyte imbalances. Also, check her urine for glucose and acetone. To correct metabolic abnormalities, administer carbohydrates or insulin, as ordered.

Patient teaching

Any patient with chronic heart failure and malnutrition has complex diet needs that can be complicated to teach. That's why you may want to seek assistance from a dietitian, who can perform a complete nutritional assessment, formulate a nutritional plan, and help teach the patient how to implement the plan. Remember that your patient probably feels weak and fatigued; whenever possible, include her family in your teaching sessions so that they can help implement your advice.

When teaching about the patient's diet plan, discuss the salt substitutes she can and can't use. Suggest herbs she can use to flavor her foods in place of salt. Encourage her to eat frequent, high-calorie meals, preferably in a social setting with family or friends. Emphasize the importance of oral hygiene to help make meals more palatable. If financial constraints threaten your patient's ability to follow her diet plan, obtain a referral for social services.

If your patient needs enteral feeding or TPN, spend time explaining why she needs it, the equipment required to administer it, and the monitoring and care procedures it requires.

Home care

The home care nurse will reinforce diet teaching begun in the hospital, assess the patient for additional learning needs, review the patient's diet diary, and meet with family members who buy and prepare the patient's meals. If the patient lives alone, the nurse will assess her ability to shop and prepare meals and will make appropriate community referrals for assistance with shopping, food preparation, or meal delivery.

The home care nurse will also provide ongoing assessment of the patient's nutritional status by monitoring such factors as diet intake, wound healing, and weight, skin, and hair changes.

Thromboembolism

Patients with chronic heart failure have an increased risk of thromboembolism. Sluggish blood flow caused by ventricular failure or atrial fibrillation can cause clots to form. Also, atria that don't contract properly raise the risk. An embolus can cause ischemia or infarction of varying severity in tissues distal to the occlusion. If those tissues happen to be cerebral or pulmonary, the embolism may be life threatening.

Systemic and cerebral emboli may originate from blood clots in the left atrium and ventricle that break free and travel through the arterial circulation. Venous thrombosis results from thrombus formation in the venous circulation, usually in the deep veins of the legs. From there, however, the clot may dislodge and travel through the vena cava to the right side of the heart, eventually wedging in the pulmonary vasculature.

Signs and symptoms

The clinical evidence of thromboembolism depends on its size and location. Acute arterial embolism in a limb causes sudden pain, pallor, and coldness in the limb; reduced or absent pulses; and paresthesia or paralysis.

A cerebral embolism may cause weakness or paralysis on one side of the body, aphasia, and an altered level of consciousness. Specific signs and symptoms depend on which cerebral artery becomes obstructed and which side of the brain it affects.

When a thrombus forms in a vein, the patient may develop inflammation, pain, tenderness, and redness at the site. A patient with deep vein thrombosis may have a positive Homans' sign—pain with dorsiflexion of the foot—although this sign isn't specific for the disorder. You'll also note edema, warmth, and pain on palpation.

A pulmonary embolism causes sudden dyspnea, tachypnea, and tachycardia as well as a cough, chest pain, crackles, hemoptysis, and an altered level of consciousness. The patient may feel a sense of impending doom.

Diagnostic tests

Atrial and ventricular thrombi can be detected with an echocardiogram using high-frequency sound waves. They also can be detected by ventriculography, which involves injection of a contrast medium into the ventricles during cardiac catheterization.

Pulmonary embolism will show up as a mismatch between ventilation and perfusion on a ventilation-perfusion scan. Pulmonary arteriography also may be used to confirm the diagnosis. It involves inserting a catheter into a vein, advancing it to the pulmonary artery, and injecting a contrast medium that produces a picture of the pulmonary vasculature.

Peripheral arteriography can reveal arterial embolism in the leg. It involves injecting a radiopaque dye into the patient's femoral artery and then taking a series of X-rays.

Many tests are available to detect venous thrombosis. For example, venography, also called phlebography, involves injection of a radiopaque dye into a foot vein, followed by a series of X-rays. If it shows obstructed or slow venous filling, the patient may have venous thrombosis.

Doppler ultrasound uses a transducer that emits an ultrasound beam. If the vein it tests is occluded, the device won't detect the normal sound of blood moving through the vessel.

Plethysmography, a noninvasive test used to detect deep vein thrombosis, involves applying pressure cuffs to the patient's leg and then attaching them to a pulse volume recorder. The proximal cuff, closest to the heart, inflates until it occludes venous flow. The distal cuff then records the rise in venous volume. When the proximal cuff deflates, venous volume should return to baseline. If venous outflow is obstructed, however, the return to baseline will take longer than normal.

Treatment

Most patients with heart failure don't take anticoagulants. However, a patient who faces a high risk of thrombus formation—from atrial fibrillation, for example—typically takes warfarin. The goal is to keep the patient's PT at 1.5 to 2.0 times the control or her INR at 2.0 to 3.0 times the control. If your patient develops an acute arterial occlusion from an embolism, she may be treated with heparin I.V. to keep her partial thromboplastin time (PTT) 1.5 to 2.0 times the control.

Thrombolytic therapy with streptokinase or urokinase may be administered to dissolve the clot. If she needs immediate restoration of blood flow, she may undergo an embolectomy to remove the clot.

Treatment for deep vein thrombosis involves bed rest to control edema and pain, continuous infusion of heparin for 7 to 10 days to prevent extension of the thrombus and embolization to the lungs, and possible thrombolytic therapy. Several days before heparin therapy stops, the patient will start taking an oral anticoagulant.

A thrombectomy may be needed if she's at high risk for pulmonary embolism or if venous drainage is severely impaired. A filter may be inserted in the patient's vena cava to trap larger emboli before they reach her lungs.

Treatment for a pulmonary embolism may involve mechanical ventilation and cardiopulmonary support. The ABG measurements reveal whether she needs supplemental oxygen. She'll receive a continuous infusion of heparin, followed by oral warfarin started a few days before I.V. therapy stops. For a massive embolus, the patient may receive thrombolytic therapy. Surgical management may include an embolectomy or insertion of a filter in her vena cava.

Nursing considerations

When caring for a patient with heart failure, stay alert for signs and symptoms of thromboembolism. Also, take measures to prevent deep vein thrombosis. Encourage your patient to walk if her condition allows. If she's on bed rest or too dyspneic to walk, teach her to perform passive and active exercises that involve the calf muscles. Don't place pillows under her knees or use the bed's knee gatch because they'll obstruct venous flow. Apply antiembolism stockings, if ordered; make sure they fit properly.

If your patient has deep vein thrombosis, she may be confined to bed rest for several days. If she complains of pain or discomfort at the site, apply a warm, moist pack. Monitor her edema by measuring her leg circumferences at marked locations on her calf and thigh.

If your patient receives anticoagulation therapy, she'll have an increased risk of bleeding. Check her PT, PTT, or INR values routinely and report any abnormalities. Also, assess her for bleeding and take measures to prevent injury.

Because pulmonary embolism is a potentially life-threatening complication of deep vein throm-bosis, you'll need to assess your patient frequently for its signs and symptoms. If pulmonary embolism develops, give oxygen as ordered and anticipate endotracheal intubation and mechanical ventilation, if necessary.

Patient teaching

Teach your patient the importance of mobility to help prevent an embolism. If she must stay in bed, show her how to perform range-of-motion or ankle-pumping exercises.

If a physician prescribed antiembolism stockings for her, explain their purpose and how to put them on properly. Discuss the signs and symptoms of deep vein thrombosis and tell your patient to notify her physician if they occur. Stress the importance of not standing for long periods of time and not crossing her legs when sitting. Also, caution the patient to avoid constrictive clothing.

Inform your patient and her family that sudden pallor, anxiety, coughing up blood, chest pain, shortness of breath, and palpitations may warn of a pulmonary embolism and require emergency care.

If your patient takes an anticoagulant, teach her how to take it properly to avoid bleeding.

Home care

During home visits, a nurse will assess the patient thoroughly for atrial fibrillation and signs and symptoms of thrombosis and embolization. The home care nurse also will reinforce the correct way to take a pulse and will determine whether the patient can detect irregular rhythms. And the nurse will reinforce the proper use of antiembolism stockings, review activity guidelines, emphasize warfarin precautions, and monitor the patient's laboratory values, including PT or INR levels.

HEART FAILURE

Suggested Readings

Baas LS, Fontana JA, Bhat G. Relationships between self-care resources and the quality of life of persons with heart failure: a comparison of treatment groups. *Prog Cardiovasc Nurs.* 1997;12(1):25-38.

Braunwald E, Colucci W, Grossman W. Clinical aspects of heart failure: high-output heart failure; pulmonary edema. In Braunwald E, ed. *Heart Disease: A Textbook of Cardiovascular Medicine.* 5th ed. Philadelphia: WB Saunders Co; 1996.

Cash LA. Heart failure from diastolic dysfunction. *Dimens Crit Care Nurs.* 1996;15(4):170-177.

Colucci WS, Packer M, Bristow MR, et al. Carvedilol inhibits clinical progression in patient with mild symptoms of heart failure. US carvedilol heart failure study group. *Circulation.* 1996;94(11):2800-2806.

Fontana JA. The emergence of the person-environment reaction in a descriptive study of vigor in heart failure. *ANS Adv Nurs Sci.* 1996; 18(4):70-82.

Funk M, Krumholz HM. Epidemiologic and economic impact of advanced heart failure. *J Cardiovasc Nurs.* 1996;10(2):1-10.

Koilpillai C, Quinones MA, Greenberg B, et al. Relation of ventricular size and function to heart failure status and ventricular dysrhythmia in patients with severe left ventricular dysfunction. *Am J Cardiol.* 1996;77(8):606-611.

Konstam M, et al. *Heart Failure: Evaluation and Care of Patients with Left-Ventricular Systolic Dysfunction.* Clinical practice guideline No 11. Rockville, Md: US Department of Health and Human Services, Public Health Service, Agency for Health Care Policy and Research; June 1994. AHCPR Publication 94-0612.

Koukounas E. You gotta have heart. *Nurs Spectr.* 1997;6(15):4-5.

Lewis SM, Collier IC. *Medical-Surgical Nursing: Assessment and Management of Clinical Problems.* 4th ed. St Louis: Mosby, Inc; 1995.

Massie B. Heart. In: Tierney LM, McPhee SJ, Papadakis MA. *Current Medical Diagnosis and Treatment, 1998.* 34th ed. Stamford, Conn: Appleton & Lange; 1997.

Moser DK. Maximizing therapy in the advanced heart failure patient. *J Cardiovasc Nurs.* 1996; 10(2):29-46.

Quaife RA, Gilbert EM, Christian PE, et al. Effects of carvedilol on systolic and diastolic left ventricular performance in idiopathic dilated cardiomyopathy or ischemic cardiomyopathy. *Am J Cardiol.* 1996;78(7):779-784.

Skidmore-Roth L, McKenry L. *Mosby's Drug Guide for Nurses.* St Louis: Mosby, Inc; 1997.

Specialty Update. Home sweet home. *Nursing.* 1997;27(5):64.

Sullivan MJ, Hawthorne MH. Nonpharmacologic interventions in the treatment of heart failure. *J Cardiovasc Nurs.* 1996;10(2):47-57.

Wood SL. *Cardiac Nursing.* 3rd ed. Philadelphia: Lippincott-Raven Pubs; 1995.

Index

---

i indicates an illustration; t indicates a table.

Asystole, 104, 145
Atenolol. *See also* Beta-blockers.
   for angina, 75t
   for MI, 128
Atherectomy, 88, 88i
Atherosclerotic lesions, development of, 47, 48i
Atorvastatin, 67t
Atria, 1, 2i
Atrial fibrillation, 138-139, 139i
Atrial flutter, 138-139, 139i
Atrial gallop, 20
Atrial kick, 5, 5i
Atrial myxoma as heart failure cause, 160
Atrial natriuretic factor as counterregulatory substance, 163
Atrioventricular blocks, 143
   treatment of, 143-145
   types of, 143, 144i
Atrioventricular node, 6i, 7
Atrioventricular valves, 2i, 3-4, 4i
Atropine, 101
Auscultation
   for heart failure, 168
   precordial 19-22
Autonomic regulation of heart, 7-8

B

Bachmann's bundle, 6i, 7
Balloon counterpulsation, 97, 148, 149i
Baroreceptors, 8
Basic cardiac life-support measures, 99, 101i
Benzothiazepines, 77. *See also* Calcium channel blockers.
Bepridil, 77-78
Beta-blockers
   adverse effects of, 76, 127-128, 182
   for angina, 72-77
   candidates for, 72, 73-74
   contraindications for, 73-74, 77, 127
   drug interactions and, 182, 182t
   elderly patient and, 77
   for heart failure, 181-183
   lipid solubility and, 75t, 76
   for MI, 127-129
   nursing considerations for, 76-77, 128-129, 182-183
   patient teaching for, 183
   pharmacodynamics of, 72-74
   receptor selectivity and, 75-76, 75t
   for unstable angina, 96t
Bile acid–binding resins, 66, 67t, 68
Biliary colic in cholelithiasis, chest pain in, 112t
Biofeedback as stress reduction technique, 65
Bisoprolol, 75t. *See also* Beta-blockers.
Bleeding, heparin therapy and, 131
Bleeding time, 32
Blood pressure, measuring, 18
Blood tests, 26-33, 27t, 30-31t
   for cardiogenic shock, 146
   for MI, 118
Blood urea nitrogen levels, implications of, 29
Body system review, health history and, 13

Bradyarrhythmias
   as heart failure trigger, 163
   MI and, 141-145, 143i, 144i
Bretylium, 102
Bronchospastic disease, beta-blockers and, 76
Bundle branches, 6i, 7
Bundle of His, 6i, 7
Bupropion, smoking cessation and, 58-59

C

CABG, 89-91
CAD. *See* Coronary artery disease.
Calcium channel blockers, 78t
   adverse effects of, 78, 79
   for angina, 77-79
   categories of, 77
   contraindications for, 78
   drug interactions with, 79
   nursing considerations for, 78-79
Canadian Cardiovascular Society Classification, angina and, 55
Capillary refill time, assessing, 26
Captopril. *See also* Angiotensin-converting enzyme inhibitors.
   for heart failure, 180, 181
   for MI, 132t
Carbon monoxide, CAD and, 51
Cardiac arrest
   pathophysiology of, 98-99
   treatment of, 99, 100i, 101-104, 101i, 103i
Cardiac catheterization, 43-44
   MI and, 118
Cardiac circulation, 8-9, 9i
Cardiac conduction, 6-7, 6i
Cardiac cycle, 5-6, 5i
Cardiac disorders, risk factors for, 14-15. *See also specific disorder.*
Cardiac enzyme and isoenzyme levels, implications of, 27-28
   in MI, 117-118, 118t
Cardiac infection as heart failure trigger, 163
Cardiac inflammation as heart failure trigger, 163
Cardiac muscle cells, 6
Cardiac rehabilitation
   activity planning and, 134-135
   determining patient's risk of complications from, 135
   lifestyle changes and, 136
   outpatient activities and, 134-136
   patient teaching for, 134
   self-monitoring and, 135-136
Cardiac risk factors. *See also specific disorder.*
   modifiable, 14-15
   nonmodifiable, 14
Cardiogenic shock as MI complication
   diagnostic tests for, 146
   nursing considerations for, 148
   pathophysiology of, 145
   signs and symptoms of, 145-146
   treatment of, 146, 147t, 148
Cardiomyopathy as heart failure cause, 158, 159i

i indicates an illustration; t indicates a table.

Hepatojugular reflux, assessing for, 167-168
Hiatal hernia, chest pain in, 113t
High-density lipoproteins, 28-29, 49t, 50
High-output states as heart failure cause, 160, 163-164
Holter monitoring, 36
Hormonal changes as CAD risk factor, 53
Hormone therapy, CAD and, 62
Hydration, assessing, 26
Hyperlipidemia
    beta-blockers and, 76
    as CAD risk factor, 49-50, 49t
Hypertension
    as CAD risk factor, 50-51
    as heart failure trigger, 163
Hypertension control as CAD treatment, 69-70
Hyperthyroidism as heart failure trigger, 164
Hypertrophic cardiomyopathy, 158, 159i

I J

Idioventricular rhythm, 103-104
Imagery, stress reduction and, 64
Inferior vena cava, 9-10
Inferior-wall myocardial infarction, 111, 111t, 113. *See also* Myocardial infarction.
Inotropic drugs
    adverse effects of, 177, 178, 178t
    categories of, 176-177
    contraindications for, 177-178
    drug interactions and, 177
    nursing considerations for, 178-179
    patient teaching for, 179-180
Inspection
    for heart failure, 166-167
    precordial, 18
Insulin resistance syndrome, 52
Integumentary assessment, 26
Intermittent claudication. *See* Claudication.
Internal mammary artery graft, 90i. *See also* Coronary artery bypass grafting.
International normalized ratio, 32
Internodal pathways, 6i, 7
Interventricular grooves, 4
Intra-aortic balloon counterpulsation, 97, 148, 149i
Intracoronary stent, 88
    nursing considerations for placement of, 89
    placement of, 88-89, 89i
Ischemia, platelet aggregation and, 82, 82i
Ischemic cardiomyopathy, 158
Isosorbide dinitrate, 80, 81t. *See also* Nitrates.
Isosorbide mononitrate, 80, 81t. *See also* Nitrates.
Jugular veins, assessing, 22-24, 23i
Jugular venous pulse, observing, 23, 23i

L

Labetalol, 75t. *See also* Beta-blockers.
Language barrier, overcoming, 17
Laser angioplasty, 87-88
    mechanics of, 87

Laser angioplasty—continued
    nursing considerations for, 87-88
Late potentials, implications of, 35, 36i
Lateral-wall myocardial infarction, 111t, 113. *See also* Myocardial infarction.
Left bundle branch, 6i, 7
Left coronary artery, 8-9, 9i
Left ventricular heart failure, 157-158. *See also* Heart failure.
Lidocaine, 102
Lifestyle as risk factor, 14
    for CAD, 52
Lifestyle modification as CAD treatment, 57-62, 64-65
Lipid level reduction as CAD treatment, 65-69, 67t
Lipid profile
    implications of, 28, 29
    patient teaching for, 51
Lipoproteins, 28-29, 49-50, 49t
Lisinopril, 132t. *See also* Angiotensin-converting enzyme inhibitors.
Loop diuretics, 173-174, 174i, 176, 176t. *See also* Diuretics.
Lovastatin, 67t. *See also* Cholesterol synthesis inhibitors.
Low-density lipoprotein, 28, 49t, 50
Low-sodium diet, patient teaching for, 186
Lung fields, auscultating, 25

M

Magnesium sulfate, 102
Magnetic resonance imaging, 40
Massage therapy, stress reduction and, 65
Meditation as stress reduction technique, 64
Metabolic acidosis, arterial blood gas levels in, 31t
Metabolic alkalosis, arterial blood gas levels in, 31t
Metabolic equivalents
    activities and, 63t
    heart failure classification and, 158
    oxygen uptake measurement and, 55-56
Metabolic impairment, 202-204
    home care for, 204
    nursing considerations for, 204
    patient teaching for, 204
    signs and symptoms of, 203, 203i
    treatment of, 203-204
Metoprolol. *See also* Beta-blockers.
    adverse effects of, 182
    for angina, 75t
    contraindications for, 182
    drug interactions and, 182t
    for MI, 128
    nursing considerations for, 182
    pharmacokinetics of, 181
MI. *See* Myocardial infarction.
Minimally invasive direct coronary artery bypass, 91
Mitral stenosis as heart failure cause, 160
Mitral valve, 2i, 3, 4, 4i
Morphine
    adverse effects of, 122-123
    counteracting, 123t
    for MI, 122-124
    nursing considerations for, 123-124

i indicates an illustration; t indicates a table.

Morphine—continued
  for stable angina, 71
  for unstable angina, 96t
Multiple-gated acquisition scan, 39-40
Myocardial cells, 6
Myocardial hibernation, 158
Myocardial infarction, 107-154
  anger as precipitating factor in, 64
  assessing, 113-116
  caring for patient during and after, 120-121t
  chest pain in, 12, 114-115
  circadian rhythms and, 107-108
  classifying, 110-111, 110i, 113
  completion of, 109
  complications of, 137-154
  diagnostic tests for, 116-118, 117i, 118t
  evolution of, 108-109
  factors that may trigger, 107, 108
  incidence and prevalence of, 107
  locating, 111, 111t, 113
  mortality rate for, 107
  pathophysiology of, 107-109
  recovery after, 134-136
  repair process and, 109
  signs and symptoms of, 114-116
  silent, 115
  thrombus formation as cause of, 108
  treatment of, 119, 122-136, 123t, 126t, 132t
  unstable angina as risk factor for, 98
  women and, 114
Myocardial perfusion studies without exercise, 38
Myocardial repair, process of, 109
Myocardial rupture as MI complication, 148-150
Myocardial stunning, 158
Myocardium, 2i, 3
Myoglobin levels, implications of, 28
  in MI, 118

N

Nadolol, 75t. *See also* Beta-blockers.
New York Heart Association
  angina classification and, 55
  heart failure classification and, 158
Niacin, 67t, 68-69
Niacin flush, 69
Nicardipine, 78t. *See also* Calcium channel blockers.
Nicotine, CAD and, 51
Nicotine replacement therapy, 58, 59
Nicotinic acid, 67t, 68-69
Nifedipine, 77, 78t
Nitrates. *See also* Nitroglycerin.
  adverse effects of, 80-82, 169
  contraindications for, 82, 172
  for heart failure, 169, 172-173
  interactions with, 169
  nursing considerations for, 80-82
  pharmacodynamics of, 79-80
  for stable angina, 79-82
  types of, 80, 81t
  for unstable angina, 96t

Nitroglycerin. *See also* Nitrates.
  administering, 74
  adverse effects of, 129
  for cardiogenic shock, 146, 147t
  effects of, 129
  for heart failure, 169, 172
  for MI, 122, 129-130
  nursing considerations for, 129-130
  patient teaching for, 173
  for stable angina, 71, 81t
Nocturia
  assessing for, 13
  as heart failure sign, 166
Nonselective beta-blockers, 75t
Norepinephrine, 147t, 148
Nutrition as risk factor, 14-15
Nutritional changes as heart failure trigger, 164

O

Obesity as risk factor, 15
  for CAD, 52
Opening snap as heart sound, 20
Orthopnea
  assessing for, 12
  as heart failure symptom, 166
Oxygen therapy
  for angina, 71
  for cardiac arrest, 101
  for MI, 119, 122

P

Pacemaker, indications for, 143-144
Pacemaker cells, 6
Palpation
  for heart failure, 167-168, 167i
  precordial, 18-19
Papillary muscle rupture as MI complication, 149-150
Papillary muscles, 2i, 3, 4, 4i
Paradoxical pulse, assessing for, 24
Parasympathetic nervous system, cardiac regulation and, 7-8
Paroxysmal nocturnal dyspnea
  assessing for, 12
  as heart failure symptom, 166
Passive smoking, 51
Past illnesses, health history and, 13
Patient Self-Determination Act, 16
Percussion for heart failure, 168
Percutaneous transluminal coronary angioplasty, 85-87
  candidates for, 86
  complications of, 86
  mechanics of, 86, 86i
  as MI treatment, 132-133
  nursing considerations for, 87, 133
Pericardial friction rub, 20, 25
Pericardial sac, 3
Pericardial space, 2i, 3
Pericardial window procedure, 151

i indicates an illustration; t indicates a table.

Sinus tachycardia, 138, 138i
Skin turgor, assessing, 26
Smoking as risk factor, 14, 58
    for CAD, 51
Smoking cessation
    as CAD treatment, 57-59
    strategies for, 58
    withdrawal signs and symptoms and, 58
Sodium bicarbonate, 102
Sodium nitroprusside
    for cardiogenic shock, 146, 147t
    for heart failure, 172
Sodium restriction as CAD treatment, 60
Sodium-water imbalance as heart failure trigger, 164
Spirituality, assessing role of, in patient's life, 16
Stable angina. *See also* Angina *and* Unstable angina.
    complications of, 93-104
    health history and, 70
    initial response to, 70-71
    invasive interventions for, 84-91, 86i, 88i, 89i, 90i
    oxygen therapy for, 71
    patient teaching for, 85, 91-92
    prophylactic drugs for, 71-84, 75t, 78t, 81t, 85
    signs and symptoms of, 70-71
    symptoms of, 54
    treatment of, 71, 74
Statins, 66, 67t
Streptokinase, 125, 126, 126t
Stress as CAD risk factor, 53
Stress echocardiography, 41-42
Stress reduction as CAD treatment, 64-65
Summation gallop, 20
Superior vena cava, 9-10
Sympathetic nervous system, cardiac regulation and, 7, 8
Sympathetic stimulation as compensatory mechanism, 160-161
Syncope, assessing for, 13
Syndrome X, 52
Systemic circulation, 8-9, 9i
Systemic hypertension as heart failure cause, 160
Systole, 5-6, 5i
Systolic heart failure, 157. *See also* Heart failure.

T

Tachyarrhythmias
    as heart failure trigger, 163
    MI and, 137-141, 138i, 139i, 140i
Technetium 99m imaging, 39
    in MI, 118
Technetium Tc 99m sestamibi imaging, 38-39
Thallium-201 imaging, 37-39
    foods and drugs to avoid before, 39
    in MI, 118
Thiazide diuretics, 173, 174, 174i, 176, 176t
Third-degree block, 143, 144i. *See also* Atrioventricular blocks.
Thoracic landmarks, 19i
Thromboembolism as heart failure complication, 204
    diagnostic tests for, 205
    home care for, 206

Thromboembolism—continued
    nursing considerations for, 206
    patient teaching for, 206
    signs and symptoms of, 205
    treatment of, 205-206
Thrombolytic therapy
    adverse effects of, 126
    candidates for, 125
    contraindications for, 125
    doses for, 126t
    drug options in, 125
    nursing considerations for, 126-127
Thrombus formation as cause of MI, 108
Thyrotoxicosis as heart failure trigger, 164
Ticlopidine, 83
Timolol, 75t. *See also* Beta-blockers.
Tirofiban, 95, 96t
Torsades de pointes, 140i, 141
Transesophageal echocardiography, 42, 43i
Transtelephonic cardiac event recording, 36-37
Tricuspid stenosis as heart failure cause, 160
Tricuspid valve, 2i, 3, 4, 4i
Triglycerides, 28, 49t
Troponin T levels, implications of, 28
    in MI, 118

U

Ultrafast computed tomography, 40
Unstable angina. *See also* Angina *and* Stable angina.
    assessing, 94-95
    characteristics of, 93, 94
    conditions that mimic, 95
    ECG changes in, 94
    incidence and prevalence of, 93
    initial response to, 93
    nursing considerations for, 97
    pathophysiology of, 93-94
    patient teaching for, 97-98
    as risk factor for MI, 98
    treatment of, 95, 96t, 97

V

VAD, 187-188, 188i
Valve insufficiency as heart failure cause, 159-160
Valve stenosis as heart failure cause, 160
Vasoactive drugs, 146, 147t, 148
Vasovagal syncope, catheter-based interventions and, 84-85
Venous return, 10
Ventricles, 1, 2i, 3
Ventricular aneurysm as MI complication
    nursing considerations for, 152
    signs and symptoms of, 151
    treatment of, 152
Ventricular assist devices, 187-188, 188i
Ventricular enlargement as compensatory mechanism, 161
Ventricular escape, 103-104
Ventricular fibrillation, 102-103, 139-141, 140i

W

i indicates an illustration; t indicates a table.